# Obstetrics, Gynecology, & Infertility

## Handbook for Clinicians
### 6th Edition

**John David Gordon, M.D.**
Co-Director
Dominion Fertility
Arlington, Virginia
Clinical Professor
Department of Obstetrics and Gynecology
The George Washington University

**Jan T. Rydfors, M.D.**
Clinical Adjunct Professor
Department of Gynecology and Obstetrics
Stanford University Medical Center
Stanford, California

**Maurice L. Druzin, M.D.**
Professor of Gynecology and Obstetrics
Director of Obstetrics
Stanford University Medical Center

**Yona Tadir, M.D.**
Professor of Obstetrics and Gynecology
Medical Director, Beckman Lase Institute and
Medical Clinic
University of California, Irvine
Irvine, California

**Yasser El-Sayed, M.D.**
Associate Professor
Division of Maternal Fetal Medicine
Department of Gynecology and Obstetrics
Stanford University Medical Center

**John Chan, M.D.**
Assistant Professor
Director, Division of Gynecologic Oncology
University of California, San Francisco
San Francisco, CA

**Dan Israel Lebovic, M.D., M.A.**
Associate Professor
Reproductive Endocrinology and Infertility
Department of Obstetrics and Gynecology
University of Michigan
Ann Arbor, MI

**Elizabeth Langen, M.D.**
Resident
Department of Gynecology and Obstetrics
Stanford University Medical Center

**Katherine Fuh, M.D.**
Resident
Department of Gynecology and Obstetrics
Stanford University Medical Center

Technical and Computer Support:

**Bill Gillespie**
Director of Computer Operations
Stanford University Medical Center

Scrub Hill Press, Inc.
46 S. Glebe Road, Suite 301
Arlington, VA 22204
(301) 469-8854
www.scrubhill.com

W9-AZR-443

ISBN 978-0-9645467-7-6

The opinions expressed in this book represent a broad range of opinions, including those of the full-time and volunteer clinical faculty of the Department of Gynecology and Obstetrics at Stanford University. These opinions are not meant to represent a "standard of care" or a "protocol" but rather a guide to common clinical conditions. Use of these guidelines is obviously influenced by local factors, varying clinical circumstances, and honest differences of opinion.

The indications and dosages of all drugs in this book have been recommended in the medical literature and conform to the practices of the general medical community. The medications described do not necessarily have specific approval by the U.S. Food and Drug Administration for use in the diseases and dosages for which they are recommended. The package insert for each drug should be consulted for use and dosage approved by the Food and Drug Administration. Because standards for usage change, it is advisable to keep abreast of revised recommendations, particularly those concerning new drugs.

Publisher: Scrub Hill Press, Inc.
Senior Editor: John David Gordon, MD
Editorial Assistance: Fran Faircloth, Silverchair Science + Communications, Inc.
Cover Design: George Foster

Cover sculpture used courtesy of Mr. Lado Goudjabidze. For information about purchasing this sculpture, please visit http://www.sculpturesbyartdeluxe.com.

First Edition – July 1991            Fourth Edition – January 1995
Second Edition – February 1993       Revised Fourth Edition – October 1997
Third Edition – September 1993       Fifth Edition – July 2001

Library of Congress Cataloging-in-Publication Data
Obstetrics, gynecology & infertility : handbook for clinicians : resident survival guide /
John David Gordon ... [et al]. -- 6th ed.
    p. ; cm.
  Includes bibliographical references and index.
  ISBN 978-0-9645467-7-6 (alk. paper : alk. paper) 1. Gynecology--Handbooks, manuals,
etc. 2. Obstetrics--Handbooks, manuals, etc. 3. Infertility--Handbooks, manuals, etc. 4.
Residents (Medicine)--Handbooks, manuals, etc. I. Gordon, John D. (John David) II. Title:
Obstetrics, gynecology, and infertility.
  [DNLM: 1. Pregnancy Complications--Handbooks. 2. Genital Diseases, Female--
Handbooks. 3. Infertility--Handbooks. WQ 39 O14 2007]

RG110.O28 2007
618--dc22
                                    2007025584

*This book is dedicated to H. Allison Smith, Ph.D. She is my best friend, my loving wife, and the mother of our wonderful children.*

JDG

The authors would like to thank all of the publishers and authors for their permission to reproduce various tables and figures in this book. Special thanks to

Advanced Technology Laboratories
Advanstar Communications, Inc.
The American College of Obstetricians and Gynecologists
The American College of Surgeons
The American Cancer Society
The American Society of Reproductive Medicine
The American Heart Association
The American Medical Association
Appleton & Lange
The Association of Professors of Gynecology and Obstetrics
Blackwell Scientific Publishing
Churchill-Livingston
Dowden Publishing Company
Elsevier Scientific
The Female Patient
Hospital Practice Publishing
Johns Hopkins University Press
The Journal of Reproductive Medicine
Keck School of Medicine of the University of Southern California
Lippincott Williams & Wilkins
Little, Brown and Company
The McGraw-Hill Companies
McMahon Publishing Group
Medical Economics Company
Mosby Year Book
The New England Journal of Medicine
OBG Management
Oxford University Press
Springer Verlag
Thieme Medical Publishers
W.B. Saunders

Dr. Ricardo Asch
Dr. Emily Baker
Dr. Paul Barash
Dr. Arie Bergman
Dr. John Bonnar
Dr. Frank Chervenak
Dr. Steven Clark
Dr. Robert Creasy
Dr. Gary Cunningham
Dr. Richard Dorr
Dr. Arthur Fleischer
Dr. Mark Glezerman
Dr. Leonard Gomella
Dr. Neville Hacker
Dr. Vaclav Insler
Dr. Sidney Joel-Cohen
Dr. Howard Jones, III
Dr. Bruno Lunenfeld
Dr. Fred Miyazaki
Dr. Keith Moore
Dr. John Rock
Dr. James Scott
Dr. Phillip Sarrel
Dr. Lourdes Scheerer
Dr. Leonard Speroff
Dr. Alan Trounson
Dr. Richard Sweet
Dr. Frederick Zuspan
Dr. James Carter
Dr. David Halbert

Dr. Gordon extends his great appreciation to the following physicians for their contributions to this handbook since it was first published:

Sunil Balgobin
Alvaro Cuadros
LeRoy Heinrichs
Shirley Tom
Hal Holbrook
Emmet Lamb
David Grimes
Amin Milki
Linda Giudice
Katherine O'Hanlan
Giuliana Songster

Julie Neidich
Natalie Sohn
David Halbert
Clifford Goldstein
Jennifer Lublin
Laurie Swaim
Khoa Lai
James Carter
Usha Chitkara
Nelson Teng

Carl Levinson
John Arpels
Susan Ballahh
Michael Katz
Gretchen Flanagan
Ian Hardy
Babak Edraki
Michael Ross
Dennis Siegler
Mary Lake Polan
Vicki Seltzer

# CONTENTS

# CONTENTS

## GENETICS                                                      **194**

## ULTRASOUND                                                    **218**

# CONTENTS

# CONTENTS

# CONTENTS

# CONTENTS

# CONTENTS

# FOREWORD

The 6th edition of the "Red Book" (*Obstetrics, Gynecology, and Infertility*) is a marked improvement over the previous five editions, even though they have set the standard for a handbook for clinicians. The reason is that multiple new charts and grafts have been added, and the scope of the book in general has grown, as has the field. The responsibilities of the practicing Obstetrician/Gynecologist have widened so that this book is essential. This edition is entirely rewritten and not only geared to OB/GYNs. Any provider who is involved in women's health will find this a critical part of their armamentarium.

The Primary Care section deals with a large spectrum of problems, many of which are quite topical, including management of type 2 diabetes; an extremely helpful chart of various medications for this condition is included. With the large proportion of the population suffering from type 2 diabetes, this is an excellent example how the "Red Book" has grown in scope and practicality.

Every topic in Obstetrics is covered in a distinctive way and brought up to date in a very current fashion. This is best exemplified by the chart illustrating anti-hypertensive medication in pregnancy that details when they are indicated, when they are not indicated, and those to avoid.

As Genetics and Ultrasound become part of a necessary body of knowledge for which the clinician is responsible, these are handled extremely well in a very helpful fashion. The section on Infectious Disease is well constructed and provides easy access to appropriate antibiotic therapy.

The Gynecology portion addresses the usual diseases, such as abnormal uterine bleeding, and also includes Menopause, Contraception, Infertility, and Oncology, with information that is easy to access. Just to attest to the thoroughness of this book, sample Operative Reports are included as well as a Spanish Primer (glossary).

Charts and tables with ready access are an extremely important format in this age of information overload. Concise material is necessary, and in the "Red Book" (*Obstetrics, Gynecology, and Infertility*) it is contained.

This is a superb contribution that is essential for the practice of OB/GYN and women's health in today's setting. As hard as I tried, I could not find anything that was missing. This is a treasure.

*Alan DeCherney, M.D.*
Chief
Reproductive Biology and Medicine Branch
National Institute of Child Health and Human Development
National Institutes of Health

This handbook was initially designed by residents for residents in an attempt to ease the transition between medical school and internship; however, it has proven useful to a wide range of medical professionals, and it is with great pleasure that I present this 6th edition. At 704 pages it is more than ten times longer than the 1st edition, and I sincerely hope that you, the reader, will not come to the conclusion that "more is less" as you use this book.

I remain grateful to all of the residents, fellows, and physicians with whom I have worked for their understanding and emotional support, especially Henry, Dave, Mack, Pamela, and Laurie at UT-Houston; Yasser, Ron, Jean, Dennis, Debbie, Thomas, and Anjali at Stanford; and Russell, Collin, and Jan at UCSF.

I wish to express my sincere thanks to Fran Faircloth, Elizabeth Willingham, Jane McQueen, and the outstanding staff at Silverchair Science and Communications. Without their outstanding efforts, this new edition would not have been possible.

Over the past years, a number of people have contributed to the success of this project and the formation of Scrub Hill Press, Inc. In particular, I would like to thank Becky Morris (and the staff of Stanford Publication Services), Jean Williams, Randy Winn, Donna Troyna, Peter Shearer, John Hardee, Fred Peterson, Robert Howard, Chris Carbone, and Dan Poyner.

My co-editors have remained enthusiastic and supportive over the years. Dr. Yona Tadir's contributions significantly improved the quality of the 4th Edition, and I am grateful to him for all of his hard work. Dr. Jan Rydfors has been a part of this project since it was conceived, and I appreciate his outstanding contribution to the content of the guide. Finally, Dr. Maurice Druzin has been my mentor since residency at Stanford, and, although we live on opposite coasts, I know that his wisdom and sage advice are always just a phone call away.

For this 6th edition, I am very pleased to have had input from five additional editors. Dr. Daniel Lebovic was my co-author on the *Reproductive Endocrinology & Infertility* handbook and provided some outstanding additions to those sections as well as anything else that I asked him. My good friend, Dr. Yasser El-Sayed was instrumental in revising the Obstetrics section and helping me stay up to date on part of our field that I deal with only rarely. Dr. John Chan provided a great deal of new information to the Gyn-Oncology section and I am pleased that he was able to participate in this project. Finally, two current Stanford residents, Dr. Elizabeth Langen and Dr. Katherine Fuh, worked very hard to keep the book focused and made sure that the book remained true to its heritage. I know how tired one gets during training, and I appreciate all that they did to improve this book.

It has been my fortune to have trained under a series of outstanding department chairmen: Dr. Charles Hammond, Dr. Robert Creasy, Dr. Mary Lake Polan, and Dr. Robert Jaffe. I am forever indebted to them for their patience in dealing with the author of this book.

In addition, I would like to thank my partner at Dominion Fertility: Dr. Michael DiMattina. He is the best partner that any physician could ever ask for, and he has remained supportive of my publishing activities during all the years of working side by side at Dominion Fertility.

This project would not have been possible without the generous financial and emotional support of my parents, Dr. and Mrs. Edward T. Gordon.

Finally, this 6th edition of the handbook remains dedicated to H. Allison Smith, my loving wife and best friend, for all of her support through medical school, two internships, residency, fellowship training, and beyond. I hope that our next 20 years of marriage will be as wonderful as the first 20 years.

*John David Gordon, M.D.*
Co-Director Dominion Fertility & Endocrinology
Clinical Professor
The George Washington University
Department of Obstetrics and Gynecology

## CANCER SCREENING

### Recommended Cancer Screening Protocols: Women at Average Risk

| Group | Modality | Frequency of Screening | Age at Initiation of Screening, yrs |
|---|---|---|---|
| *Breast Cancer* | | | |
| U.S. Preventive Services Task Force | Mammography | 1–2 yrs | ≥40 |
| American Cancer Society | Mammography | Annually | ≥40 |
| | Breast self-examination | Discuss risks and benefits with patient | ≥20 |
| | Clinical breast examination | Every 3 yrs | 20–39 |
| | | Annually | ≥40 |
| American College of Obstetricians and Gynecologists | Mammography | 1–2 yrs | 40–49 |
| | | Annually | ≥50 |
| *Colon Cancer* | | | |
| American Cancer Society | FOBT *or* | Annually | ≥50 |
| | Flexible sigmoidoscopy *or* | Every 5 yrs | |
| | FOBT + sigmoidoscopy *or* | FOBT—annually Sigmoidoscopy— every 5 yrs | |
| | Double-contrast barium enema *or* | Every 5 yrs | |
| | Colonoscopy | Every 10 yrs | |
| *Cervical Cancer* | | | |
| American College of Obstetricians and Gynecologists | Pap smear/HPV cytology | Annually | 21, or 3 yrs after vaginal sex (until age 30) |
| | | Every 2–3 yrs[a] | |
| American Cancer Society | Pap smear | Annually | 21, or 3 yrs after vaginal sex (until age 30) |
| | | Every 2–3 yrs[a] | |
| | HPV cytology | Every 2 yrs | |

**FOBT,** fecal occult blood test; **HPV,** human papillomavirus; **Pap,** Papanicolaou.

[a]After age 30 and with 3 consecutive negative Pap/HPV results; HIV-negative; no history of cervical disease. Reproduced with permission from Poyner EA. The latest information on cancer screening. *OB/GYN Special Edition.* 2005:25–28.

## ACOG CANCER SCREENING

**Estimated Number and Lifetime Risk of Women Who Will Develop or Die from Various Types of Cancer in 2006**

| Type of Cancer | Number of New Cases | Lifetime Risk of Developing, 1 in | Number of Deaths | Lifetime Risk of Dying from, 1 in |
|---|---|---|---|---|
| Breast | 212,920 | 8 | 40,970 | 34 |
| Lung | 81,770 | 17 | 72,130 | 20 |
| Colorectal | 75,810 | 18 | 27,300 | 45 |
| Endometrial | 41,200 | 38 | 7350 | 196 |
| Skin | 30,420 | 77 | 3720 | 500 |
| Ovarian | 20,180 | 68 | 15,310 | 95 |
| Cervical | 9710 | 135 | 3700 | 385 |

Reproduced with permission from Routine cancer screening. ACOG Committee Opinion. *Obstet Gynecol.* 2006;108(6):1611–1613.

## Suggested Routine Cancer Screening Guidelines

| Topic | Guideline |
|---|---|
| General health counseling and cancer evaluation | All women should have a general health evaluation annually or as appropriate that should include evaluation for cancer and examination, as indicated, to detect signs of premalignant or malignant conditions. |
| Breast cancer | Mammography should be performed every 1–2 yrs beginning at age 40 yrs and yearly beginning at age 50 yr. All women should have an annual clinical breast examination as part of the physical examination. Despite a lack of definitive data for or against breast self-examination, breast self-examination has the potential to detect palpable breast cancer and can be recommended. |
| Cervical cancer | Cervical cytology should be performed annually beginning at approximately 3 yrs after initiation of sexual intercourse but no later than age 21 yrs. Cervical cytology screening can be performed every 2–3 yrs after three consecutive negative test results if the patient is aged 30 yrs or older with no history of cervical intraepithelial neoplasia 2 or 3, immunosuppression, human immunodeficiency virus (HIV) infection, or diethylstilbestrol exposure in utero. Annual cervical cytology also is an option for women aged 30 yrs and older. The use of a combination of cervical cytology and HPV DNA screening is appropriate for women aged 30 yrs and older. If this combination is used, women who receive negative results on both tests should be rescreened no more frequently than every 3 yrs. |

| Topic | Guideline |
|-------|-----------|
| Colorectal cancer | Beginning at age 50 yrs, one of five screening options should be selected:<br>1) Yearly patient-collected fecal occult blood testing (FOBT) or fecal immunochemical testing (FIT)[a] or<br>2) Flexible sigmoidoscopy every 5 yrs or<br>3) Yearly patient-collected FOBT or FIT[a] plus flexible sigmoidoscopy every 5 yrs or<br>4) Double-contrast barium enema every 5 yrs or<br>5) Colonoscopy every 10 yrs |
| Endometrial cancer | Screening asymptomatic women for endometrial cancer and its precursors is not recommended at this time. |
| Lung cancer | Available screening techniques are not cost-effective and have not been shown to reduce mortality from lung cancer. Accordingly, routine lung cancer screening is not recommended. |
| Ovarian cancer | Currently, there are no effective techniques for the routine screening of asymptomatic, low-risk women for ovarian cancer. It appears that the best way to detect early ovarian cancer is for both the patient and her clinician to have a high index of suspicion of the diagnosis in the symptomatic woman, and both should be aware of the symptoms commonly associated with ovarian cancer. Persistent symptoms such as an increase in abdominal size, abdominal bloating, fatigue, abdominal pain, indigestion, inability to eat normally, urinary frequency, pelvic pain, constipation, back pain, urinary incontinence of recent onset, or unexplained weight loss should be evaluated with ovarian cancer being included in the differential diagnosis. |
| Skin cancer | Evaluate and counsel regarding exposure to ultraviolet rays. |

[a]Both FOBT and FIT require two or three samples of stool collected by the patient at home and returned for analysis. A single stool sample for FOBT or FIT obtained by digital rectal examination is not adequate for the detection of colorectal cancer.
Reproduced with permission from Routine cancer screening. ACOG Committee Opinion. *Obstet Gynecol.* 2006;108(6):1611–1613.

## NUTRITION

### Vitamin and Mineral Recommendations

| Vitamin | Current RDI[a] | New DRI[b] | UL[c] |
|---|---|---|---|
| Vitamin A | 5000 IU | 900 mcg (3000 IU) | 3000 mcg (10,000 IU) |
| Vitamin C | 60 mg | 90 mg | 2000 mg |
| Vitamin D | 400 IU (10 mcg) | 15 mcg (600 IU) | 50 mcg (2000 IU) |
| Vitamin E | 30 IU (20 mg) | 15 mg[d] | 1000 mg |
| Vitamin K | 80 mcg | 120 mcg | ND |
| Thiamin | 1.5 mg | 1.2 mg | ND |
| Riboflavin | 1.7 mg | 1.3 mg | ND |
| Niacin | 20 mg | 16 mg | 35 mg |
| Vitamin B6 | 2 mg | 1.7 mg | 100 mg |
| Folate | 400 mg (0.4 mg) | 400 mcg from food, 200 mcg synthetic[e] | 1000 mcg synthetic |
| Vitamin B12 | 6 mcg | 2.4 mcg[f] | ND |
| Biotin | 300 mcg | 30 mcg | ND |
| Pantothenic acid | 10 mg | 5 mg | ND |
| Choline | Not established | 550 mg | 3500 mg |

[a]The Reference Daily Intake (RDI) is the value established by the Food and Drug Administration (FDA) for use in nutrition labeling. It is based initially on the highest 1968 Recommended Dietary Allowance (RDA) for each nutrient, to assure that needs were met for all age groups.

[b]The Dietary Reference Intakes (DRI) are the most recent set of dietary recommendations established by the Food and Nutrition Board of the Institute of Medicine, 1997–2001. They replace previous RDAs, and may be the basis for eventually updating the RDIs. The value shown here is the highest DRI for each nutrient.

[c]The Upper Limit (UL) is the upper level of intake considered to be **safe** for use by adults, incorporating a safety factor. In some cases, lower ULs have been established for children.

[d]Historic vitamin E conversion factors were amended in the DRI report, so that 15 mg is defined as the equivalent of 22 IU of natural vitamin E or 33 IU of synthetic vitamin E.

[e]It is recommended that women of childbearing age obtain 400 mcg of synthetic folic acid from fortified breakfast cereals or dietary supplements, in addition to dietary folate.

[f]It is recommended that people over 50 meet the B12 recommendation through fortified foods or supplements, to improve bioavailability.

*ND,* upper limit not determined. No adverse effects observed from high intakes of the nutrient.

*Source:* Council for Responsible Nutrition. The Science Behind the Supplements. Accessed at http//www.crnvsa.org. March 2007.

## Vitamin and Mineral Recommendations

| Mineral | Current RDI[a] | New DRI[b] | UL[c] |
|---|---|---|---|
| Calcium | 1000 mg | 1300 mg | 2500 mg |
| Iron | 18 mg | 18 mg | 45 mg |
| Phosphorus | 1000 mg | 1250 mg | 4000 mg |
| Iodine | 150 mcg | 150 mcg | 1100 mcg |
| Magnesium | 400 mg | 420 mg | 350 mg[d] |
| Zinc | 15 mg | 11 mg | 40 mg |
| Selenium | 70 mcg | 55 mcg | 400 mcg |
| Copper | 2 mg | 0.9 mg | 10 mg |
| Manganese | 2 mg | 2.3 mg | 11 mg |
| Chromium | 120 mcg | 35 mcg | ND |
| Molybdenum | 75 mcg | 45 mcg | 2000 mcg |

[a]The Reference Daily Intake (RDI) is the value established by the Food and Drug Administration (FDA) for use in nutrition labeling. It was based initially on the highest 1968 Recommended Dietary Allowance (RDA) for each nutrient, to assure that needs were met for all age groups.

[b]The Dietary Reference Intakes (DRI) are the most recent set of dietary recommendations established by the Food and Nutrition Board of the Institute of Medicine, 1997–2001. They replace previous RDAs, and may be the basis for eventually updating the RDIs. The value shown here is the highest DRI for each nutrient.

[c]The Upper Limit (UL) is the upper level of intake considered to be **safe** for use by adults, incorporating a safety factor. In some cases, lower ULs have been established for children.

[d]Upper limit for magnesium applies to intakes from dietary supplements or pharmaceutical products, not including intakes from food and water.

ND, upper limit not determined. No adverse effects observed from high intakes of the nutrient.

*Source:* Council for Responsible Nutrition. The Science Behind the Supplements. Accessed at http//www.crnvsa.org. March 2007.

# PRIMARY CARE

## BODY MASS INDEX

### Nomogram

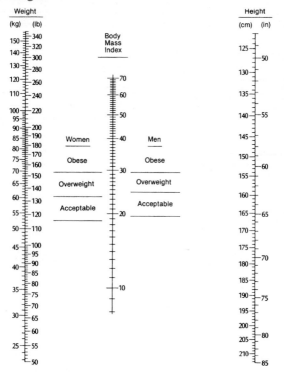

*Source*: Speroff L, Glass RH, Kase NG. Obesity. In: *Clinical Gynecologic Endocrinology and Infertility.* 6th ed. Philadelphia: Lippincott Williams & Wilkins, 1999. Reproduced with the permission of the publisher.

## Body Mass Index Table

Body Weight (lb)

| Height (in) | Normal | | | | | | Overweight | | | | | Obese | | | | | | | | | | Extreme Obesity | | | | | | | | | | | | | | |
|---|---|---|---|---|---|---|---|---|---|---|---|---|---|---|---|---|---|---|---|---|---|---|---|---|---|---|---|---|---|---|---|---|---|---|---|---|
| BMI | 19 | 20 | 21 | 22 | 23 | 24 | 25 | 26 | 27 | 28 | 29 | 30 | 31 | 32 | 33 | 34 | 35 | 36 | 37 | 38 | 39 | 40 | 41 | 42 | 43 | 44 | 45 | 46 | 47 | 48 | 49 | 50 | 51 | 52 | 53 | 54 |
| 58 | 91 | 96 | 100 | 105 | 110 | 115 | 119 | 124 | 129 | 134 | 138 | 143 | 148 | 153 | 158 | 162 | 167 | 172 | 177 | 181 | 186 | 191 | 196 | 201 | 205 | 210 | 215 | 220 | 224 | 229 | 234 | 239 | 244 | 248 | 253 | 258 |
| 59 | 94 | 99 | 104 | 109 | 114 | 119 | 124 | 128 | 133 | 138 | 143 | 148 | 153 | 158 | 163 | 168 | 173 | 178 | 183 | 188 | 193 | 198 | 203 | 208 | 212 | 217 | 222 | 227 | 232 | 237 | 242 | 247 | 252 | 257 | 262 | 267 |
| 60 | 97 | 102 | 107 | 112 | 118 | 123 | 128 | 133 | 138 | 143 | 148 | 153 | 158 | 163 | 168 | 174 | 179 | 184 | 189 | 194 | 199 | 204 | 209 | 215 | 220 | 225 | 230 | 235 | 240 | 245 | 250 | 255 | 261 | 266 | 271 | 276 |
| 61 | 100 | 106 | 111 | 116 | 122 | 127 | 132 | 137 | 143 | 148 | 153 | 158 | 164 | 169 | 174 | 180 | 185 | 190 | 195 | 201 | 206 | 211 | 217 | 222 | 227 | 232 | 238 | 243 | 248 | 254 | 259 | 264 | 269 | 275 | 280 | 285 |
| 62 | 104 | 109 | 115 | 120 | 126 | 131 | 136 | 142 | 147 | 153 | 158 | 164 | 169 | 175 | 180 | 186 | 191 | 196 | 202 | 207 | 213 | 218 | 224 | 229 | 235 | 240 | 246 | 251 | 256 | 262 | 267 | 273 | 278 | 284 | 289 | 295 |
| 63 | 107 | 113 | 118 | 124 | 130 | 135 | 141 | 146 | 152 | 158 | 163 | 169 | 175 | 180 | 186 | 191 | 197 | 203 | 208 | 214 | 220 | 225 | 231 | 237 | 242 | 248 | 254 | 259 | 265 | 270 | 278 | 282 | 287 | 293 | 299 | 304 |
| 64 | 110 | 116 | 122 | 128 | 134 | 140 | 145 | 151 | 157 | 163 | 169 | 174 | 180 | 186 | 192 | 197 | 204 | 209 | 215 | 221 | 227 | 232 | 238 | 244 | 250 | 256 | 262 | 267 | 273 | 279 | 285 | 291 | 296 | 302 | 308 | 314 |
| 65 | 114 | 120 | 126 | 132 | 138 | 144 | 150 | 156 | 162 | 168 | 174 | 180 | 186 | 192 | 198 | 204 | 210 | 216 | 222 | 228 | 234 | 240 | 246 | 252 | 258 | 264 | 270 | 276 | 282 | 288 | 294 | 300 | 306 | 312 | 318 | 324 |
| 66 | 118 | 124 | 130 | 136 | 142 | 148 | 155 | 161 | 167 | 173 | 179 | 186 | 192 | 198 | 204 | 210 | 216 | 223 | 229 | 235 | 241 | 247 | 253 | 260 | 266 | 272 | 278 | 284 | 291 | 297 | 303 | 309 | 315 | 322 | 328 | 334 |
| 67 | 121 | 127 | 134 | 140 | 146 | 153 | 159 | 166 | 172 | 178 | 185 | 191 | 198 | 204 | 211 | 217 | 223 | 230 | 236 | 242 | 249 | 255 | 261 | 268 | 274 | 280 | 287 | 293 | 299 | 306 | 312 | 319 | 325 | 331 | 338 | 344 |
| 68 | 125 | 131 | 138 | 144 | 151 | 158 | 164 | 171 | 177 | 184 | 190 | 197 | 203 | 210 | 216 | 223 | 230 | 236 | 243 | 249 | 256 | 262 | 269 | 276 | 282 | 289 | 295 | 302 | 308 | 315 | 322 | 328 | 335 | 341 | 348 | 354 |
| 69 | 128 | 135 | 142 | 149 | 155 | 162 | 169 | 176 | 182 | 189 | 196 | 203 | 209 | 216 | 223 | 230 | 236 | 243 | 250 | 257 | 263 | 270 | 277 | 284 | 291 | 297 | 304 | 311 | 318 | 324 | 331 | 338 | 345 | 351 | 358 | 365 |
| 70 | 132 | 139 | 146 | 153 | 160 | 167 | 174 | 181 | 188 | 195 | 202 | 209 | 216 | 222 | 229 | 236 | 243 | 250 | 257 | 264 | 271 | 278 | 285 | 292 | 299 | 306 | 313 | 320 | 327 | 334 | 341 | 348 | 355 | 362 | 369 | 376 |
| 71 | 136 | 143 | 150 | 157 | 165 | 172 | 179 | 186 | 193 | 200 | 208 | 215 | 222 | 229 | 236 | 243 | 250 | 257 | 265 | 272 | 279 | 286 | 293 | 301 | 308 | 315 | 322 | 329 | 338 | 343 | 351 | 358 | 365 | 372 | 379 | 386 |
| 72 | 140 | 147 | 154 | 162 | 169 | 177 | 184 | 191 | 199 | 206 | 213 | 221 | 228 | 235 | 242 | 250 | 258 | 265 | 272 | 279 | 287 | 294 | 302 | 309 | 316 | 324 | 331 | 338 | 346 | 353 | 361 | 368 | 375 | 383 | 390 | 397 |
| 73 | 144 | 151 | 159 | 166 | 174 | 182 | 189 | 197 | 204 | 212 | 219 | 227 | 235 | 242 | 250 | 257 | 265 | 272 | 280 | 288 | 295 | 302 | 310 | 318 | 325 | 333 | 340 | 348 | 355 | 363 | 371 | 378 | 386 | 393 | 401 | 408 |
| 74 | 148 | 155 | 163 | 171 | 179 | 186 | 194 | 202 | 210 | 218 | 225 | 233 | 241 | 249 | 256 | 264 | 272 | 280 | 287 | 295 | 303 | 311 | 319 | 326 | 334 | 342 | 350 | 358 | 365 | 373 | 381 | 389 | 396 | 404 | 412 | 420 |
| 75 | 152 | 160 | 168 | 176 | 184 | 192 | 200 | 208 | 216 | 224 | 232 | 240 | 248 | 256 | 264 | 272 | 279 | 287 | 295 | 303 | 311 | 319 | 327 | 335 | 343 | 351 | 359 | 367 | 375 | 383 | 391 | 399 | 407 | 415 | 423 | 431 |
| 76 | 156 | 164 | 172 | 180 | 189 | 197 | 205 | 213 | 221 | 230 | 238 | 246 | 254 | 263 | 271 | 279 | 287 | 295 | 304 | 312 | 320 | 328 | 336 | 344 | 353 | 361 | 369 | 377 | 385 | 394 | 402 | 410 | 418 | 426 | 435 | 443 |

| Weight category | BMI |
|---|---|
| Underweight | <18.5 |
| Normal weight | 18.5–24.9 |
| Overweight | 25–29.9 |
| Obesity (Class I) | 30–34.9 |
| Obesity (Class II) | 35–39.9 |
| Extreme Obesity (Class III) | ≥40 |

Reproduced with permission from The role of the obstetrician-gynecologist in the assessment and management of obesity. ACOG Committee Opinion. *Obstet Gynecol.* 2005;106(4): 895–897.

## CARDIOVASCULAR DISEASE IN WOMEN

### Classification of CVD Risk in Women

| Risk Status | Criteria |
| --- | --- |
| High risk | Established coronary heart disease |
| | Cerebrovascular disease |
| | Peripheral arterial disease |
| | Abdominal aortic aneurysm |
| | End-stage or chronic renal disease |
| | Diabetes mellitus |
| | 10-Year Framingham global risk >20%[a] |
| At risk | ≥1 major risk factor for CVD, including |
| |   Cigarette smoking |
| |   Poor diet |
| |   Physical inactivity |
| |   Obesity, especially central adiposity |
| |   Family history of premature CVD (CVD at <55 yrs of age in male relative and <65 yrs of age in female relative) |
| |   Hypertension |
| |   Dyslipidemia |
| | Evidence of subclinical vascular disease (e.g., coronary calcification) |
| | Metabolic syndrome |
| | Poor exercise capacity on treadmill test and/or abnormal heart rate recovery after stopping exercise |
| Optimal risk | Framingham global risk <10% and a healthy lifestyle with no risk factors |

CVD, cardiovascular disease.

[a]Or at risk on the basis of another population-adapted tool used to assess global risk.

Reproduced with permission from Evidence-based guidelines for cardiovascular disease prevention in women: 2007 update. *J Am Coll Cardiol*. 2007;49(11):1230–1250.

## Algorithm for Cardiovascular Preventative Care

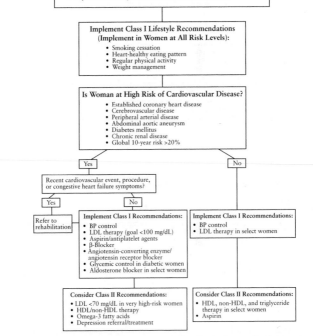

Labs, laboratory tests; BP, blood pressure; LDL, low-density lipoprotein cholesterol; and HDL, high-density lipoprotein cholesterol. Reproduced with permission from Evidence-based guidelines for cardiovascular disease prevention in women: 2007 update. *J Am Coll Cardiol.* 2007;49(11):1230–1250.

## Guidelines for Prevention of CVD in Women: Clinical Recommendations

### Lifestyle interventions

#### Cigarette smoking

- Women should not smoke and should avoid environmental tobacco smoke. Provide counseling, nicotine replacement, and other pharmacotherapy as indicated in conjunction with a behavioral program or formal smoking cessation program *(Class I, Level B)*.

#### Physical activity

- Women should accumulate a minimum of 30 mins of moderate-intensity physical activity (e.g., brisk walking) on most, and preferably all, days of the wk *(Class I, Level B)*.
- Women who need to lose weight or sustain weight loss should accumulate a minimum of 60–90 mins of moderate-intensity physical activity (e.g., brisk walking) on most, and preferably all, days of the wk *(Class I, Level C)*.

#### Rehabilitation

- A comprehensive risk-reduction regimen, such as cardiovascular or stroke rehabilitation or a physician-guided home- or community-based exercise training program, should be recommended to women with a recent acute coronary syndrome or coronary intervention, new-onset or chronic angina, recent cerebrovascular event, peripheral arterial disease *(Class I, Level A)*, or current/prior symptoms of heart failure and an LVEF <40% *(Class I, Level B)*.

#### Dietary intake

- Women should consume a diet rich in fruits and vegetables; choose whole-grain, high-fiber food; consume fish, especially oily fish,[a] at least twice a wk; limit intake of saturated fat to <10% of energy, and if possible to <7%, cholesterol to <300 mg/day, alcohol intake to no more than 1 drink per day,[b] and sodium intake to <2.3 g/day (approximately 1 tsp salt). Consumption of trans-fatty acids should be as low as possible (e.g., <1% of energy) *(Class I, Level B)*.

#### Weight maintenance/reduction

- Women should maintain or lose weight through an appropriate balance of physical activity, caloric intake, and formal behavioral programs when indicated to maintain/achieve a BMI between 18.5 and 24.9 kg/m$^3$ and a waist circumference ≤35 in *(Class I, Level B)*.

#### Omega-3 fatty acids

- As an adjunct to diet, omega-3 fatty acids in capsule form (approximately 850–1000 mg of EPA and DHA) may be considered in women with CHD, and higher does (2–4 g) may be used for treatment of women with high triglyceride levels *(Class IIb, Level B)*.

#### Depression

- Consider screening women with CHD for depression and refer/treat when indicated *(Class IIa, Level B)*.

### Major risk factor interventions

#### Blood pressure—optimal level and lifestyle

- Encourage an optimal blood pressure of <120/80 mm Hg through lifestyle approaches such as weight control, increased physical activity, alcohol moderation, sodium restriction, and increased consumption of fresh fruits, vegetables, and low-fat dairy products *(Class I, Level B)*.

## Guidelines for Prevention of CVD in Women: Clinical Recommendations

### Blood pressure—pharmacotherapy

• Pharmacotherapy is indicated when blood pressure is ≥140/90 mm Hg or at even lower blood pressure in the setting of chronic kidney disease or diabetes (≥130/80 mm Hg). Thiazide diuretics should be part of the drug regimen for most patients unless contraindicated or if there are compelling indications for other agents in specific vascular disease. Initial treatment of high-risk women[c] should be with β-blockers and/or ACE inhibitors/ARBs, with addition of other drugs such as thiazides as needed to achieve goal blood pressure *(Class I, Level A).*

### Lipid and lipoprotein levels—optimal levels and lifestyle

• The following levels of lipids and lipoproteins in women should be encouraged through lifestyle approaches: LDL-C <100 mg/dL, HDL-C >50 mg/dL, triglycerides <150 mg/dL, and non–HDL-C (total cholesterol minus HDL cholesterol) <130 mg/dL *(Class I, Level B).* If a woman is at high risk[c] or has hypercholesterolemia, intake of saturated fat should be <7% and cholesterol intake <200 mg/dL *(Class I, Level B).*

### Lipids—pharmacotherapy for LDL lowering, high-risk women

• Utilize LDL-C–lowering drug therapy simultaneously with lifestyle therapy in women in CHD to achieve an LDL-C <100 mg/dL *(Class I, Level A)* and similarly in women with other atherosclerotic CVD or diabetes mellitus or 10-year absolute risk >20% *(Class I, Level B).*

• A reduction to <70 mg/dL is reasonable in very-high-risk women[d] with CHD and may require an LDL-lowering drug combination *(Class IIa, Level B).*

### Lipids—pharmacotherapy for LDL lowering, other at-risk women

• Utilize LDL-C–lowering therapy if LDL-C level is ≥130 mg/dL with lifestyle therapy and there are multiple risk factors and 10-yr absolute risk 10–20% *(Class I, Level B).*

• Utilize LDL-C–lowering therapy if LDL-C level is ≥160 mg/dL with lifestyle therapy and multiple risk factors, even if 10-yr absolute risk is <10% *(Class I, Level B).*

• Utilize LDL-C–lowering therapy if LDL-C level is ≥190 mg/dL regardless of the presence or absence of other risk factors or CVD on lifestyle therapy *(Class I, Level B).*

### Lipids—pharmacotherapy for low HDL or elevated non-HDL, high-risk women

• Utilize niacin[e] or fibrate therapy when HDL-C is low or non–HDL-C is elevated in high risk women[e] after LDL-C goal is reached *(Class IIb, Level B).*

### Lipids—pharmacotherapy for low HDL or elevated non-HDL, other at-risk women

• Consider niacin[f] or fibrate therapy when HDL-C is low or non–HDL-C is elevated after LDL-C goal is reached in women with multiple risk factors and a 10-yr absolute risk 10–20% *(Class IIb, Level B).*

### Diabetes mellitus

• Lifestyle and pharmacotherapy should be used as indicated in women with diabetes *(Class I, Level B)* to achieve an $HbA_{1C}$ <7% if this can be accomplished without significant hypoglycemia *(Class I, Level C).*

*continued*

## Guidelines for Prevention of CVD in Women: Clinical Recommendations

---

**Preventive drug interventions**

**Aspirin, high risk**

- Aspirin therapy (75–325 mg/d) should be used in high-risk[c] women unless contraindicated *(Class I, Level A)*.
- If a high risk[c] woman is intolerant of aspirin therapy, clopidogrel should be substituted *(Class I, Level B)*.

**Aspirin—other at-risk or healthy women**

- In women ≥65 yrs of age, consider aspirin therapy (81 mg daily or 100 mg every other day) if blood pressure is controlled and benefit for ischemic stroke and MI prevention is likely to outweigh risk of gastrointestinal bleeding and hemorrhagic stroke *(Class IIa, Level B)* and in women <65 yrs of age when benefit for ischemic stroke is likely to outweigh adverse effects of therapy *(Class IIb, Level B)*.

**β-Blockers**

- β-Blockers should be used indefinitely in all women after MI, acute coronary syndrome, or left ventricular dysfunction with or without heart failure symptoms, unless contraindicated *(Class I, Level A)*.

**ACE inhibitors/ARBs**

- ACE inhibitors should be used (unless contraindicated) in women after MI and in those with clinical evidence of heart failure or an LVEF ≤40% or with diabetes mellitus *(Class I, Level A)*. In women after MI and in those with clinical evidence of heart failure or an LVEF ≤40% or with diabetes mellitus who are intolerant of ACE inhibitors, ARBs should be used instead *(Class I, Level B)*.

**Aldosterone blockade**

- Use aldosterone blockade after MI in women who do not have significant renal dysfunction or hyperkalemia who are already receiving therapeutic doses of an ACE inhibitor and β-blocker, and have LVEF ≤40% with symptomatic heart failure *(Class I, Level B)*.

---

LVEF, left ventricular ejection fraction; BMI, body mass index; EPA, eicosapentaenoic acid; DHA, docosahexaenoic acid; CHD, coronary heart disease; ACE, angiotensin-converting enzyme; ARB, angiotensin receptor blocker; LDL-C, low-density lipoprotein cholesterol; HDL-C, high-density lipoprotein cholesterol; CVD, cardiovascular disease; MI, myocardial infarction.

[a]Pregnant and lactating women should avoid eating fish potentially high in methylmercury (e.g., shark, swordfish, king mackerel, or tile fish) and should eat up to 12 oz/wk of a variety of fish and shellfish low in mercury and check the Environmental Protection Agency and the U.S. Food and Drug Administration's Web sites for updates and local advisories about safety of local catch.

[b]A drink equivalent is equal to a 12-oz bottle of beer, a 5-oz glass of wine, or a 1.5-oz shot of 80-proof spirit.

[c]Criteria for high risk includes established CHD, cerebrovascular disease, peripheral arterial disease, abdominal aortic aneurysm, end-stage or chronic renal disease, diabetes mellitus, and 10-yr Framingham risk >20%.

[d]Criteria for very high risk include established CVD plus any of the following: multiple major risk factors, severe and poorly controlled risk factors, diabetes mellitus.

[e]Dietary supplemental niacin should not be used as a substitute for prescription niacin.

[f]After percutaneous intervention with stent placement or coronary artery bypass grafting within previous year and in women with noncoronary forms of CVD, use current guidelines for aspirin and clopidogrel. Reproduced with permission from Evidence-based guidelines for cardiovascular disease prevention in women: 2007 update. *J Am Coll Cardiol.* 2007;49(11):1230–1250.

## HYPERCHOLESTEROLEMIA TREATMENT

Reproduced from the National Cholesterol Education Program Expert Panel on Detection, Evaluation and Treatment of High Blood Cholesterol in Adults (Adult Treatment Panel III).

### ATP III Recommendations

**Step 1: Determine lipoprotein levels—obtain complete lipoprotein profile after 9- to 12-hour fast:**

| LDL Cholesterol—Primary Target of Therapy | |
| --- | --- |
| <100 | Optimal |
| 100–129 | Near optimal/above optimal |
| 130–159 | Borderline high |
| 160–189 | High |
| ≥190 | Very high |
| **Total Cholesterol** | |
| <200 | Desirable |
| 200–239 | Borderline high |
| ≥240 | High |
| **HDL Cholesterol** | |
| <40 | Low |
| ≥60 | High |

**Step 2: Identify presence of clinical atherosclerotic disease that confers high risk for coronary heart disease (CHD) events (CHD risk equivalent):**

- Clinical CHD
- Symptomatic carotid artery disease
- Peripheral artery disease
- Abdominal aortic aneurysm

**Step 3: Determine the presence of major risk factors (other than LDL):**

- Cigarette smoking
- Hypertension (BP ≥140/90 mm Hg or on antihypertensive therapy)
- Low HDL cholesterol (<40 mg/dL)*
- Family history of premature CHD (male first degree relative <55 years, female first degree relative <65 years)
- Age (men ≥45 years; women ≥55 years)

**Step 4: If 2+ risk factors (other than LDL) are present without CHD or CHD risk equivalent, assess 10-year (short-term) CHD risk (see Framingham tables). Three levels of 10-year risk:**

- >20%—CHD risk equivalent
- 10–20%
- <10%

*HDL cholesterol ≥60 mg/dL counts as "negative" risk factor; its presence removes one risk factor from total count.
NOTE: In ATP III, diabetes is regarded as a CHD risk equivalent.

# PRIMARY CARE

## Step 5: Determine risk category:
- Establish LDL goal of therapy
- Determine need for therapeutic lifestyle changes (TLC)
- Determine level for drug consideration

| Risk Category | Initiate TLC[a] | Consider Drug Therapy |
|---|---|---|
| **High risk:** | | |
| CHD or CHD risk equivalents (10-year risk >20%) | ≥100 mg/dL[b] | ≥100 mg/dL (<100 mg/dL: consider drug options)[c] |
| **Moderately high risk:** | | |
| ≥2 risk factors (10-year risk 10–20%) | ≥130 mg/dL[b] | ≥130 mg/dL (100–129 mg/dL: consider drug options)[d] |
| **Moderate risk:** | | |
| ≥2 risk factors (10-year risk <10%) | ≥130 mg/dL | ≥160 mg/dL |
| **Lower risk:** | | |
| 0–2 risk factors | ≥160 mg/dL | ≥190 mg/dL (160–189 mg/dL: LDL-Cl–lowering drug optional) |

[a]Therapeutic lifestyle changes.
[b]Any person at high risk or moderately high risk who has lifestyle-related risk factors (obesity, physical inactivity, elevated triglycerides, low HDL-C, or metabolic syndrome) is a candidate for TLC to modify these risk factors regardless of LDL-C level.
[c]If baseline LDL-C is <100 mg/dL, institution of an LDL-lowering drug is a therapeutic option on the basis of available clinical trial results. If a high-risk person has high triglycerides and low HDL-C, combining a fibrate or nicotinic acid with an LDL-C lowering drug can be considered.
[d]For moderately high-risk persons, when LDL-C level is 100–120 mg/dL, at baseline or on lifestyle therapy, initiation of an LDL-C lowering drug to achieve an LDL-C level <100 mg/dL is a therapeutic option on the basis of available clinical trial results.
Third Report of the Expert Panel on Detection, Evaluation, and Treatment of High Blood Cholesterol in Adults (Adult Treatment Panel III). Bethesda, MD: National Institutes of Health, National Heart, Lung, and Blood Institute; 2001. NIH Publication 01-3095. Updated with: Grundy SM, Cleeman JI, Merz CNB, et al. Implications of Recent Clinical Trials for the National Cholesterol Education Program Adult Treatment Panel III Guidelines. Circulation. 2004;110:227–239.

## Step 6: Initiate therapeutic lifestyle changes (TLC) if LDL is above goal:
*TLC Features*

| Nutrient | Recommended Intake |
|---|---|
| Saturated fat[a] | <7% of total calories |
| Polyunsaturated fat | Up to 10% of total calories |
| Monounsaturated fat | Up to 20% of total calories |
| Total fat | 25–35% of total calories |
| Carbohydrate (especially complex carbohydrates) | 50–60% of total calories |
| Fiber | 20–30 g/d |
| Protein | ~15% of total calories |
| Cholesterol | <200 mg/d |

[a]Trans fatty acids also raise low-density lipoprotein cholesterol and should be kept at a low intake.
Note: Regarding total calories, balance energy intake and expenditure to maintain desirable body weight.
*Source:* From the Third Report of the Expert Panel on Detection, Evaluation, and Treatment of High Blood Cholesterol in Adults (Adult Treatment Panel III). Bethesda, MD: National Institutes of Health, National Heart, Lung, and Blood Institute; 2001. NIH Publication 01-3095.

## Step 7: Consider adding drug therapy if LDL exceeds levels shown in Step 5 table:

- Consider drug simultaneously with TLC for CHD and CHD equivalents
- Consider adding drug to TLC after 3 months for other risk categories

| Class of Drug | Typical Daily Dose | Lipid/ Lipoprotein Effects | Side Effects | Contraindications |
|---|---|---|---|---|
| **HMG CoA reductase inhibitors ("statins")** | | | | |
| Atorvastatin (Lipitor) | 10–80 mg | LDL-C ↓ 18–55% | Myopathy | Absolute |
| Lovastatin (Mevacor) | 20 mg | HDL-C ↑ 5–15% | Increased liver enzymes | Active or chronic liver disease |
| Simvastatin (Zocor) | 20–80 mg | TG ↓ 7–30% | | Relative |
| Pravastatin (Pravachol) | 20–40 mg | | | Concomitant use of certain drugs[a] |
| Fluvastatin (Lescol) | 20–80 mg | | | |
| Cerivastatin | 0.4–0.8 mg | | | |
| **Bile acid sequestrants or resins** | | | | |
| Cholestyramine (Questran) | 4–16 g | LDL-C ↓ 15–30% | Gastrointestinal distress | Absolute |
| Colestipol (Colestid) | 5–20 g | HDL-C ↑ 3–5% | Constipation | • Dysbetalipoproteinemia |
| Colesevelam (Welchol) | 2.6–3.8 g | TG No change | Decreased absorption of other drugs | • TG >400 mg/dL |
| | | | | Relative |
| | | | | • TG >200 mg/dL |
| **Nicotinic acid** | | | | |
| Niacin (Niacor) | 1 g tid | LDL-C ↓ 5–25% | Flushing | Absolute |
| | | HDL-C ↑ 15–35% | Hyperglycemia | • Chronic liver disease |
| | | TG ↓ 20–50% | Hyperuricemia (or gout) | • Severe gout |
| | | | Upper GI distress | Relative |
| | | | Hepatotoxicity | • Diabetes |
| | | | | • Hyperuricemia |
| | | | | • Peptic ulcer disease |
| **Fibric acid** | | | | |
| Gemfibrozil (Lopid) | 600 mg bid | LDL-C ↓ 5–20% (may be increased in patients with high TG) | Dyspepsia | Absolute |
| Clofibrate (Atromid) | 1 g bid | | Gallstones | • Severe renal disease |
| Fenofibrate | 200 mg | | Myopathy | • Severe hepatic disease |
| | | HDL-C ↑ 10–20% | | |
| | | TG ↓ 20–50% | | |

[a]Cyclosporine, macrolide antibiotics, various anti-fungal agents, and cytochrome P-450 inhibitors (fibrates and niacin should be used with appropriate caution).

# PRIMARY CARE

## Procedure for Implementing Therapeutic Lifestyle Changes (TLC)

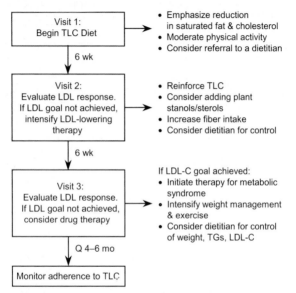

Visit 1:
Begin TLC Diet

- Emphasize reduction in saturated fat & cholesterol
- Moderate physical activity
- Consider referral to a dietitian

6 wk

Visit 2:
Evaluate LDL response. If LDL goal not achieved, intensify LDL-lowering therapy

- Reinforce TLC
- Consider adding plant stanols/sterols
- Increase fiber intake
- Consider dietitian for control

6 wk

Visit 3:
Evaluate LDL response. If LDL goal not achieved, consider drug therapy

If LDL-C goal achieved:
- Initiate therapy for metabolic syndrome
- Intensify weight management & exercise
- Consider dietitian for control of weight, TGs, LDL-C

Q 4–6 mo

Monitor adherence to TLC

*Source:* Third Report of the Expert Panel on Detection, Evaluation, and Treatment of High Blood Cholesterol in Adults (Adult Treatment Panel III). Bethesda, Md: National Institutes of Health, National Heart, Lung, and Blood Institute; 2001. NIH Publication 01-3095.

**Procedure for Implementing Drug Therapy to Treat Lipid Abnormalities**

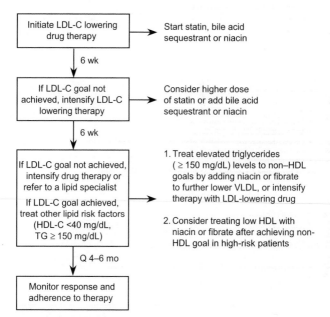

Initiate LDL-C lowering drug therapy → Start statin, bile acid sequestrant or niacin

↓ 6 wk

If LDL-C goal not achieved, intensify LDL-C lowering therapy → Consider higher dose of statin or add bile acid sequestrant or niacin

↓ 6 wk

If LDL-C goal not achieved, intensify drug therapy or refer to a lipid specialist

If LDL-C goal achieved, treat other lipid risk factors (HDL-C <40 mg/dL, TG ≥ 150 mg/dL) →

1. Treat elevated triglycerides ( ≥ 150 mg/dL) levels to non–HDL goals by adding niacin or fibrate to further lower VLDL, or intensify therapy with LDL-lowering drug

2. Consider treating low HDL with niacin or fibrate after achieving non-HDL goal in high-risk patients

↓ Q 4–6 mo

Monitor response and adherence to therapy

*Source:* Third Report of the Expert Panel on Detection, Evaluation, and Treatment of High Blood Cholesterol in Adults (Adult Treatment Panel III). Bethesda, Md: National Institutes of Health, National Heart, Lung, and Blood Institute; 2001. NIH Publication 01-3095.

# PRIMARY CARE

## HYPERTENSION
### Evaluation

#### Classification of Blood Pressure (BP)[a]

| Category | SBP mm Hg | | DBP mm Hg |
|----------|-----------|-----|-----------|
| Normal | <120 | and | <80 |
| Prehypertension | 120–139 | or | 80–89 |
| Hypertension, Stage 1 | 140–159 | or | 90–99 |
| Hypertension, Stage 2 | ≥160 | or | ≥100 |

[a]See *Blood Pressure Measurement Techniques* (below).
SBP, systolic blood pressure; DBP, diastolic blood pressure.

#### Diagnosis Workup of Hypertension

- Assess risk factors and comorbidities.
- Reseal identifiable causes of hypertension.
- Assess presence of target organ damage.
- Conduct history and physical examination.
- Obtain laboratory tests: urinalysis, blood glucose, hematocrit and lipid panel, serum potassium, creatinine, and calcium. Optional: urinary albumin/creatinine ratio.
- Obtain electrocardiogram.

#### Assess for Major Cardiovascular Disease (CVD) Risk Factors

- Hypertension
- Obesity (body mass index ≥30 kg/m²)
- Dyslipidemia
- Diabetes mellitus
- Cigarette smoking

- Physical activity
- Microalbuminuria, estimated glomerular filtration rate <60 mL/min
- Age (>55 for men, >65 for women)
- Family history of premature CVD (men age <55, women age <65)

#### Assess for Identifiable Causes of Hypertension

- Sleep apnea
- Drug induced/related
- Chronic kidney disease
- Primary aldosteronism
- Renovascular disease

- Cushing's syndrome or steroid therapy
- Pheochromocytoma
- Coarctation of aorta
- Thyroid/parathyroid disease

Reproduced from U.S. Department of Health and Human Services. NIH Publication No. 03-5231, May 2003.

## Principles of Hypertension Treatment

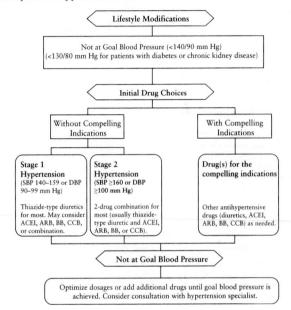

ACEI, angiotension converting enzyme inhibitors; ARB, angiotensin receptor blocker; BB, beta blocker; CCB, calcium channel blocker; DBP, diastolic blood pressure; SBP, systolic blood pressure.

Reproduced from U.S. Department of Health and Human Services. NIH Publication No. 03-5231, May 2003.

# PRIMARY CARE

## Blood Pressure Measurement Techniques

| Method | Notes |
|--------|-------|
| In-office | Two readings, 5 mins apart, sitting in chair. Confirm elevated reading in contralateral arm. |
| Ambulatory BP monitoring | Indicated for evaluation of "white coat hypertension." Absence of 10–20% BP decrease during sleep may indicate increased CVD risk. |
| Patient self-check | Provides information on response to therapy. May help improve adherence to therapy and is useful for evaluating "white coat hypertension." |

## Causes of Resistant Hypertension

- Improper BP measurement
- Excess sodium intake
- Inadequate diuretic therapy
- Medication
  - Inadequate doses
  - Drug actions and interactions (e.g., nonsteroidal anti-inflammatory drugs [NSAIDs], illicit drugs, sympathomimetics, oral contraceptives)
  - Over-the-counter (OTC) drugs and herbal supplements
- Excess alcohol intake
- Identifiable causes of hypertension (see related table above)

## Compelling Indications for Individual Drug Classes

| Compelling Indication | Initial Therapy Options |
|----------------------|------------------------|
| • Heart failure | THIAZ, BB, ACEI, ARB, ALDO ANT |
| • Post myocardial infarction | BB, ACEI, ALDO ANT |
| • High CVD risk | THIAZ, BB, ACEI, CCB |
| • Diabetes | THIAZ, BB, ACEI, ARB, CCB |
| • Chronic kidney disease | ACEI, ARB |
| • Recurrent stroke prevention | THIAZ, ACEI |

ACEI, angiotensin converting enzyme inhibitor; ALDO ANT, aldosterone antagonist; ARB, angiotensin receptor blocker; BB, β-blocker; CCB, calcium channel blocker; THIAZ, thiazide diuretic.

## Clinical Trial and Guideline Basis for Compelling Indications for Individual Drug Classes

| Compelling Indication[a] | Recommended Drugs | | | | | | Clinical Trial Basis[b] |
|---|---|---|---|---|---|---|---|
| | Diuretic | BB | ACEI | ARB | CCB | Aldo ANT | |
| Heart failure | • | • | • | • | | • | ACC/AHA Heart Failure Guideline, MERIT-HF, COPERNICUS, CIBIS, SOLVD, AIRE, TRACE, ValHEFT, RALES, CHARM |
| Postmyocardial infarction | | • | • | | | • | ACC/AHA Post-MI Guideline, BHAT, SAVE, Capricorn, EPHESUS |
| High coronary disease risk | • | • | • | | • | | ALLHAT, HOPE, ANBP₂, LIFE, CONVINCE, EUROPA, INVEST |
| Diabetes | • | • | • | • | • | | NKF-ADA Guideline, UKPOS, ALLHAT |
| Chronic kidney disease | | | • | • | | | NFK Guideline, Captopril Trial, RENAAL, IDNT, REIN, AASK |
| Recurrent stroke prevention | • | | • | | | | PROGRESS |

AASK, African American Study of Kidney Disease and Hypertension; ACC/AHA, American College of Cardiology/American Heart Association; ACEI, angiotensin converting enzyme inhibitor; AIRE, Acute Infarction Ramipril Efficacy; Aldo ANT, aldosterone antagonist; ALLHAT, Antihypertensive and Lipid-Lowering Treatment to Prevent Heart Attack Trial; ANBP₂, Second Australian National Blood Pressure Study; ARB, angiotensin receptor blocker; BB, β-blocker; BHAT, β-Blocker Heart Attack Trial; Capricorn, Carvedilol Post-Infarct Survival Control in Left Ventricular Dysfunction; CCB, calcium channel blocker; CHARM, Candesartan in Heart Failure Assessment of Reduction in Mortality and Morbidity; CIBIS, Cardiac Insufficiency Bisoprolol Study; CONVINCE, Controlled Onset Verapamil Investigation of Cardiovascular End Points; COPERNICUS, Carvedilol Prospective Randomized Cumulative Survival Study; EPHESUS, Eplerenone Post-Acute Myocardial Infarction Heart Failure Efficacy and Survival Study; EUROPA, European Trial on Reduction of Cardiac Events with Perindopril in Stable Coronary Artery Disease; HOPE, Heart Outcomes Prevention Evaluation Study; IDNT, Irbesartan Diabetic Neuropathy Trial; INVEST, The International Verapamil-Trandolapril Study; LIFE, Losartan Intervention for Endpoint Reduction in Hypertension Study; MERIT-HF, Metoprolol CR/XL Randomized Intervention Trial in Congestive Heart Failure; NKF-ADA, National Kidney Foundation-American Diabetes Association; PROGRESS, Perindopril Protection Against Recurrent Stroke Study; RALES, Randomized Aldactone Evaluation Study; REIN, Ramipril Efficacy in Nephropathy Study; RENAAL, Reduction of Endpoints in Non-Insulin Dependent Diabetes Mellitus with the Angiotensin II Antagonist Losartan Study; SAVE, Survival and Ventricular Enlargement Study; SOLVD, Studies of Left Ventricular Dysfunction; TRACE, Trandolapril Cardiac Evaluation Study; UKPDS, United Kingdom Prospective Diabetes Study; ValHEFT, Valsartan Heart Failure Trial.

[a]Compelling indications for antihypertensive drugs are based on benefits from outcome studies or existing clinical guidelines; the compelling indication is managed in parallel with the BP.

[b]Conditions for which clinical trials demonstrate the benefit of specific classes of antihypertensive drugs used as part of an antihypertensive regimen to achieve BP goal to test outcomes.

Reproduced with permission from The seventh report of the joint national committee on prevention, detection, evaluation, and treatment of high blood pressure. *JAMA*. May 2003;289(19):2568.

# PRIMARY CARE

## Principles of Lifestyle Modifications

- Encourage healthy lifestyles for all individuals.
- Prescribe lifestyle modifications for all patients with prehypertension and hypertension.
- Components of lifestyle modifications include weight reduction. DASH eating plan, dietary sodium reduction, aerobic physical activity, and moderation of alcohol consumption.

## Lifestyle Modification Recommendations

| Modification | Recommendation | Avg. SBP Reduction Range[a] |
|---|---|---|
| Weight reduction | Maintain normal body weight (body mass index 18.5–24.9 kg/m$^2$). | 5–20 mm Hg/10 kg |
| DASH eating plan | Adopt a diet rich in fruits, vegetables, and low-fat dairy products with reduced content of saturated and total fat. | 8–14 mm Hg |
| Dietary sodium reduction | Reduce dietary sodium intake to ≤100 mmol per day (2.4 g sodium or 6 g sodium chloride). | 2–8 mm Hg |
| Aerobic physical activity | Regular aerobic physical activity (e.g., brisk walking) at least 30 mins per day, most days of the week. | 4–9 mm Hg |
| Moderation of alcohol consumption | Men: limit to ≤2 drinks[b] per day. | 2–4 mm Hg |
| | Women and lighter weight persons: limit to ≤1 drink[b] per day. | |

[a]Effects are dose and time dependent.
[b]1 drink = 1/2 oz or 15 mL ethanol (e.g., 12 oz beer, 5 oz wine, 1.5 oz 80 proof whiskey).
Reproduced from U.S. Department of Health and Human Services. NIH Publication No. 03-5231, May 2003.

## Combination Drugs for Hypertension

| Combination Type[a] | Fixed-Dose Combination, MG[b] | Trade Name |
|---|---|---|
| | Amlodipine-benazepril hydrochloride (2.5/10, 5/10, 5/20, 10/20) | Lotrel |
| | Enalapril-felodipine (5/5) | Lexxel |
| | Trandolapril-verapamil (2/180, 1/240, 2/240, 4/240) | Tarka |
| ACEIs and diuretics | Benazepril-hydrochlorothiazide (5/6.25, 10/12.5, 20/12.5, 20/25) | Lotensin HCT |
| | Captopril-hydrochlorothiazide (25/15, 25/25, 50/15, 50/25) | Capozide |
| | Enalapril-hydrochlorothiazide (5/12.5, 10/25) | Vaseretic |
| | Fosinopril-hydrochlorothiazide (10/12.5, 20/12.5) | Monopril/HCT |
| | Lisinopril-hydrochlorothiazide (10/12.5, 20/12.5, 20/25) | Prinzide, Zestoretic |
| | Moexipril-hydrochlorothiazide (7.5/12.5, 15/25) | Uniretic |
| | Quinapril-hydrochlorothiazide (10/12.5, 20/12.5, 20/25) | Accuretic |
| ARBs and diuretics | Candesartan-hydrochlorothiazide (16/12.5, 32/12.5) | Atacand HCT |
| | Eprosartan-hydrochlorothiazide (600/12.5, 600/25) | Teveten-HCT |
| | Irbesartan-hydrochlorothiazide (150/12.5, 300/12.5) | Avalide |
| | Losartan-hydrochlorothiazide (50/12.5, 100/25) | Hyzaar |
| | Olmesartan medoxomil-hydrochlorothiazide (20/12.5, 40/12.5, 40/25) | Benicar HCT |
| | Telmisartan-hydrochlorothiazide (40/12.5, 80/12.5) | Micardis-HCT |
| | Valsartan-hydrochlorothiazide (80/12.5, 160/12.5, 160/25) | Diovan-HCT |
| BBs and diuretics | Atenolol-chlorthalidone (50/25, 100/25) | Tenoretic |
| | Bisoprolol-hydrochlorothiazide (2.5/6.25, 5/6.25, 10/6.25) | Ziac |
| | Metoprolol-hydrochlorothiazide (50/25, 100/25) | Lopressor HCT |
| | Nadolol-bendroflumethiazide (40/5, 80/5) | Corzide |
| | Propranolol LA-hydrochlorothiazide (40/25, 80/25) | Inderide LA |
| | Timolol-hydrochlorothiazide (10/25) | Timolide |

*(continued)*

## Combination Drugs for Hypertension *(continued)*

| Combination Type[a] | Fixed-Dose Combination, MG[b] | Trade Name |
|---|---|---|
| Centrally acting drug and diuretic | Methyldopa-hydrochlorothiazide (250/15, 250/25, 500/30, 500/50) | Aldoril |
| | Reserpine-chlorthalidone (0.125/250, 0.25/50) | Demi-Regroton, Regroton |
| | Reserpine/chlorothiazide (0.125/250, 0.25/500) | Diupres |
| | Reserpine-hydrochlorothiazide (0.125/25, 0.125/50) | Hydropres |
| Diuretic and diuretic | Amiloride-hydrochlorothiazide (5/50) | Moduretic |
| | Spirolactone-hydrochlorothiazide (25/25, 50/50) | Aldactazide |
| | Triamterene-hydrochlorothiazide (37.5/25, 75/50) | Dyazide, Maxzide |

[a]ACEIs, angiotensin converting enzyme inhibitors; ARBs, angiotensin receptor blockers; BBs, β-blockers; CCBs, calcium channel blockers.

[b]Some drug combinations are available in multiple fixed doses. Each drug dose is reported in milligrams. Reproduced with permission from The seventh report of the joint national committee on prevention, detection, evaluation, and treatment of high blood pressure. *JAMA.* May 2003;289(19):2567.

## MANAGING TYPE 2 DIABETES

### Fast Facts

- Type 2 diabetes results in enormous human suffering and economic cost.
- Complications can be reduced by achieving non-diabetic glucose levels.
- First line of treatment is lifestyle modification and metformin.
- Early addition of insulin is recommended if goals not achieved.

| | Summary of Antidiabetic Interventions as Monotherapy | | |
|---|---|---|---|
| Intervention | Expected Decrease in Hemoglobin A1C (%) | Advantages | Disadvantages |
| Step 1: | | | |
| Decrease weight and increase activity | 1–2 | Low cost, many benefits | Fails for most in first yr |
| Metformin | 1.5 | Weight neutral, cheap | GI side effects, rare lactic acidosis |
| Step 2: (additional therapy) | | | |
| Insulin | 1.5–2.5 | No dose limit, cheap, improved lipid profile | Injections, monitoring, weight gain |
| Sulfonylureas | 1.5 | Cheap | Weight gain, hypoglycemia |
| TZDs | 0.5–1.4 | Improved lipid profile | Fluid retention, weight gain, expensive |
| Alpha-glucosidase inhibitors | 0.5–0.8 | Weight neutral | GI side effects, TID dosing, expensive |
| Exenatide | 0.5–1.0 | Weight loss | Injections, GI side effects, expensive, little experience |
| Glinides | 1–1.5 | Short duration | TID dosing, expensive |
| Pramlintide | 0.5–1.0 | Weight loss | Injections, TID dosing, GI side effects, expensive, little experience |

*Source:* Adapted from Nathan et al. Management of hyperglycemia in type 2 diabetes: A consensus algorithm for the initiation and adjustment of therapy. *Diabetes Care.* 2006;29(8):1963–1972. (Copyright, 2006 by the American Diabetes Association).

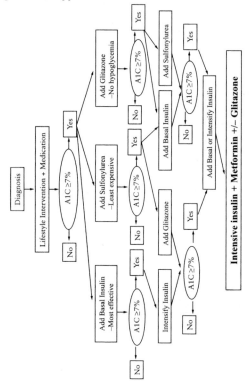

A1C, glycosylated hemoglobin.

*Source:* Adapted from Nathan et al. Management of hyperglycemia in type 2 diabetes: A consensus algorithm for the initiation and adjustment of therapy. *Diabetes Care.* 2006;29(8):1963–1972. (Copyright, 2006 by the American Diabetes Association).

## Initiating Insulin Therapy

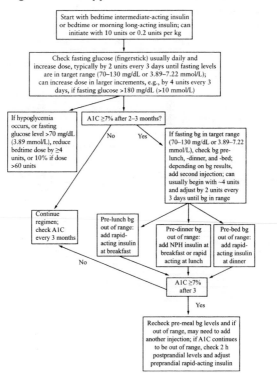

A1C, glycosylated hemoglobin; bg, blood glucose; NPH, neutral protamine hagedorn.
*Source:* Adapted from Nathan et al. Management of hyperglycemia in type 2 diabetes: A consensus algorithm for the initiation and adjustment of therapy. *Diabetes Care.* 2006;29(8):1963–1972. (Copyright, 2006 by the American Diabetes Association).

## SMOKING CESSATION

### Agents to Help Smokers Quit

| Factor | Bupropion hydrochloride SR (Zyban®, Wellbutrin®) | Patch (Various) | Gum (Nicorette®) |
|---|---|---|---|
| Treatment Period | 7–12 wks<br>Take for 1–2 wks before quitting smoking<br>May use for maintenance for up to 6 mos | 6–8 wks | Up to 12 wks<br>May use for longer time as needed |
| Dosage | Days 1–3: 150-mg tablet each morning<br>Days 4–end: 150-mg tablet in morning and evening | One patch each day<br>Taper dose if using: 21 mg for 4 wks<br>14 mg for 2 wks<br>7 mg for 2 wks<br>No taper if using 15 mg for 8 wks<br>Light smokers (≤10 cigarettes/day) can start with lower dose | 2 mg<br>4 mg (heavy smokers)<br>Chew one piece every 1–2 hrs (10–15 pieces/day)<br>Many people do not use enough gum—chew gum whenever you need it! |
| Pros | Easy to use<br>Reduces urges to smoke | Easy to use<br>Steady dose of nicotine | Can control your own dose<br>Helps with predictable urges (e.g., after meals)<br>Keeps mouth busy |
| Cons | May disturb sleep<br>May cause dry mouth | May irritate skin<br>May disturb sleep<br>Cannot adjust amount of nicotine in response to urges | Need to chew correctly—"chew and park"<br>May stick to dentures<br>Should not drink acidic beverages while chewing gum |
| Availability | Prescription only | Over the counter | Over the counter |

Reproduced with permission from Anderson JE, Jorenby DE, Scott WJ, Fiore MC. Treating tobacco use and dependence: an evidence-based clinical practice guideline for tobacco cessation. *Chest*. 2002;121:932–941.

| Inhaler (Nicotrol®) | Nasal Spray (Nicotrol®) | Lozenge (Commit™) |
|---|---|---|
| 3–6 mos<br>Taper use over last few wks | 3–6 mos<br>Taper use over last few wks | 12 wks |
| 6–16 cartridges/day<br>Need to inhale about 80 times to use up cartridge<br>Can use part of cartridge, save rest for later that day | One dose equals one squirt to each nostril<br>Dose 1–2 times/hr as needed<br>Minimum = 8 doses/day<br>Maximum = 40 doses/day | Take one 2-mg lozenge (if you smoke first cigarette more than 30 mins after waking up) or one 4-mg lozenge (if you smoke first cigarette within 30 mins of waking up) every 1–2 hr/day (wks 1–6); every 2–4 hrs (wks 7–9); every 4–8 hrs (wks 10–12) |
| Can control your own dose<br>Helps with predictable urges<br>Keeps hands and mouth busy | Can control your own dose<br>Fastest acting for relief of urges | Easy to use<br>Takes about 20–30 mins to dissolve completely |
| May irritate mouth and throat (improves with use)<br>Does not work well <40°F<br>Should not drink acidic beverages while using inhaler | Need to use correctly (do not inhale it)<br>May irritate nose (improves with use)<br>May cause dependence | May cause hiccups, heartburn, nausea, or other side effects if used continuously<br>Do not chew or swallow lozenge<br>Cannot eat or drink 15 mins before using or while lozenge is in mouth |
| Prescription only | Prescription only | Over the counter |

# PRIMARY CARE

## MIGRAINE HEADACHES

### Fast Facts

- Acute abortive therapy for migraine should be migraine specific and should be used early in the course of the migraine for best results.
- Narcotic pain relieving medications are not indicated for first-line treatment of migraine attacks.
- Use of acute symptomatic therapies for migraine more than 2 days per week, especially analgesics, may lead to medication overuse headache (rebound headache).
- Non-treatment or delayed treatment of migraine attacks may lead to central sensitization, making the attacks more refractory to treatment.

### Available Triptans and Their Doses

| Generic | Tablet Strength | Optimum Dose[a] | Maximum Daily Dose | Additional Formulations |
|---|---|---|---|---|
| Almotriptan | 6.25 & 12.5 mg | 12.5 mg | 25 mg | — |
| Eletriptan | 20 & 40 mg | 40 mg | 80 mg | — |
| Frovatriptan | 2.5 mg | 2.5 mg | 7.5 mg | — |
| Naratriptan | 1 & 2.5 mg | 2.5 mg | 5 mg | — |
| Rizatriptan | 5 & 10 mg | 10 mg | 30 mg | ODT |
| Sumatriptan | 25, 50, & 100 mg | 50 or 100 mg | 200 mg | SC, NS, PR |
| Zolmitriptan | 2.5 & 5 mg | 2.5 or 5 mg | 10 mg | ODT, NS |

NS, nasal spray; ODT, orally disintegrating tablet; PR, per rectum (suppository); SC, subcutaneous.

[a]Optimum dose derived from data showing the highest effective dose with the least side-effects. Some studies with early intervention treatment schemes suggest higher doses to be more beneficial when taken early without increasing side effects.

*Source:* Curtis P. Schreiber, MD. *Clinics in Family Practice* Volume 7, Number 3, September 2005. From the Headache Care Center, Springfield, Missouri.

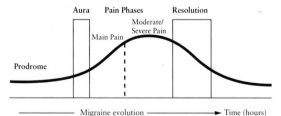

*Source:* The clinical phases of migraine. *Clinics in Family Practice.* 2005;7(3). Adapted from Smith TR. Copyright © 2005 W. B. Saunders Company.

## Characteristics of Migraine, Cluster, and Tension-Type Headache

| Characteristic | Migraine | Cluster | Tension-Type |
|---|---|---|---|
| Onset | Peak incidence in adolescence | 30s or 40s | Variable, generally problematic in the 20s or beyond |
| Frequency | 1 or 2 attacks per mo, often with menses | 1 or more attacks per day for 6 to 8 wks | *Episodic*—less than 15 days per mo<br>*Chronic*—more than 15 days per mo |
| Location | Unilateral > bilateral<br>Fronto-temporal or orbital | 100% unilateral; generally orbito-temporal | Bifrontal, biooccipital, neck |
| Description | Throbbing or intense pressure | Nonthrobbing, excruciating, boring, penetrating | Squeezing, pressing, aching |
| Duration | 4–72 hrs, usually 12–24 hrs | 30 mins to 2 hrs, usually 45–90 mins | *Episodic*—several hrs<br>*Chronic*—all day |
| Prodrome | Changes in mood, energy, appetite | May include brief mild burning in the ipsilateral inner canthus or internal nares | None |
| Aura | Up to 60 mins, usually 20 mins, often visual | None | None |
| Associated symptoms | Nausea, vomiting, sonophobia and photophobia, sensitivity, occasional ptosis | Ipsilateral ptosis-miosis, conjunctival injection, lacrimation; ipsilateral stuffed and running nostril | *Episodic*—loss of appetite, either light or sound sensitivity<br>*Chronic*—light or sound sensitivity or presence of nausea |
| Behavior | Retreat to a dark, quiet room (hibernate) | Frenetic pacing, rocking | Generally not affected; may have mild reduction in functional capacity |

Reproduced with permission from Marks DR, Rapoport AM. Practical evaluation and diagnosis of headache. Semin Neurol. 1997;17:309.

## Selected Drugs Used in the Acute Treatment and Prophylaxis of Migraine[a]

| Drug Class | Type of Drug | Drug Used, with Dose | Acute Rx for Migraine | Prophy-laxis for Migraine |
|---|---|---|---|---|
| Analgesics | NSAIDs | Ibuprofen, 400–800 mg, orally OTC or Rx | • | • |
| | | Naproxen, 250–500 mg, orally OTC or Rx | | |
| | | Indomethacin, 50 mg orally | • | |
| | Acetaminophen | Acetaminophen, 1000 mg orally OTC | • | |
| | Opioids | Codeine, 30 mg orally | • | |
| | Opiate antagonist | Butorphanol, 1 mg, NS | • | |
| | Combination analgesics | Esgic, 1–2 tablets orally (butalbital, 50 mg, acetaminophen, 325 mg, caffeine, 40 mg) | | |
| | | Fioricet, 1–2 tablets orally (butalbital, 50 mg, acetaminophen, 325 mg, caffeine, 40 mg) | | |
| Vasoactive agents | Dihydroergota-mine mesylate | Dihydroergotamine mesylate, 1 mg IM, SQ, IV | • | |
| | Other combina-tion agents | Midrin, 2 capsules orally, then 1 each hr up to 6 capsules (isometheptene mucate, 65 mg dichloralphenazone, 100 mg, acetaminophen, 325 mg) | • | |
| | 5-HT agonists[b] | Sumatriptan, 6 mg SQ, 25–100 mg orally, 20 mg NS | | • |
| | | Naratriptan, 1.0–2.5 mg orally | | |
| | | Rizatriptan, 5–10 mg orally | | |
| | | Zolmitriptan, 1.25–2.5 mg orally | | |
| | Ergotamine | Ergotamine, 2 mg orally | • | |
| | | Various combinations of ergota-mine and caffeine, orally and rectally | | |
| β-Blockers | | Propranolol, 80–240 mg orally, once daily | | • |
| | | Metoprolol, 50–100 mg orally, once daily | | |

## Selected Drugs Used in the Acute Treatment and Prophylaxis of Migraine[a]

| Drug Class | Type of Drug | Drug Used, with Dose | Acute Rx for Migraine | Prophy-laxis for Migraine |
|---|---|---|---|---|
| Antidepres-sants | Tricyclic antide-pressants | Amitriptyline, 25–100 mg orally, once daily | | • |
| | | Doxepin, 175–300 mg | | |
| | Selective seroto-nin reuptake inhibitors | Fluoxetine, 20–80 mg orally, daily (others may be effective) | | • |
| Calcium channel blockers | | Verapamil, 80–480 mg, daily | | • |
| | | Nimodipine, 30 mg 3 times daily | | |
| Anticonvul-sants | | Valproic acid, 250–500 mg orally, daily | | |

DHE, dihydroergotamine; 5-HT, 5-hydroxytryptamine; IM, intramuscularly; IV, intravenously; NS, nasal spray; NSAIDs, nonsteroidal antiinflammatory drugs; OTC, over the counter; Rx, prescription; SO, sub-cutaneously.

[a]Consult the manufacturer or other information for a complete list of therapeutic precautions, contraindi-cations, and drug interactions.

[b]The maximum to be administered in 24 hrs is 2 doses of any formula with at least 2 hrs between doses.

•Indicates drug is preferred for tension headache prophylaxis. All drugs listed for migraine prophylaxis may have some efficacy.

Reproduced with permission from Kieu A, Saxton E. Approach to the patient with headache. In: Pregler JP, DeCheney AH, eds. *Women's Health: Principles and Clinical Practice*. Hamilton (ON): BC Decker Inc; 2002: 722–723.

# PRIMARY CARE

## LOW BACK PAIN

### Fast Facts

- One of the leading causes of MD clinic visits.
- Most of the time, it is self-limiting.
- 90% are pain free within 3 months, and, of those, 90% are pain free in 4 weeks.
- Important to rule out serious causes such as malignancy, infection, trauma, or significant neurological compromise.
- Positive straight leg test (SLT) often indicates disc herniation.
- Location on pain with SLT will often indicate the anatomical location of the lesion.
- Laboratory tests are rarely needed.
- Activity, NSAIDs, Ultram, physical therapy are useful for uncomplicated low back pain.

### Strength and Motor Testing to Evaluate Different Nerve Roots

| Nerve Root | Reflex | Muscle | Test |
|------------|--------|--------|------|
| L4 | Knee jerk | Quadriceps | Leg extension weakness |
| L5 | Hamstrings | Extensor hallucis longus | Weakness of great toe extension |
| | | Tibialis anterior | Weakness of ankle dorsiflexion (possible footdrop) |
| S1 | Ankle jerk | Gluteus maximus | Affected gait, pelvic tilt, weakness of hip external rotator |
| | | Flexor digitorum | Weakness of toe flexors |
| | | Gastrocnemius | Weakness of plantar flexion, weakness of heel-raise |

From: Clinics in Family Practice. Volume 7, Number 2, June 2005. Copyright © 2005 W. B. Saunders Company. Marc I. Harwood, MD, Bradley J. Smith, MD. From the Department of Family Medicine, Jefferson Medical College, Thomas Jefferson University, Philadelphia, Pennsylvania (MIH, BBJS); and the Sports Medicine Fellowship Program, Jefferson Medical College, Thomas Jefferson University, Philadelphia, Pennsylvania (MIH).

**Diagnostic Evaluation of Back Pain**

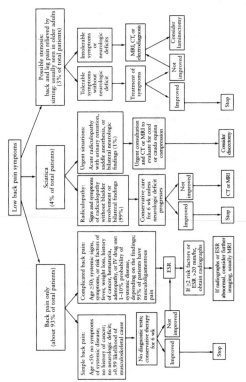

CT, computed tomography; ESR, erythrocyte sedimentation rate; MRI, magnetic resonance imaging. (*From:* Jarvik J, Deyo R. Diagnostic evaluation of low back pain with emphasis on imaging. *Ann Intern Med.* 2002;137:586–595; with permission.)

## Summary of the Nonsurgical Treatment Options for Low Back Pain

| Treatment Modality | Recommendation | Grade | Comment |
|---|---|---|---|
| Bed rest | To be avoided | A | Bed rest should be avoided; patients should be instructed to remain as active as possible within the limits of their pain. |
| Lifestyle modification: weight loss, tobacco cessation, exercise program | Recommended | C | Limited evidence as these non-medical therapies do not lend themselves to easy comparison and analysis via RCT. |
| Physical therapy | Recommended | D | Limited evidence to document efficacy, but most clinicians agree that PT should be routinely recommended. |
| NSAIDs | Recommended | A | Drugs of choice for management of acute LBP. |
| Acetaminophen | Not routinely recommended | B | Inconsistent evidence suggests that NSAIDs may be superior to acetaminophen. |
| COX-2 inhibitors | Not recommended | B | No more efficacious than traditional NSAIDs. Have been touted for their beneficial GI side-effect profile; however, new data regarding prothrombotic risk is concerning. |
| Muscle relaxants | May be helpful for bothersome night symptoms | B | Can be helpful for short courses, but the benefit arises with significant side effects, particularly sedation. |
| Narcotic analgesics | Recommended only for severe LBP | C | Studies comparing narcotics to NSAIDs and acetaminophen are of low quality. Narcotic analgesics may be helpful for severe cases of LBP with marked functional limitations. |
| Tramadol | Recommended for moderate to severe pain | A | Tramadol can be used as an adjunct to NSAIDs. |
| Epidural steroid injections | Recommended in carefully selected patients | D | Limited evidence for utility, but low methodologic quality of studies. |

| Treatment Modality | Recommendation | Grade | Comment |
|---|---|---|---|
| Spinal manipulation | Not routinely recommended | C | No documented benefit, but a generally safe modality. |
| Chiropractic manipulation | Not routinely recommended | D | Not more effective than other treatment modalities, but patient satisfaction is high with chiropractic treatment. |
| TENS | Not routinely recommended | B | Limited evidence to support its use, but a safe modality. |
| Prolotherapy | Not recommended | D | Evidence is lacking, and there are limited long-term data to document safety. |
| Acupuncture/ massage | Not routinely recommended | B | No high-quality evidence available to support its use, but a generally safe modality. |
| Back school | Reserved for patients with chronic LBP with marked functional impairment | B | Cost-effectiveness data unavailable. |
| Heat or cryotherapy | Recommended | C | No high-quality evidence to support its use. Safe, minimally invasive modality. |

LBP, low back pain; NSAID, nonsteroidal anti-inflammatory drug; PT, physical therapy; RCT, randomized control trial.
*Source:* Adapted from Harwood MI, Smith BJ. *Clinics in Family Practice.* 2005;7(2). © 2005 W.B. Saunders Company.

# PRIMARY CARE

## TOPICAL STEROIDS

The following potency chart categorizes brand-name topical steroid medications along with the name of the corresponding generic drug. The list positions these medications according to their potency. The list may not be comprehensive.

| Brand Name | Generic Name |
| --- | --- |
| **CLASS 1—Superpotent** | |
| Clobex Lotion, 0.05% | Clobetasol propionate |
| Cormax Cream/Solution, 0.05% | Clobetasol propionate |
| Diprolene Gel/Ointment, 0.05% | Betamethasone dipropionate |
| Olux Foam, 0.05% | Clobetasol propionate |
| Psorcon Ointment, 0.05% | Diflorasone diacetate |
| Temovate Cream/Ointment/Solution, 0.05% | Clobetasol propionate |
| Ultravate Cream/Ointment, 0.05% | Halobetasol propionate |
| **CLASS 2—Potent** | |
| Cyclocort Ointment, 0.1% | Amcinonide |
| Diprolene Cream AF, 0.05% | Betamethasone dipropionate |
| Diprosone Ointment, 0.05% | Betamethasone dipropionate |
| Elocon Ointment, 0.1% | Mometasone furoate |
| Florone Ointment, 0.05% | Diflorasone diacetate |
| Halog Ointment/Cream, 0.1% | Halcinonide |
| Lidex Cream/Gel/Ointment, 0.05% | Fluocinonide |
| Maxiflor Ointment, 0.05% | Diflorasone diacetate |
| Maxivate Ointment, 0.05% | Betamethasone dipropionate |
| Psorcon Cream 0.05% | Diflorasone diacetate |
| Topicort Cream/Ointment, 0.25% | Desoximetasone |
| Topicort Gel, 0.05% | Desoximetasone |
| **CLASS 3—Upper Mid-Strength** | |
| Aristocort A Ointment, 0.1% | Triamcinolone acetonide |
| Cutivate Ointment, 0.005% | Fluticasone propionate |
| Cyclocort Cream/Lotion, 0.1% | Amcinonide |
| Diprosone Cream, 0.05% | Betamethasone dipropionate |
| Florone Cream, 0.05% | Diflorasone diacetate |
| Lidex-E Cream, 0.05% | Fluocinonide |
| Luxiq Foam, 0.12% | Betamethasone valerate |
| Maxiflor Cream, 0.05% | Diflorasone diacetate |
| Maxivate Cream/Lotion, 0.05% | Betamethasone dipropionate |
| Topicort Cream, 0.05% | Desoximetasone |

| Brand Name | Generic Name |
|---|---|
| Valisone Ointment, 0.1% | Betamethasone valerate |
| **CLASS 4—Mid-Strength** | |
| Aristocort Cream, 0.1% | Triamcinolone acetonide |
| Cordran Ointment, 0.05% | Flurandrenolide |
| Derma-Smoothe/FS Oil, 0.01% | Fluocinolone acetonide |
| Elocon Cream, 0.1% | Mometasone furoate |
| Kenalog Cream/Ointment/Spray, 0.1% | Triamcinolone acetonide |
| Synalar Ointment, 0.025% | Fluocinolone acetonide |
| Uticort Gel, 0.025% | Betamethasone benzoate |
| Westcort Ointment, 0.2% | Hydrocortisone valerate |
| **CLASS 5—Lower Mid-Strength** | |
| Cordran Cream/Lotion/Tape, 0.05% | Flurandrenolide |
| Cutivate Cream, 0.05% | Fluticasone propionate |
| Dermatop Cream, 0.1% | Prednicarbate |
| DesOwen Ointment, 0.05% | Desonide |
| Diprosone Lotion, 0.05% | Betamethasone dipropionate |
| Kenalog Lotion, 0.1% | Triamcinolone acetonide |
| Locoid Cream, 0.1% | Hydrocortisone butyrate |
| Pandel Cream 0.1% | Hydrocortisone probutate |
| Synalar Cream, 0.025% | Fluocinolone acetonide |
| Uticort Cream/Lotion, 0.025% | Betamethasone benzoate |
| Valisone Cream/Ointment, 0.1% | Betamethasone valerate |
| Westcort Cream, 0.2% | Hydrocortisone valerate |
| **CLASS 6—Mild** | |
| Aclovate Cream/Ointment, 0.05% | Alclometasone dipropionate |
| DesOwen Cream, 0.05% | Desonide |
| Synalar Cream/Solution, 0.01% | Fluocinolone acetonide |
| Tridesilon Cream, 0.05% | Desonide |
| Valisone Lotion, 0.1% | Betamethasone valerate |
| **CLASS 7—Least Potent** | |
| Topicals with hydrocortisone, dexamethasone, methylprednisolone and prednisolone | |

Source: Adapted from the National Psoriasis Foundation). http://www.psoriasis.org/treatment/psoriasis/steroids/potency.php.

# PRIMARY CARE

## SINUSITIS

**Fast Facts**

### Four types of sinusitis
- Acute sinusitis (<4 weeks)
- Subacute sinusitis (a.k.a., partially treated) (4–8 weeks)
- Chronic sinusitis (>8 weeks)
- Recurrent sinusitis (≥3 per year)

### 1. Acute sinusitis
- Symptoms purulent rhinorrhea, postnasal drainage, pain over sinuses.
- Often preceded by viral infection.
- Mostly caused by *S. pneumoniae*, *H. influenzae*, and *M. catarrhalis*.
- Wait to treatment 7–10 days unless severe symptoms, then treatment sooner.
- Treatment consists of 10–14 days of antibiotics:
  Ampicillin 500 mg bid, Augmentin 500–875 mg bid, cefuroxime 250–500 mg bid.
- Nasal corticosteroids and saline nasal sprays/lavage might be helpful.

### 2. Subacute sinusitis (partial response)
- Consider another 10–14 days of antibiotics and consider using stronger antibiotics.
- If still not improved, consider CT scan and referral to allergist and/or ENT.

### 3. Chronic sinusitis
- Symptoms similar to acute sinusitis but more subtle.
- Often caused by noninfectious reasons.
- If infectious component, mostly caused by *S. aureus*, gram-negative enteric bacteria, anaerobes.
- Consider referral to allergist and/or ENT.

## Evaluation of Sinusitis

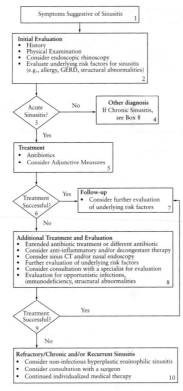

```
                    ┌─────────────────────────────────────┐
                    │ Symptoms Suggestive of Sinusitis   1 │
                    └─────────────────────────────────────┘
                                    │
    ┌───────────────────────────────────────────────────────┐
    │ Initial Evaluation                                     │
    │   • History                                            │
    │   • Physical Examination                               │
    │   • Consider endoscopic rhinoscopy                     │
    │   • Evaluate underlying risk factors for sinusitis     │
    │     (e.g., allergy, GERD, structural abnormalities)  2 │
    └───────────────────────────────────────────────────────┘
                                    │
                  ╱─────────╲   No    ┌──────────────────────┐
                 ╱  Acute    ╲───────▶│ Other diagnosis      │
                 ╲ Sinusitis? ╱       │ If Chronic Sinusitis,│
                  ╲    3    ╱          │ see Box 8          4 │
                   ╲───────╱          └──────────────────────┘
                       │ Yes
    ┌───────────────────────────────────┐
    │ Treatment                         │
    │   • Antibiotics                   │
    │   • Consider Adjunctive Measures 5│
    └───────────────────────────────────┘
                       │
                  ╱─────────╲   Yes   ┌──────────────────────────┐
                 ╱ Treatment ╲───────▶│ Follow-up                │
                 ╲Successful? ╱       │  • Consider further      │
                  ╲    6    ╱          │    evaluation of         │
                   ╲───────╱          │    underlying risk       │
                       │ No           │    factors             7 │
                                      └──────────────────────────┘
    ┌─────────────────────────────────────────────────────────────┐
    │ Additional Treatment and Evaluation                          │
    │   • Extended antibiotic treatment or different antibiotic    │
    │   • Consider anti-inflammatory and/or decongestant therapy   │
    │   • Consider sinus CT and/or nasal endoscopy                 │
    │   • Further evaluation of underlying risk factors            │
    │   • Consider consultation with a specialist for evaluation   │
    │   • Evaluation for opportunistic infections,                 │
    │     immunodeficiency, structural abnormalities             8 │
    └─────────────────────────────────────────────────────────────┘
                       │
                  ╱─────────╲   Yes
                 ╱ Treatment ╲───────▶
                 ╲Successful? ╱
                  ╲    9    ╱
                   ╲───────╱
                       │ No
    ┌─────────────────────────────────────────────────────────────────┐
    │ Refractory/Chronic and/or Recurrent Sinusitis                    │
    │   • Consider non-infectious hyperplastic eosinophilic sinusitis  │
    │   • Consider consultation with a surgeon                         │
    │   • Continued individualized medical therapy                  10 │
    └─────────────────────────────────────────────────────────────────┘
```

CT, computed tomography; GERD, gastroesophageal reflux disease.

*Source:* Slavin RG, Spector SL, Bernstein L. The diagnosis and management of sinusitis: a practice parameter update. *Journal of Allergy and Clinical Immunology.* 2005:116(6)suppl. © 2005 Mosby, Inc.

# PRIMARY CARE

## ALTERNATIVE MEDICINE/BOTANICALS

### Common Alternative Medications by Use and Toxic or Adverse Effect

| Name | Common Use | Toxic/Adverse Effects | Drug Interaction |
|------|-----------|----------------------|------------------|
| St. John's wort | Reduces depression and nervousness | Headache, restlessness, photosensitization | Reacts with SSRIs and other antidepressants, digoxin (Lanoxin), human immunodeficiency virus drugs, theophylline, cyclosporine, and oral contraceptives |
| Ephedra | Increases alertness, improves breathing, may reduce weight | Increased risk of heart attacks, rhythm disorders, strokes, seizures, or death | Interacts with caffeine, decongestants, stimulants, and antidepressants |
| Kava | Reduces stress and anxiety; also used as a muscle relaxant, sedative, or diuretic | Addictive effect, deep sedation or coma | Interacts with sedatives, sleeping pills, antipsychotics, and alcohol |
| Flaxseed (phytoestrogen) | Relieves menopausal symptoms, lowers low-density-lipoprotein cholesterol | May slow absorption of other oral medications, contains omega-3 fatty acids | Interacts with warfarin and aspirin to increase bleeding |
| Fish oils | Decreases risk of cardiovascular disease | Increases INR, may cause hemorrhage | Interacts with warfarin, aspirin, and NSAIDs |
| Gingko biloba | Enhances cognitive function, delays memory loss | May increase INR, cause excessive bleeding, and have a specific platelet effect | Interacts with warfarin, aspirin, and NSAIDs |

INR, international normalized ratio; NSAID, nonsteroidal antiinflammatory drug; SSRI, selective serotonin reuptake inhibitor.

*Source:* American College of Obstetricians and Gynecologists. PROLOG: Gynecologic oncology and critical care. 5th ed. Washington, DC: ACOG; 2006.

## Botanicals: Potential for Interactions with Drugs

| Drug Class | Herb | Potential Interactions |
|---|---|---|
| Anticoagulants | Bilberry | Increased risk of bleeding (high dose) |
| | Chamomile | Increased risk of bleeding |
| | Co-enzyme Q10 | Decreased effectiveness of anticoagulants |
| | Danshen | Increased risk of bleeding |
| | Dong quai | Increased risk of bleeding |
| | Feverfew | Increased risk of bleeding |
| | Garlic | Increased risk of bleeding |
| | Ginger | Increased risk of bleeding |
| | Ginkgo | Increased risk of bleeding |
| | Ginseng | Increased risk of bleeding |
| | Kava | Increased risk of bleeding |
| | St. John's wort | Decreased effectiveness of anticoagulants |
| Anticonvulsants | Borage | Decreased seizure threshold |
| | Comfrey | Increased risk of phenobarbital toxicity |
| | Evening primrose oil | Decreased seizure threshold |
| | Valerian | Increased effects of barbiturates |
| Antidepressants | Ephedra | Increased effect of monoamine oxidase inhibitors |
| | Ginseng | Increased effect of monoamine oxidase inhibitors |
| | Kava | Hypertension |
| | St. John's wort | Monoamine oxidase inhibitors—increased blood pressure level |
| | Yohimbine | Tricyclics—hypertension; selective serotonin reuptake inhibitors—increased serotonin levels |
| Diuretics | Aloe | Increased risk of hypokalemia |
| | Cascara sagrada | Increased risk of hypokalemia |
| | Licorice | Increased risk of hypokalemia |
| | Senna | Increased risk of hypokalemia |
| Hypoglycemic agents | Aloe | Risk of hypoglycemia |
| | Ginseng | Risk of hypoglycemia |
| | Stinging nettle | Potential elevation of blood glucose level |
| Sedatives | Chamomile | Increased drowsiness |
| | Kava | Increased risk of sedation |
| | Valerian | Increased risk of sedation |

Reproduced with permission from O'Mathuna DP. Herb-drug interactions. *Altern Med Alert.* 2003;6(4):37–43.

# PRIMARY CARE

## Commonly Used Botanicals and Vitamins and Their Possible Effects in the Surgical Patient

| Substance | Potential Negative Effect |
|---|---|
| Chaparral | Hepatotoxicity |
| Chondroitin | Anticoagulative properties |
| Chromium | Hypoglycemia |
| Dong quai | Anticoagulative properties |
| Echinacea | Hepatotoxicity |
| Feverfew | Anticoagulative properties |
| Garlic | Anticoagulative properties |
| Ginger | Anticoagulative properties |
| Ginkgo | Anticoagulative properties |
| Ginseng | Anticoagulative properties; hypertension; hypoglycemia |
| Goldenseal | Can reduce effect of antihypertensives |
| Kava | Potentiates the sedative effects of anesthetics; hepatotoxicity |
| Licorice root | Hypertension; hyperkalemia; hypokalemia; hypernatremia; edema |
| Ma huang (ephedra) | Arrhythmias; hypertension |
| Red yeast rice | Hepatotoxicity |
| St. John's wort | Prolongs anesthetic effects; inhibits reuptake of serotonin, dopamine, and noradrenaline |
| Valerian | Prolongs anesthetic effects; hepatotoxicity |
| Vitamin E | Anticoagulative properties |

Reproduced with permission from ACOG: Clinical Updates in Women's Health Care: Complementary and Alternative Medicine. October 2004:3(5);55.

# OUTPATIENT MANAGEMENT

## Charting Pearls

**Each visit document**

- Fetal heart tones and fetal movement.
- √ Blood pressure, urine dipstick protein.
- Outstanding lab results.
- Presentation and fundal height.
- Estimated gestational age.
- Date of return visit.
- Confirm and note type of uterine incision if previous cesarean section (C/S).
- Confirm and note discussion regarding postpartum contraception.
- Confirm and note discussion of vaginal birth after cesarean (VBAC) if previous low transverse C/S.
  - Consider VBAC consent form.
- Cervical exam, possible cervical length, ultrasound, and/or a fibronectin if preterm labor symptoms present (see flowchart on page 145).
- Presence or absence of preterm labor symptoms, bleeding, vaginal discharge, or spontaneous rupture of membranes.
- Presence or absence of symptoms of preeclampsia.
  - Blurred vision
  - Scotoma
  - Headache
  - Rapid weight gain and edema

# OBSTETRICS

## Routine Prenatal Laboratories

| First Visit | Comments |
|---|---|
| Type and screen | |
| Cystic fibrosis | |
| Rubella | Administer vaccine postpartum |
| VDRL | Same as RPR |
| HBsAg | |
| HIV | |
| Pap smear | |
| Cervical cultures for GC and chlamydia | Include Group B strep depending on clinic protocol |
| Complete blood count | |
| Hemoglobin electrophoresis | Where indicated |
| PPD | |
| Discuss genetic screening | e.g., Tay-Sachs, Canavan's, cystic fibrosis, risk for aneuploidy and CVS vs. amniocentesis |
| **9–14 wks gestation** | |
| Offer first trimester genetic screening | PAPP-A, free β-hCG and nuchal translucency screening (See page 202) |
| **15–20 wks gestation** | |
| Offer MSAFP or "triple screen" | Triple screen = AFP + estriol + free B-HCG |
| Offer "quad screen" genetic screening | β-hCG, estrogen, AFP, inhibin (See page 202) |
| **18–20 wks gestation** | |
| Ultrasound examination | As indicated |
| **24–28 wks gestation** | |
| 1 hr glucose challenge | See comments on page 112 |
| **28–30 wks gestation** | |
| RhoGAM administration | Must have negative antibody screen prior to RhoGAM |
| **35–37 wks gestation** | |
| Group B strep culture | |
| Repeat CBC | |
| **34–40 wks gestation** | |
| Repeat VDRL (RPR) and HIV | In high-risk patients |

AFP, alpha-fetoprotein; β-hCG, β human chorionic gonadotrophin; GC, neisseria gonorrhoeae; HIV, human immunodeficiency virus; MSAFP, maternal serum alpha-fetal protein; RPR, rapid plasma reagin; VDRL, Venereal Disease Research Laboratory test of syphilis.

## NAUSEA AND VOMITING IN PREGNANCY

| Therapy | Route of Administration/Dose | Efficacy | Comments |
|---------|------------------------------|----------|----------|
| **Anti-emetics** | | | |
| Metaclopramide (Reglan) | PO (10–30 mg qid) IM/IV (10 mg q4–6hr) | Effective | Concern over possible teratogenic effects not well founded in humans, often given with hydroxyzine (Aterax), 25–50 mg q4–6hr |
| Ondansetron (Zofran) | PO (4–8 mg q4–8hr) IV (8 mg q4–8hr) | Probably effective | A serotonin receptor antagonist, common side effects include mild sedation and headache |
| Droperidol (Inapsine) | IV/IM (2.5 mg q3–6hr) IV continuous infusion (1–2.5 mg/hr) | Probably effective | No known teratogenicity |
| **Phenothiazines/Antipsychotics** | | | |
| Promethazine (Phenergan) | PO/PR/IM (12.5–50 mg q4–6hr) | Effective | No known teratogenicity, may cause extrapyramidal (Parkinsonian) side effects, hypertension, sedation |
| Prochlorperazine (Compazine) | PO/IV/IM (5–10 mg q4–6hr) PR (25 mg q12hr) | Probably effective | No known teratogenicity |
| Chlorpromazine (Thorazine) | PO/IM (10–50 mg q6–8hr) | Probably effective | No known teratogenicity |
| **Antihistamines** | | | |
| Doxylamine succinate (Unisom) | PO (12.5–25 mg daily) | Probably effective | No known teratogenicity |
| Doxylamine succinate 10 mg + pyridoxine 10 mg (Bendectin) | PO (1–2 tablets q6–8hr) | Effective | Initial concern over teratogenic effects not well founded in humans |
| Meclizine (Antivert) | PO (25–100 mg daily) | Possibly effective | No known teratogenicity |
| Chlorpheniramine (Chlor-Trimeton) | PO (8–12 mg daily) | Possibly effective | No known teratogenicity |
| Diphenhydramine (Dramamine) | PO/IM/IV (50–75 mg q4–6hr) | Possibly effective | No known teratogenicity |
| Trimethobenzamide (Tigan) | PO (250 mg tid/qid) PR/IM (200 mg q6–8hr) | Possibly effective | No known teratogenicity |

Source: Modified from Erick, M. Hyperemesis gravidarum: a practical management strategy. *OBG Management*, November 2000, 25–35. Reproduced with permission of Dr. Errol Norwitz, Department of Maternal Fetal Medicine, Brigham and Women's Hospital, Boston, MA.

# OBSTETRICS

## Nausea and Vomiting in Pregnancy

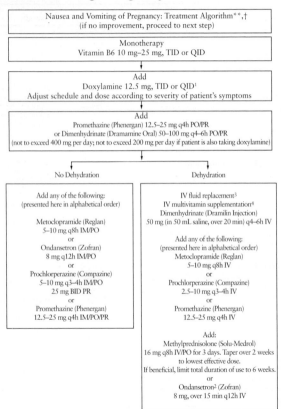

Nausea and Vomiting of Pregnancy: Treatment Algorithm**,†
(if no improvement, proceed to next step)

Monotherapy
Vitamin B6 10 mg–25 mg, TID or QID

Add
Doxylamine 12.5 mg, TID or QID[1]
Adjust schedule and dose according to severity of patient's symptoms

Add
Promethazine (Phenergan) 12.5–25 mg q4h PO/PR
or Dimenhydrinate (Dramamine) 50–100 mg q4–6h PO/PR
(not to exceed 400 mg per day; not to exceed 200 mg per day if patient is also taking doxylamine)

**No Dehydration**

Add any of the following:
(presented here in alphabetical order)

Metoclopramide (Reglan)
5–10 mg q8h IM/PO
or
Ondansetron (Zofran)
8 mg q12h IM/PO
or
Prochlorperazine (Compazine)
5–10 mg q3–4h IM/PO
25 mg BID PR
or
Promethazine (Phenergan)
12.5–25 mg q4h IM/PO/PR

**Dehydration**

IV fluid replacement[3]
IV multivitamin supplementation[4]
Dimenhydrinate (Dramilin Injection)
50 mg (in 50 mL saline, over 20 min) q4–6h IV

Add any of the following:
(presented here in alphabetical order)
Metoclopramide (Reglan)
5–10 mg q8h IV
or
Prochlorperazine (Compazine)
2.5–10 mg q3–4h IV
or
Promethazine (Phenergan)
12.5–25 mg q4h IV

Add:
Methylprednisolone (Solu-Medrol)
16 mg q8h IV/PO for 3 days. Taper over 2 weeks
to lowest effective dose.
If beneficial, limit total duration of use to 6 weeks.
or
Ondansetron[2] (Zofran)
8 mg, over 15 min q12h IV

[1]In the United States, doxylamine is available as the active ingredient in Unisom® Sleep Tabs™; one half of a scored 25-mg tablet can be used to provide a 12.5-mg dose of doxylamine. Diclectin® (doxylamine 10 mg and pyridoxine 10 mg) is presently available only in Canada in a delayed-release formulation that is typically prescribed 3–4 times daily.

[2]Safety, particularly in the first trimester of pregnancy, not yet determined; has no effect on nausea.

[3]No study has compared different fluid replacements for nausea and vomiting of pregnancy.

[4]100 mg thiamin IV daily for 2–3 days (followed by IV multivitamin) is recommended for every woman who requires IV hydration and has vomited for more than 3 wks.

[5]Steroids may increase risk for oral clefts in first 10 wks of gestation.

**The use of this algorithm assumes that other causes of nausea and vomiting have been ruled out.

†At any step, consider parenteral nutrition, if indicated.

*Source:* Reproduced with permission from Levichek Z, Atanackovic G, Oepkes D, et al. *Can Fam Physician.* 2002;48:267–268, 277.

# OBSTETRICS

## NUTRITION

### Weight Gain
- Recommendations based on body mass index (BMI) or IBW.
- Prepregnancy values are the only values with documented clinical significance.
- Adolescents should strive for gains at the upper end of the range.
- Short women (<157 cm or 62 in) should aim for the lower end of the range.
- Obese women should gain at least 6 kg.

| Prepregnancy Weight | IBW (%) | BMI | Recommended Net Weight Gain |
|---|---|---|---|
| Underweight | <90 | <19.8 | 12–18 kg |
| Acceptable | 90–120 | 19.8–26.0 | 11–16 kg |
| Overweight | 121–135 | 26.0–29.0 | 7–11 kg |
| Severely overweight | >135 | >29.0 | 7 kg |
| Excessive weight gain | >1.5 kg/mo | | |
| Inadequate weight gain | <0.25 kg/wk or <1 kg/mo | | |

### Caloric Requirements
- 1st and early 2nd trimester      25–30 kcal/kg IBW
- Late 2nd and early 3rd trimester      25–35 kcal/kg IBW

### Iron Supplementation
- Total iron requirement during pregnancy = 1000 mg
  - 30 mg of elemental iron/day recommended (U.S. Centers for Disease Control and Prevention recommends starting at the first prenatal visit)
    ⇨ 150 mg ferrous sulfate or
    ⇨ 300 mg ferrous gluconate or
    ⇨ 100 mg ferrous fumarate

### Folate Supplementation
- Routine supplementation is now recommended for all women of reproductive age (0.4 mg/day = amount in most prenatal vitamins)
- History of neural tube defects
  - Begin prepregnancy (*Source: MMWR 40: 513–16, 1991*)
  - 4 mg daily

### Special Needs
- Vitamin D—10 mcg (400 IU) daily for complete vegetarians
- Vitamin B12—2 mcg daily for complete vegetarians
- Calcium—1300 mg daily for women <19 years old, 1000 mg daily for women 19–50 years old

## CLINICAL PELVIMETRY

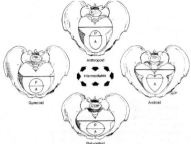

*Source:* Cunningham FG, MacDonald PC, Gant NF et al. Anatomy of the female reproductive tract. In: *Williams Obstetrics.* 22nd ed. New York: McGraw-Hill, 2005. Reproduced with permission of the publisher.

| Classification | Forepelvis | Sidewalk | Sacrum Inclination | Sacrosciatic Notch | Ischial Spines | Arch |
|---|---|---|---|---|---|---|
| Gynecoid | wide | straight | medium | medium | not prominent | wide |
| Android | narrow | convergent | forward | narrow | prominent | narrow |
| Anthropoid | narrow | divergent | backward | wide | not prominent | medium |
| Platypelloid | wide | straight | forward | narrow | not prominent | medium |

| Pelvic Plane | Diameter | Average Length (cm) |
|---|---|---|
| Inlet | True conjugate | 11.5 |
| | Obstetric conjugate | 11 |
| | Transverse | 13.5 |
| | Oblique | 12.5 |
| | | 4.5 |
| Greatest diameter | A-P | 12.75 |
| | Transverse | 12.5 |
| Mid-plane | A-P | 12 |
| | Bispinous | 10 |
| | Posterior sagittal | 4.5-5 |
| Outlet | Anatomic A-P | 9.5 |
| | Obstetric A-P | 11.5 |
| | Bituberous | 11 |
| | Posterior sagittal | 7.5 |

*Source:* Bochner C. Anatomic characteristics of the fetal head and maternal pelvis. In: Hacker NF, Moore JG, ed. *Essentials of Obstetrics and Gynecology.* 2nd ed. Philadelphia: Saunders, 1992. Reproduced with permission of the publisher.

# OBSTETRICS

## INDUCTION OF LABOR

### Fast Facts
- Overall rate of induction has increased to 20.6% of all births in 2002.
- Induction indicated for various maternal/fetal conditions.
- Bishop score ≥6 favorable for success.
- All prostaglandins should be discouraged in women with a history of prior C/S, but pitocin and/or foley bulb can be considered. (See ACOG Practice Bulletin, Vaginal Birth after Previous Cesarean Delivery, Number 54, July 2004.)

### Attributes of Commercially Available Prostaglandin Analogues

|  | Dinoprostone (GE2 Cervical Gel) | Dinoprostone (PGE2 Vaginal Insert) | Misoprostol (PGE1 Analogue) |
|---|---|---|---|
| Description | Sterile, semitranslucent viscous preparation for endocervical application of 0.5 mg PGE2 per 3.0 g, in syringe | Thin, flat polymeric slab of 10 mg dinoprostone pessary contained within knitted polyester retrieval system | 100 or 200 mcg oral tablets, divided in the pharmacy into 25- and 50-mcg doses; intravaginal use more preferable than oral |
| FDA status | FDA approved for cervical ripening | FDA approved for cervical ripening | FDA approved as an ulcer medication; Class X drug with black box warning contraindicating use by pregnant women; documented abortifacient properties |
| Pharmacokinetics | Half-life <5 mins; extensively metabolized in the lungs; rapidly absorbed; $T_{max}$ of 0.5–0.75 hrs | 2.5–5-min half-life; 95% is cleared on first pass through pulmonary circulation; controlled release of approximately 0.3 mg/hr in vivo | 20–40-min half-life; no industry standard dosing schedule |
| Initial dose | 0.5 mg | 10 mg | 25–50 mcg |
| Route | Intracervical | Intravaginal | Intravaginal |
| Maximum number of doses | 3 doses per 24 hrs | 1 dose | 6 doses per 24 hrs |
| Mechanisms of action | Softens the cervix; relaxes cervical smooth muscle; causes uterine contractions | Softens the cervix; relaxes cervical smooth muscle; causes uterine contractions | Causes uterine contractions |

## Attributes of Commercially Available Prostaglandin Analogues

| | Dinoprostone (GE2 Cervical Gel) | Dinoprostone (PGE2 Vaginal Insert) | Misoprostol (PGE1 Analogue) |
|---|---|---|---|
| Use in VBAC | Implicated in the literature for increased risk of uterine rupture | Implicated in the literature for increased risk of uterine rupture | Specifically contraindicated by ACOG due to risk of uterine rupture |
| Price per dose | Approximately $150; usually requires more than 1 dose | Approximately $175; only 1 dose needed | Approximately $1.00 |
| Refrigeration | Required | Required | Not required |
| Uterine hyperstimulation | Tocolytic agents must be administered | Resolves immediately upon removal of vaginal pessary | Tocolytic agents must be administered |
| Oxytocin administration | 6–12 hrs after administration of the last dose of the gel | 30–60 mins after removal of pessary | Minimum of 3 hrs after administration of the last dose of PGE1 |
| Efficacy as cervical ripener | Comparable | Comparable | Comparable |
| Medicolegal | Labeled use precludes additional action | Labeled use precludes additional action | Off-label use requires informed consent |
| Cesarean delivery rate | No diminishment | No diminishment | No diminishment |

ACOG, American College of Obstetricians and Gynecologists; FDA, U.S. Food and Drug Administration; PGE1, prostaglandin E1; PGE2, prostaglandin E2; VBAC, vaginal birth after cesarean delivery.
Source: Witter F, Devoe L. Update on successful induction of labor. *Advanced Studies in Medicine*. Johns Hopkins University School of Medicine. 2005;5(90):5888–5897.

## Foley Catheter

- Comparable success to medical methods.
- Insert sterile speculum and clean cervix with Betadine or other antiseptic.
- Use ring forceps to insert tip of Foley catheter just beyond internal cervical os (may need to use a stylet).
- Use a 26 french catheter with 30 cc balloon.
- Fill balloon with 30–60 cc of normal saline over 1 minute.
- Retract the balloon so that it rests at the internal cervical os.
- Tape to patient's thigh with the traction in place.
- Foley will fall out when cervix has dilated to 3–4 cm in response to the pressure applied.
- May attach a 1 liter IV fluid bag to end of catheter and let hang out of the bed.
- Remove 6 hours later or at time of the rupture of membranes or spontaneous expulsion.
- May be combined with Pitocin administration.

*Source:* Culver J et al. A randomized trial comparing vaginal misoprostol versus Foley catheter with concurrent oxytocin for labor induction in nulliparous women. *Am J Perinatol* 2004;21(3):139–146.

# OBSTETRICS

## Pitocin

- Multiple protocols with either low or high dose Pitocin have been studied.
- Most institutions will have standard protocols for Pitocin augmentation.
- There is conflicting evidence regarding the use of Pitocin in women with a history of a prior C/S. Even studies that show an increase in rate of uterine rupture with use of Pitocin for induction, however, still report a rupture rate of less than 1%. (see pg. 72)

## Precautions

- Document indication, estimated fetal weight, and presentation (by ultrasound) clearly in chart.
- If elective induction, document lung maturity if <39 weeks.
- Document normal fetal heart rate (FHR) and less than 3 contractions per 10 minutes prior to placement of prostaglandins.
- Monitor FHR and uterine activity for at least 30 minutes to 2 hours after administration of gel or continuously with misoprostol.
- Use caution in patients with asthma, glaucoma, or renal, pulmonary, and hepatic disease.

## Bishop Scoring for Cervical Ripening

| Factor | 0 | 1 | 2 | 3 |
|---|---|---|---|---|
| Cervical dilation (cm) | closed | 1–2 | 3–4 | 5+ |
| Cervical effacement (%) | 0–30 | 40–50 | 60–70 | 80+ |
| Fetal station | –3 | –2 | –1 | +1, +2 |
| Cervical consistency | firm | medium | soft | • |
| Cervical position | posterior | mid | anterior | • |

Add 1 point for preeclampsia, each prior vaginal delivery.
Deduct 1 point for postdates, nulliparity, preterm or prolonged PROM.

## Predictive Value for Success

| Score | | |
|---|---|---|
| | 0–4 | 45–50% failure |
| | 5–9 | 10% failure |
| | 10–13 | 0% failure |

## FETAL LUNG MATURITY
### ACOG Committee Opinion

Fetal maturity may be assumed and amniocentesis need not be performed if **one** of the following is met:

1. Fetal heart tones have been documented for 20 weeks by non-electric fetoscope or for 30 weeks by Doppler.

2. It has been 36 weeks since a positive serum or urine human chorionic gonadotropin pregnancy test was performed by a reliable laboratory.

3. An ultrasound measurement of the crown-rump length, obtained at 6–11 weeks, supports a gestational age of >39 weeks.

4. An ultrasound, obtained at 12–20 weeks, confirms the gestational age of >39 weeks determined by clinical history and physical exam.

# OBSTETRICS

## Fetal Lung Maturity Testing

| Test | Technique | Threshold | Mature | Immature | Notes |
|---|---|---|---|---|---|
| Lecithin/sphingo-myelin ratio | Thin-layer chromatography | 2.0–3.5 | 95–100 | 33–50 | Many variations in technique; laboratory variation significant |
| Phosphatidylglyc-erol | Thin-layer chromatography | "Present" (usually means >3% of total phospho-lipid) | 95–100 | 23–53 | Not affected by blood, meconium; vaginal pool samples satisfactory |
| | Antisera | 0.5 = low positive 2.0 = high positive | 95–100 | 23–53 | Not affected by blood, meconium; vaginal pool samples satisfactory |
| Foam stability index | Ethanol added to amniotic fluid, solution shaken, presence of stable bubbles at meniscus noted | ≥47 or 48 | 95 | 51 | Affected by blood, meconium, vaginal pool debris, silicone-coated test tubes |
| Fluorescence polarization | Fluorescence polarization | ≥55 mg/g of albu-min | 96–100 | 47–61 | Minimal intraassay and interassay variability; simple testing procedure |
| Optical density (OD) at 650 nm | Spectrophotometric reading | OD ≥0.15 | 98 | 13 | Simple technique |
| Lamellar body counts | Counts using commercial hematology counter | 30,000–40,000 (still investigational) | 97–98 | 29–35 | Promising technique |

Source: American College of Obstetricians and Gynecologists. Assessment of Fetal Lung Maturity. Educational Bulletin 230. ACOG, Washington, DC © 1996. Reproduced with permission of the publisher.

## LABOR AND DELIVERY
### Labor-Normal
- Ideally each patient should be evaluated at least q2hr (with or without an exam)
- Labor is a physiologic not pathologic process
- See the Friedman curve as detailed below:

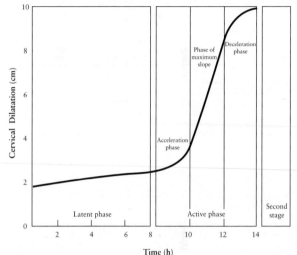

*Source:* Modified from Friedman EA. *Labor: Evaluation and Management*, 2nd edition. East Norwalk CT: Appleton-Century-Crofts, 1978.

# OBSTETRICS

Avoid unnecessary examinations and remember the following (Courtesy of S. Joel-Cohen):

| 5 Cs | 5 Ps |
|---|---|
| Clean (first) | Presentation |
| Catheterize (or empty bladder, second) | Position |
| Cervix (effacement, dilation...) | Place (station) |
| Caput (is it head or caput?) | Pelvis (clinical pelvimetry) |
| Cord (are there cord pulsations beyond membranes?) | Puncture (spontaneous rupture of membranes or need for amniotomy) |

| Pattern | Nulligravida | Multiparous | Therapeutic Interventions |
|---|---|---|---|
| Prolonged latent phase | >20 hrs | >14 hrs | Rest, oxytocin |
| Protraction disorder | | | |
| Dilation | <1.2 cm/hr | <1.5 cm/hr | AROM, oxytocin |
| Descent | <1cm/hr | <2 cm/hr | Oxytocin |
| Arrest disorder[a] | | | |
| Dilation | >2 hrs | >2 hrs | AROM, oxytocin, cesarean section |
| Descent | >2 hrs | >1 hr | Forceps, vacuum, cesarean section |
| | >3 hrs with epidural | >2 hrs with epidural | |

[a]With documented adequate uterine contractions: >200 Montevideo units/10 mins for 2 hrs. AROM, artificial rupture of membranes.

Note: The newest American College of Obstetricians and Gynecologists (ACOG) Bulletin *(Dystocia and Augmentation of Labor.* Number 49, December 2003) suggests that one can wait up to 4 hrs of adequate contractions prior to diagnosing an arrest of dilation and performing a C/S. The other therapeutic option for an arrest of descent is continued observation (if maternal and fetal status are reassuring). Average second stage 19 min multiparous and 54 min nulligravida.

Sources: ACOG: Dystocia. Technical Bulletin 137. ACOG, Washington, DC © 1989. Operative Vaginal Delivery. ACOG Practice Bulletin #17, June 2000. ACOG, Washington, DC © 2000. Reproduced with the permission of the publisher and American College of Obstetricians and Gynecologists.

## SHOULDER DYSTOCIA

### Definition

"Delivery that requires additional maneuvers following failure of gentle downward traction on the fetal head to effect delivery of the shoulders." (*Source:* ACOG practice bulletin: shoulder dystocia. Number 40, November 2002.)

### Incidence

0.6–1.4% of all deliveries.

### Risk Factors

Maternal obesity, diabetes, history of macrosomic infant, current macrosomia, history of prior shoulder dystocia

### Risk of Shoulder Dystocia (%) as a Function of Birthweight

| Reference | 2500–2999 g | 3000–3499 g | 3500–3999 g | 4000–4499 g | 4500–5000 g | >5000 g |
|---|---|---|---|---|---|---|
| Acker DB et al. *Obstet Gynecol* 1985;66(6): 762–768. | 0.2 | 0.6 | 2.3 | 10.3 | 23.9 | |
| Spellacy WN et al. *Obstet Gynecol* 1985;66(2): 158–61. | 0.3 | | N/A | | 7.3 | 14.6 |
| Benedetti TJ et al. *Obstet Gynecol* 1978;52(5): 526–529. | 1.5 | | 3.0 | | | |

- $^2/_3$ occur with birthweight <4000 g.
- Diabetic pregnancies are at higher risk.

### Warning Signs

**Anticipation is key!**

- Prolonged 2nd stage of labor
- Recoil of head on perineum (turtle sign)
- Lack of spontaneous restitution

### Treatment

1. McRobert's Maneuver—dorsiflexion of hips against abdomen and abduction.
2. Cut generous episiotomy.
3. Suprapubic pressure (**NOT** fundal pressure).
4. Constant moderate **DOWNWARD** traction to count of 30.
5. Rubin's Screw Maneuver (rotate face towards floor).
6. Attempt Wood's Screw.
7. Attempt delivery of posterior arm (may fracture humerus).
8. Zavenelli Maneuver—cephalic replacement/abdominal rescue.

# OBSTETRICS

## Fetal Complications
- Occur in 4–40% of deliveries complicated by shoulder dystocia.
- Common injuries include brachial plexus injury, clavicle fracture, and humerus fracture.
- <10% have permanent injuries.
- Increased risk of asphyxia.

## Maternal Complications
- 11% risk of postpartum hemorrhage
- 3.8% risk of 4th degree laceration

## HELPER Alogorithm
Help
Episiotomy
Leg elevated (McRobert's)
Pressure (suprapubic)
Enter vagina and attempt rotation (Wood's screw)
Reach for fetal arm

*Source:* Personal communication, Dr. Khoa Lai.

## OPERATIVE VAGINAL DELIVERY

### Criteria for Types of Forceps Delivery

| Outlet forceps |
| --- |

1. Scalp is visible at the introitus without separating the labia.
2. Fetal skull has reached the pelvic floor.
3. Sagittal suture is in an anteroposterior diameter or right or left occiput anterior or posterior position.
4. Rotation does not exceed 45°.

| Low forceps |
| --- |

Leading point of fetal skull is at station ≥ +2 cm, and not on the pelvic floor.

Rotation is 45°or less (left or right occiput anterior to occiput anterior, or left or right occiput posterior to occiput posterior.

Rotation is greater than 45°.

| Mid forceps |
| --- |

Station above +2 cm but head is engaged.

| High forceps |
| --- |

Not included in classification.

*Source:* American College of Obstetricians and Gynecologists: Operative Vaginal Delivery. ACOG Practice Bulletin #17, June 2000. ACOG, Washington, DC © 2000.

### Tips from Dr. Shirley Tom

• Have clear indication for forceps (fetal distress, prolonged 2nd stage, etc.).
• Have good anesthesia.
• Empty the bladder.
• Know fetal position precisely (feel for fetal ear helix if caput present).
• Obtain consent from the patient.

*Source:* Personal communication, Palo Alto Medical Clinic, Palo Alto, CA.

### Indications for Operative Vaginal Delivery

No indication for operative vaginal delivery is absolute. The following indications apply when the head is engaged and the cervix fully dilated.

| Prolonged second stage | |
| --- | --- |
| Nulliparous women | Lack of continuing progress for 3 hrs with regional anesthesia, or 2 hrs without regional anesthesia |
| Multiparous women | Lack of continuing progress for 2 hrs with regional anesthesia, or 1 hr without regional anesthesia |
| Suspicion of immediate or potential fetal compromise | |
| Shortening of the second stage for maternal benefit | |

*Source:* American College of Obstetricians and Gynecologists: *Operative Vaginal Delivery.* ACOG Practice Bulletin #17, June 2000. ACOG, Washington, DC © 2000. Reproduced with permission.

# OBSTETRICS

## Types of Forceps

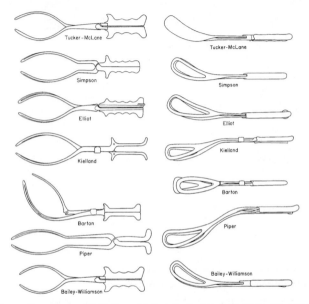

*Source:* From Zuspan FP, Quilligan EJ. Forceps. In: *Douglas-Stromme Operative Obstetrics.* 5th ed. Norwalk, Conn.: Appleton & Lange, 1988. Reproduced with the permission of the publisher.

## VACUUM EXTRACTION

### Fast Facts

- Use same indications as forceps, but ease of application has clouded judgment of some physicians.
- All cups are approximately 6 cm in diameter.
- Can result in fetal injuries similar to forceps, higher incidence of scalp injuries.
  - Cephalohematoma in 14–16% of vacuum deliveries (vs. 2% with forceps)
  - Subgaleal hematoma in 26–45/1000 vacuum deliveries
  - Retinal hemorrhages in 38% (vs. 17% with forceps)

### Application and Delivery

- Know the fetal position exactly.
- Check manufacturer's recommendations.
- Position cup symmetrically over sagittal suture 3 cm anterior to posterior fontanelle: "flexion point."
- Apply low suction (100 mm Hg), increase pressure to 500 mm Hg, and pull along pelvic curve.
- Check that no vaginal or cervical tissue is trapped by cup.
- Descent of the head must occur with each pull.
- Delivery should be accomplished with 3–5 pulls.
- Maximum of 2 "pop-offs."
- Head should be completely delivered within 15 minutes of first application.
- Do not use for rotation.
- Avoid rocking movements or excessive torque.

### Classification and Use of Vacuum Delivery Cups

| | |
|---|---|
| Soft cups—Indicated for outlet and low OA <45° assisted deliveries | Kiwi ProCup and Kiwi OmniCup |
| | Silc, Gentle Vac, and Secure Cups |
| | Silastic. Reusable and Vac-U-Nate cups |
| | Standard MityVac and Soft Touch cups |
| Rigid 'anterior' cups—Indicated for outlet and low OA <45° assisted deliveries | M-Style MityVac cup |
| | Flex cup |
| | Malmstrom, Bird, and O'Neil cups |
| Rigid 'posterior' cups— Indicated for OA >45°, OP and OT assisted deliveries | Kiwi OmniCup |
| | M-Select Mityvac cup |
| | Bird and O'Neil Posterior cups |

OA, occiput-anterior; OP, occiput-posterior; OT, occiput-transverse.
*Source:* Reproduced with permission from McQuivery RW. Vacuum-assisted delivery: a review. *The Journal of Maternal-Fetal and Neonatal Medicine.* 2003;16:171–179.

# OBSTETRICS

## Proper Placement

The center of the cup should be over the sagittal suture and about 3 cm in front of the posterior fontanelle. The cup is generally placed as far posteriorly as possible.

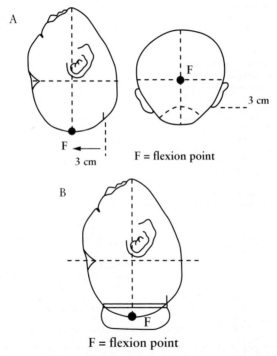

A

F ←—— 3 cm

F = flexion point

3 cm

B

F = flexion point

(A) During normal delivery condition, the mentocervical diameter emerges on the sagittal suture approximately 3 cm in front of the posterior fontanelle. (B) The center of the extraction cup has been placed over the flexion point, and axis traction is applied.

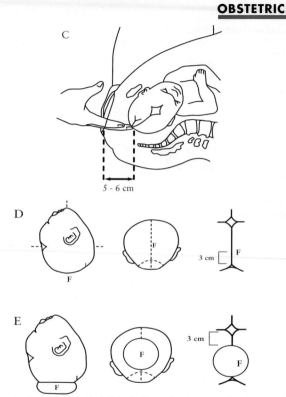

(C) Locating the flexion point and calculating the distance from the posterior fourchette using the examining finger. (D) The flexion point is situated on the sagittal suture 3 cm forward of the posterior fontanelle. (E) The center of the vacuum cup should be placed over the flexion point with the sagittal suture in the midline.

*Source:* Reproduced with permission from Vacca A. Vacuum-Assisted Delivery: Improving patient outcomes and protecting yourself against litigation. Supplement to *OBG Management*, February 2004. S1–S7.

# OBSTETRICS

## Relative Contraindications

- Prematurity (Most experts recommend against use of vacuum <34 weeks.)
- Suspected macrosomia
- Suspected fetal coagulation disorder
- Fetal scalp sampling
- Non-vertex presentation
- Fetal bone disorder

| Delivery Method | Neonatal Death | Intracranial Hemorrhage | Other[a] |
|---|---|---|---|
| Spontaneous vaginal delivery | 1/5000 | 1/1900 | 1/216 |
| Cesarean delivery during labor | 1/1250 | 1/952 | 1/71 |
| Cesarean delivery after vacuum/forceps | N/R | 1/333 | 1/38 |
| Cesarean delivery with no labor | 1/1250 | 1/2040 | 1/105 |
| Vacuum alone | 1/3333 | 1/860 | 1/122 |
| Forceps alone | 1/2000 | 1/664 | 1/76 |
| Vacuum and forceps | 1/1666 | 1/280 | 1/58 |

N/R, not reported.

[a]Facial nerve/brachial plexus injury, convulsions, central nervous system depression, mechanical ventilation

Data from Towner D. Castro MA, Eby-Wilkens E, Gilbert WM. Effect of mode of delivery in nulliparous women on neonatal intracranial brain injury. *N Engl J Med* 1999;341:1709–1714.

*Source:* American College of Obstetricians and Gynecologists: Operative Vaginal Delivery. ACOG Practice Bulletin #17, June 2000. ACOG, Washington, DC © 2000.

## CESAREAN SECTION

### Fast Facts

- Origin of term remains mysterious.
  - Method of delivery of Julius Caesar (certainly a myth)
  - *Lex cesarea*—Roman law requiring removal of fetus from dead mother
  - Derived from Latin verb *caedere* "to cut"
- Maternal mortality low (less than 1/5000).
- C/S accounted for 29.1% of births in the United States in 2004, based on information from the U.S. Center for Disease Control and Prevention.

### Indications

- Be precise; be specific.
- Write a detailed pre-operative note.

| Fetal |
| --- |
| Fetal distress (specify abnormality-recurrent late deals, bradycardia, etc.) |
| Fetal intolerance of labor |
| Inability to document fetal well-being |
| Malpresentation (breech, transverse lie) |
| Twins (non-vertex first twin, possibly for non-vertex 2nd twin) |
| Maternal HSV infection |
| Fetal congenital anomalies |

| Maternal-fetal |
| --- |
| Labor abnormalities |
| • Active phase arrest |
| • Arrest of descent |
| • Failed induction |
| • Inefficient uterine contractility unresponsive to therapy |
| Placental abruption (certain cases) |
| Placenta previa |
| Pelvic malformation (absolute pelvic disproportion) |
| Estimated fetal weight >4500 g in patients with diabetes or 5000 g in non-diabetic patients |

| Maternal |
| --- |
| Obstructive benign/malignant tumors |
| Severe vulvar condylomata |
| Cervical carcinoma |
| Abdominal cerclage |
| Prior vaginal colporrhaphy |
| Vaginal delivery contraindicated (medical indications) |

HSV, herpes simplex virus.

# OBSTETRICS

## CESAREAN DELIVERY ON MATERNAL REQUEST (CDMR)

Patient-choice cesarean is a controversial, but not contraindicated, reason for cesarean delivery.

### NIH State-of-the-Science Conference on CDMR: Summary of the Evidence-based Review

|  | Maternal | Neonatal |
|---|---|---|
| **Moderate quality evidence** |  |  |
| Favors planned **vaginal** | Reduced length of hospital stay | Less respiratory morbidity |
| Favors planned **cesarean** | Less risk of postpartum hemorrhage |  |
| **Weak quality evidence** |  |  |
| Favors planned **vaginal** | Lower infection rates | Less iatrogenic prematurity |
|  | Fewer anesthetic complications, less subsequent placenta previa | Shorter hospital stay |
|  | Higher breastfeeding rate |  |
| Favors planned **cesarean** | Less short-term stress urinary incontinence and fewer surgical complications compared to unplanned CDs | Lower fetal mortality |
|  |  | Less IVH, neonatal asphyxia, encephalopathy, brachial plexus injury, and neonatal infection |
| Sensitive to parity, family size[a] | Subsequent uterine rupture |  |
|  | Hysterectomy |  |
|  | Number of pregnancies |  |
| **Weak evidence:** Neither delivery route affords any advantages on these issues | Mortality | Mortality |
|  | Anorectal function | Long-term outcomes |
|  | Sexual function |  |
|  | Pelvic organ prolapse |  |
|  | Subsequent stillbirth |  |

[a]Subsequent uterine rupture is reduced with planned repeat CD; it is increased with planned VBAC. There is no difference in risk for hysterectomy in the first PVD vs. the first CD; there is an increased risk of hysterectomy with multiple CDs. The number of pregnancies is decreased with CD compared to vaginal delivery, but this may be voluntary.

CD, cesarean delivery; IVH, intraventricular hemorrhage; MR, maternal request; NIH, National Institutes of Health; PVD, planned vaginal delivery; VBAC, vaginal birth after cesarean.
*Source:* Reproduced with permission from Hibbard JV, Della Torre M. When mom requests a cesarean. *Cont OB/GYN*. 2006;Dec:38–50. *Cont OB/GYN* is a copyrighted publication of Advanstar Communications Inc. All rights reserved.

## What Do Professional Organizations Say?

**ACOG:** Committee on Ethics' surgical consent used CDMR as an example:

> **CDMR is justified** if OB believes overall health of patient and fetus greater with CDMR than with vaginal.

> **CDMR is not justified** if OB does not believe CDMR is beneficial over vaginal.

**SOGC:** "**Vaginal birth remains preferred approach and safest option** for most women, and carries with it less risk of complication in pregnancy and subsequent pregnancy."

**NICE/RCOG:** "**Maternal request is not on its own an indication for CS.** An individual clinician has the right to decline a request for CS in the absence of an identifiable reason...she should be offered referral for second opinion."

**FIGO (WHO):** Absence of evidence of benefit; potential drain on resources. **Not ethically justified.**

**NIH State-of-the-Science Conference:**

- Insufficient evidence to recommend one mode of delivery over the other

- Decision for CDMR should be individualized, consistent with ethical principles

- More prospective research needed

ACOG, American College of Obstetricians and Gynecologists; CDMR, cesarean delivery maternal request; CS, cesarean section; FIGO, International Federation of Gynecology and Obstetrics; NICE, National Institute for Health and Clinical Excellence; NIH, National Institutes of Health; RCOG, Royal College of Obstetricians and Gynaecologists; SOGC, Society of Obstetricians and Gynaecologists of Canada; WHO, World Health Organization.
*Source:* Reproduced with permission from Hibbard JV, Della Torre M. When mom requests a cesarean. *Cont OB/GYN.* 2006;Dec:38–50. *Cont OB/GYN* is a copyrighted publication of Advanstar Communications Inc. All rights reserved.

# OBSTETRICS

## Uterine Incision for Cesarean Section

- Most common: low transverse (see figure A below) or Kerr (see figure D below)
- Low vertical (see figure B below)
  - Premature fetus with malpresentation or poorly developed lower segment
  - Usually extends into active segment
- Classical (see figure C below)
  - Often used for delivery of premature infants as needed
  - Impacted transverse lie, cervical carcinoma

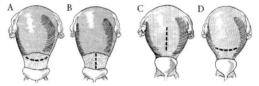

*Source:* Scott JR. Cesarean delivery. In: Scott JR, DiSaia PD, Hammond CB, Spellacy WN, ed. *Danforth's Obstetrics and Gynecology.* 7th ed. Philadelphia: Lippincott, 1994. Reproduced with the permission of the publisher.

## Druzin Splint Maneuver

- Malpresentations in premature fetus often associated with difficult delivery.
- Choose correct uterine incision.
- Druzin splint technique as detailed below to allow atraumatic delivery.
  - Breech or transverse lie
  - Intact membranes helpful

If fails, then uterine relaxants and version/extraction.

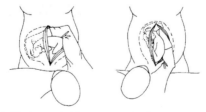

*Source:* Druzin ML. Atraumatic delivery in cases of malpresentation of the very low birth weight fetus at cesarean section: the splint technique. *Am J Obstet Gynecol* 1986;154(4): 941–942. Reproduced with the permission of the publisher, Mosby-Year Book: St. Louis.

## VAGINAL BIRTH AFTER CESAREAN
### Candidate Selection
### Criteria for Trial of Labor

| Qualifications |
| --- |
| 1 prior low-transverse cesarean section |
| Clinically adequate pelvis |
| No other uterine scars |
| **Disqualifications** |
| Prior classical or T-shaped uterine incision |
| Multiple uterine incisions |
| Previous uterine rupture |
| Contracted pelvis |
| Contraindications to vaginal birth |
| **Requirements throughout active labor** |
| Obstetrician immediately available |
| Continuous electronic monitoring of the fetal heart rate |
| Personnel skilled in interpreting fetal tracings |
| Anesthesia for emergency cesarean |
| Physician qualified for emergency cesarean |
| **Precautions** |
| Unknown uterine scars |
| Prior low vertical uterine incision |
| Uterine malformations |
| Prior single-layer uterine closure |
| Short interdelivery interval |
| Need for labor induction |
| Need for external cephalic version |
| Twin gestation |
| Suspected macrosomia |
| Maternal obesity |
| Postdates |
| Advanced maternal age |
| No prior vaginal delivery |

*Source:* Reproduced with permission from the American College of Obstetricians and Gynecologists. ACOG Practice Bulletin #54: Vaginal Birth after Previous Cesarean Delivery. Washington, DC: ACOG; July 2004.

# OBSTETRICS

## Incidence and Relative Risk of Uterine Rupture during a Second Delivery among Women with a Prior Cesarean Delivery[a]

| Type of Delivery | No. of Women | Incidence (per 1,000) | Relative Risk (95% Confidence Interval) |
|---|---|---|---|
| Repeated cesarean delivery without labor | 6980 | 1.6 | 1.0 |
| Spontaneous onset of labor | 10,789 | 5.2 | 3.3 (1.8–6.0) |
| Induction of labor without prostaglandins | 1960 | 7.7 | 4.9 (2.4–9.7) |
| Induction of labor with prostaglandins | 366 | 24.5 | 15.6 (8.1–30.0) |

[a]Incidence is expressed as the number of cases of uterine rupture per 1000 women who delivered a second singleton infant after a prior cesarean delivery. Women who had repeated cesarean delivery served as the reference group.

*Source:* Reproduced with permission from Lydon-Rochelle M, Holt VL, Easterling TR, Martin DP. The risk of uterine rupture during labor among women with a prior cesarean delivery. *N Engl J Med.* 2001;345:3. Copyright 2001 Massachusetts Medical Society.

- Use of an intrauterine pressure catheter does not predict rupture but can be useful in documenting adequate contractions in arrest disorders.
- Success rates vary with indications of previous section.
  - Non-recurrent indications (breech): 75–86% success, similar to women without a prior C/S
  - Previous arrest disorder (such as cephalopelvic disproportion): 50–80%

## POSTPARTUM HEMORRHAGE

### Definition

≥500 cc blood loss in first 24 hours after delivery

### Etiology and Risk Factors

1. *Atony*
- Grand multiparity
- Uterine overdistention
- Prolonged labor with Pitocin augmentation
- Chorioamnionitis
- General anesthesia
- $MgSO_4$ therapy for seizure prophylaxis
- Rapid labor
2. *Retained placental tissue*
- Usually delayed postpartum hemorrhage
- Placenta accreta (especially multiple prior cesareans)
- Preterm delivery
- Succenturiate lobe
- Cord avulsion
3. *Genital tract laceration*
- Precipitous labor and delivery
- Improper episiotomy repair
- Operative vaginal delivery
4. *Uterine inversion—Don't pull on that cord!*

### Blood Component Therapy

| Component | Contents | Volume | Anticipated Effect (per unit) |
|---|---|---|---|
| Packed red blood cells | RBC, WBC, plasma | 300 mL | Increase in hemoglobin by 1 g/dL |
| Platelets[a] | Platelets, RBC, WBC, plasma | 50 mL | Increase in platelet count by 7500/mm³ |
| Fresh frozen plasma | Fibrinogen, antithrombin III, clotting factors, plasma | 250 mL | Increase in fibrinogen by 10 mg/dL |
| Cryoprecipitate | Fibrinogen, factor VIII, von Willebrand factor, factor XIII | 40 mL | Increase in fibrinogen by 10 mg/dL |

[a]Always given as a pooled concentrate of 6–10 units.

*Source:* Adapted with permission from Martin SR, Strong TH Jr. Transfusion of blood components and derivatives in the obstetric intensive care patient. In: Foley MR, Strong TH Jr, Garite TJ. *Obstetric Intensive Care Manual.* 2004. McGraw-Hill Medical Publishing Division.

# OBSTETRICS

## Uterotonic Therapy

| Agent | Dose | Route | Dosing Frequency | Side Effects | Contraindications |
|---|---|---|---|---|---|
| Oxytocin (Pitocin) | 10–80 units in 1000 mL of crystalloid solution | First line: IV<br>Second line: IM or IU | Continuous | Nausea, emesis, water intoxication | None |
| Methylergonovine (Methergine) | 0.2 mg | First line: IM<br>Second line: IU or PO | Every 2–4 hrs | Hypertension, hypotension, nausea, emesis | Hypertension, preeclampsia |
| 15-methyl prostaglandin $F_{2\alpha}$ (Hemabate) | 0.25 mg | First line: IM<br>Second line: IU | Every 15–90 mins (8 dose maximum) | Nausea, emesis, diarrhea, flushing, chills | Active cardiac, pulmonary, renal, or hepatic disease |
| Prostaglandin $E_2$ (Dinoprostone) | 20 mg | PR | Every 2 hrs | Nausea, emesis, diarrhea, fever, chills, headache | Hypotension |
| Misoprostol[a] (Cytotec) | 600–1000 mcg | First line: PR<br>Second line: PO | Single dose | Nausea, emesis, diarrhea, fever, chills | None |

[a]Off-label use, not FDA-approved.

IM, intramuscular; IU, intrauterine; IV, intravenous; PO, per oral; PR, per rectum.

*Source:* Reproduced with permission from Francois K. Managing uterine atony and hemorrhagic shock. *Cont Ob/Gyn.* 2006;Feb:52–59. *Cont OB/GYN* is a copyrighted publication of Advantar Communications Inc. All rights reserved.

**Management of Atony and Hemorrhagic Shock**

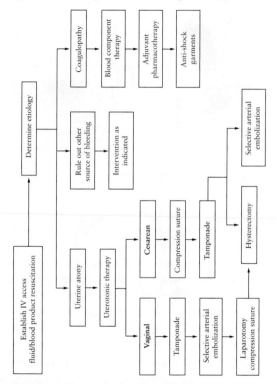

# OBSTETRICS

## Uterine Artery Ligation

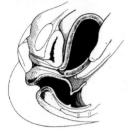

Grasp and elevate the uterus with the left hand and tilt it to expose the vessels.

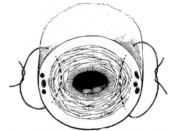

A coronal view of lower uterine segment is shown. Insert the suture into the substance of the cervix without entering the uterine cavity and medial to the blood vessels.

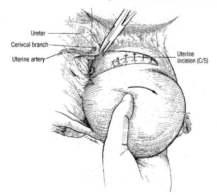

Ureter

Cerivcal branch

Uterine artery

Uterine incision (C/S)

The ligation, 2–3 cm inferior to the uterine incision, includes 2–3 cm of myometrium in the suture.

*Source:* O'Leary JA. Stop OB hemorrhage with uterine artery ligation. *Cont Ob/Gyn* Special Issue: Update on Surgery 1986. Reproduced with the permission of David A. Factor, medical illustrator.

## B-Lynch Suture for Postpartum Hemorrhage

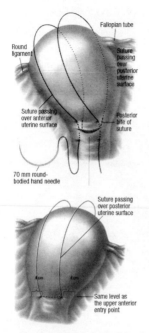

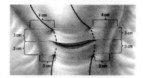

# OBSTETRICS

## Lower Uterine Segment Packing

### Foley Catheter Technique

- Insert tip of Foley through the cervix up all the way to the fundus.
- Use ring forceps if needed for placement of the tip.
- Inflate the balloon with 60 cc of normal saline (it can take that much volume).
- Check fundal location with ultrasound if available.
- Consider inserting another Foley catheter if needed.
- Leave in for 12–24 hours and treat empirically with broad-spectrum antibiotics.

### Bakri Postpartum Balloon

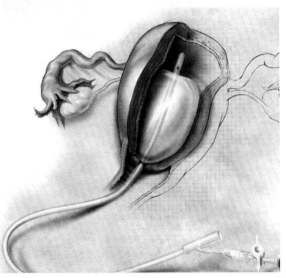

Reproduced with permission from Cook Women's Health. Spencer, Indiana.

## Gauze Packing Method

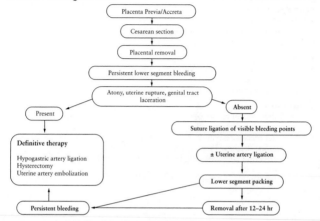

Pack with saline soaked gauze pack through uterine incision, passing into vagina and close uterus over packed area with care.

*Source:* Modified from Druzin ML. Packing of lower uterine segment for control of postcesarean bleeding in instances of placenta previa. *Surg Gynecol Obstet* 1989;169(6):543–545. Reproduced with the permission of *Surgery, Gynecology & Obstetrics,* now known as the *Journal of the American College of Surgeons.*

# OBSTETRICS
## UTERINE INVERSION
### Fast Facts
- 1/25,000 deliveries
- More common in multigravida pregnancies
- Often iatrogenic

### Presentation
- Placenta appears at introitus with mass attached.
- Shock with bradycardia 2 to vagal response.
- Excessive hemorrhage.

### Treatment
- Treat for shock and blood loss.
- Call for assistance (especially anesthesia).
- Administer uterine relaxants.
  - Terbutaline 0.25 mg IV (may repeat × 1)
  - Nitroglycerine 100–250 mcg IV up to total of 1000 mcg (watch blood pressure)
- Replace uterus.
  - "Last out; first in."
  - Pressure applied around, not at, leading point.
  - May require general anesthesia (halothane).
  - Do not remove placenta if firmly attached until uterus replaced.
- Exploratory laparotomy with replacement if all else fails.

## CERVICAL CERCLAGE
### Types of Cerclage

| Type of Cerclage | Complication | Percentage (%) |
|---|---|---|
| Elective | Rupture of membranes | 0.8–18 |
| | Chorioamnionitis | 1–6.2 |
| Urgent | Rupture of membranes | 3–65.2 |
| | Chorioamnionitis | Approximately 30–35 |
| Emergency | Rupture of membranes | 0–51 |
| | Chorioamnionitis | Approximately 9–37 |

*Source:* Reproduced with permission from Clinical Management Guidelines, Number 48, Cervical Insufficiency, Obstetrics & Gynecology 2003;102:1091–1099.

### Algorithm to Evaluate for Cerclage Placement

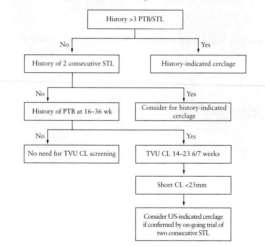

CL, cervical length; PTB, preterm birth; STL, second-trimester losses; TVU, transvaginal ultrasound.
*Source:* Reproduced with permission from Berghella V, Baxter J, Pereira L. Cerclage: Should we be doing them? *Cont Ob/Gyn.* 2005; Dec:34–41. *Cont OB/GYN* is a copyrighted publication of Advanstar Communications Inc. All rights reserved.

# OBSTETRICS
## McDonald Cerclage

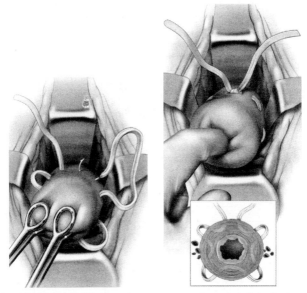

A weighted speculum and right angle retractors are used to optimized visualization of the surgical field. Starting at the vesicocervical reflection, a purse-string suture is placed in four to six passes circumferentially around the cervix. Each pass should be deep enough to contain sufficient cervical stroma to avoid "pulling through," but not too deep as to enter the endocervical canal. Taking care to avoid the uterine vessels laterally, place the suture high on the posterior aspect of the cervix, as this is the most likely site of suture displacement. The suture is tied anteriorly, tight enough to be closed at the internal os. Successive knots are placed, and the ends are left long enough to facilitate later removal.

*Source:* Reproduced with permission from Berghella V, Baxter J, Pereira L. Cerclage: Should we be doing them? *Cont Ob/Gyn.* 2005; Dec:34–41. *Cont OB/GYN* is a copyrighted publication of Advanstar Communications Inc. All rights reserved.

## Modified Shirodkar Cerclage

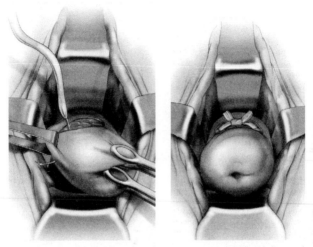

The initial transverse incision is made in the anterior cervicovaginal epithelium at the reflection of the bladder. The vesicovaginal fascia is reflected cephalad to the level of the internal os, similarly to when beginning a vaginal hysterectomy. A similar incision is made posteriorly. An Allis clamp is placed laterally with the jaws in the anterior and posterior incisions as high on the cervix as possible to minimize the cephalad dissection. Lateral traction is placed on the submucosal tissue to avoid the uterine vasculature. The suture is driven by successive passes with an atraumatic needle on each side just distal to the Allis clamp above the insertion of the cardinal ligaments. After ensuring that the suture tape lies flat posteriorly, the suture is then tied anteriorly, light enough as to be closed at the internal os. Successive knots are placed to facilitate identification and later removal. The mucosal incisions are closed over only if active bleeding is noted.

*Source:* Reproduced with permission from Berghella V, Baxter J, Pereira L. Cerclage: Should we be doing them? *Cont Ob/Gyn.* 2005; Dec:34–41. *Cont OB/GYN* is a copyrighted publication of Advanstar Communications Inc. All rights reserved.

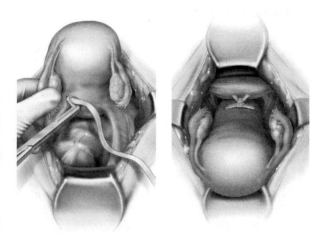

While the surgeon digitally places the uterine vessels laterally, a 5-mm Mersilene suture is guided through the broad ligament at the level of the internal os by blunt perforation with a right-angle clamp. This is completed on each side and the suture is tied anteriorly.

*Source:* Reproduced with permission from Berghella V, Baxter J, Pereira L. Cerclage: Should we be doing them? *Cont Ob/Gyn.* 2005; Dec:34–41. *Cont OB/GYN* is a copyrighted publication of Advanstar Communications Inc. All rights reserved.

# EMERGENCY CERCLAGE

## Fast Facts

- Method to perform cerclage in face of prolapsed membranes
- Heroic measure

## Inclusion Criteria

- Intact membranes
- No evidence of chorioamnionitis
- Advanced dilation
- History compatible with incompetent cervix (not preterm labor)
- No gross fetal anomalies
- Extreme prematurity

## Preparation

- Informed consent
- General or regional anesthesia
- Perineal and vaginal prep

## Technique

- Steep Trendelenburg position
- Insert Foley into bladder
- Backfill bladder with $1/2$ NS in 250 cc increments
- Membranes usually recede after 800–1000 cc
- Place cerclage (McDonald or Shirodkar)

## Post-Operative Care

- Empty bladder
- Antibiotics*
- Prophylactic tocolytics*

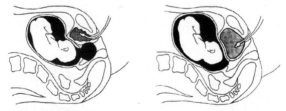

*Source:* Scheerer LJ, Lam F, Bartolucci L, et al. A new technique for reduction of prolapsed fetal membranes for emergency cervical cerclage. *Obstet Gynecol.* 1989;74(3):408–410. Reproduced with the permission of the American College of Obstetricians and Gynecologists.

*Although a common practice there is no good evidence to support this and it should be done with caution. (*Source:* ACOG bulletin, Number 48, November 2003: Cervical insufficiency. *Obstet Gynecol,* 2003;102:1091–1099.)

# OBSTETRICS

## AMNIOINFUSION

### Fast Facts

- Attempt to prevent problems in labor associated with oligohydramnios.
- Reduction in C/S rate for fetal distress by reducing variable decelerations.
- *Not* shown to reduce the risk of meconium aspiration syndrome or other complications of meconium stained fluid (*Source:* Fraser WD, et al. Amnioinfusion for the prevention of the Meconium Aspiration Syndrome. *NEJM* 2005;353:909–917).

### Candidates for Amnioinfusion

- Preterm premature rupture of membranes (PROM) with ultrasound-demonstrated oligohydramnios.
- Term labor with recurrent variable decels and decreased amniotic fluid.
- Cephalic presentation.
- Previous C/S or previous myomectomy not an absolute contraindication.
- Chorioamnionitis is a relative contraindication.

### Technique

- Document fetal presentation and oligohydramnios by ultrasound.
- Place fetal scalp electrode and intrauterine pressure catheter (preferably double lumen catheter).
- Initial bolus of 250–500 cc of normal saline (warmed) with maintenance infusion (3 cc/min).
- Rebolus as needed.
- Measure intrauterine pressure every 30 minutes or continuously (second intrauterine pressure catheter or double lumen).

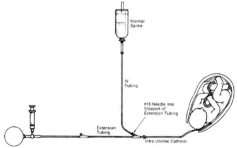

*Source:* Miyazaki FS, Nevarez F. Saline amnioinfusion for relief of repetitive variable decelerations: a prospective randomized study. *Am J Obstet Gynecol* 1985;153(3):301–306. Reproduced with the permission of the publisher, Mosby-Year Book: St. Louis.

# FETAL HEART RATE PATTERNS

## Definitions of Fetal Heart Rate Patterns

| Pattern | Definition |
| --- | --- |
| Baseline | • The mean FHR rounded to increments of 5 beats per min during a 10-min segment, excluding:<br>—Periodic or episodic changes<br>—Periods of marked FHR variability<br>—Segments of baseline that differ by more than 25 beats per min<br>• The baseline must be for a minimum of 2 mins in any 10-min segment |
| Baseline variability | • Fluctuations in the FHR of two cycles per min or greater<br>• Variability is visually quantitated as the amplitude of peak-to-trough in beats per min<br>—Absent—amplitude range undetectable<br>—Minimal—amplitude range detectable but 5 beats per min or fewer<br>—Moderate (normal)—amplitude range 6–25 beats per min<br>—Marked—amplitude range greater than 25 beats per min |
| Acceleration | • A visually apparent increase (onset to peak in less than 30 secs) in the FHR from the most recently calculated baseline<br>• The duration of an acceleration is defined as the time from the initial change in FHR from the baseline to the return of the FHR to the baseline<br>• At 32 wks of gestation and beyond, an acceleration has an acme of 15 beats per min or more above baseline, with a duration of 15 secs or more but less than 2 mins<br>• Before 32 wks of gestation, an acceleration has an acme of 10 beats per min or more above baseline, with a duration of 10 secs or more but less than 2 mins<br>• Prolonged acceleration lasts 2 mins or more but less than 10 mins<br>• If an acceleration lasts 10 mins or longer, it is a baseline change |
| Bradycardia | • Baseline FHR less than 110 beats per min |
| Early deceleration | • In association with a uterine contraction, a visually apparent, gradual (onset to nadir 30 secs or more) decrease in FHR with return to baseline<br>• Nadir of the deceleration occurs at the same time as the peak of the contraction |
| Late deceleration | • In association with a uterine contraction, a visually apparent, gradual (onset to nadir 30 secs or more) decrease in FHR with return to baseline<br>• Onset, nadir, and recovery of the deceleration occur after the beginning, peak, and end of the contraction, respectively |

# OBSTETRICS

## Definitions of Fetal Heart Rate Patterns

| Pattern | Definition |
|---------|-----------|
| Tachycardia | • Baseline FHR greater than 160 beats per min |
| Variable deceleration | • An abrupt (onset to nadir less than 30 secs), visually apparent decrease in the FHR below the baseline |
| | • The decrease in FHR is 15 beats per min or more, with a duration of 15 secs or more but less than 2 mins |
| Prolonged deceleration | • Visually apparent decrease in the FHR below the baseline |
| | • Deceleration is 15 beats per min or more, lasting 2 mins or more but less than 10 mins from onset to return to baseline |

FHR, fetal heart rate.

*Source:* Reproduced with permission from *Am J Obstet Gynecol*, Vol 177, Electronic fetal heart rate monitoring: research guidelines for interpretation, National Institute of Child Health and Human Development Research Planning Workshop, 1385–1390. Copyright 1997.

## Effects of Medications on Fetal Heart Rate Patterns

| Medications | Reference | Study Design | Effect on Fetal Heart Rate |
|---|---|---|---|
| Butorphanol | Hatjis 1986[1] | Case–control | Transient sinusoidal FHR pattern |
| Cocaine | Chazotte 1991[2] | Case–control | No characteristic changes in FHR pattern |
| Corticosteroid | Senat 1998[3] | Randomized clinical trial | Decrease in FHR variability with betamethasone but not dexamethasone |
| Magnesium sulfate | Hallak 1999[4] and Wright 1996[5] | Randomized clinical trial and retrospective | A significant decrease in the FHR baseline and variability; inhibits the increase in accelerations with advancing gestational age |
| Meperidine | Giannina 1995[6] | Randomized clinical trial | No characteristic changes in FHR pattern |
| Morphine | Kopecky 2000[7] | Case–control | Decreased number of accelerations |
| Nalbuphine | Giannina 1995[6] | Randomized clinical trial | Decreased the number of accelerations, long- and short-term variation |
| Terbutaline | Tejani 1983[8] | Retrospective | Abolishment or decrease in frequency of late and variable decelerations |
| Zidovudine | Blackwell 2001[9] | Case–control | No difference in the FHR baseline, variability, number of accelerations or decelerations |

FHR, fetal heart rate.

[1]Hatjis CG, Meis PJ. Sinusoidal fetal heart rate pattern associated with butorphanol administration. *Obstet Gynecol* 1986;67:377–380.

[2]Chazotte C, Forman L, Gandhi J. Heart rate patterns in fetuses exposed to cocaine. *Obstet Gynecol* 1991;78:323–325.

[3]Senat MV, Minoui S, Mutton O, Fernandez H, Frydman R, Ville Y. Effect of dexamethasone and betamethasone on the fetal heart rate variability in preterm labour: a randomised study. *Br J Obstet Gynaecol* 1998;105:749–755.

[4]Hallak M, Martinez-Poyer I, Kruger ML, Hassan S, Blackwell SC, Sorokin Y. The effect of magnesium sulfate on fetal heart rate parameters: a randomized, placebo-controlled trial. *Am J Obstet Gynecol* 1999;181:1122–1127.

[5]Wright JW, Ridgway LE, Wright BD, Covington DL, Bobitt JR. Effect of MgSO$_4$ on heart rate monitoring in the preterm fetus. *J Reprod Med* 1996;41:605–608.

[6]Giannina G, Guzman ER, Lai YL, Lake MF, Cernadas M, Vintzileos AM. Comparison of the effects of meperidine and nalbuphine on intrapartum fetal heart rate tracings. *Obstet Gynecol* 1995;86:441–445.

[7]Kopecky EA, Ryan ML, Barrett JF, Seaward PG, Ryan G, Koren G, et al. Fetal response to maternally administered morphine. *Am J Obstet Gynecol* 2000;183:424–430.

[8]Tejani NA, Verma UL, Chatterjee S, Mittelmann S. Terbutaline in the management of acute intrapartum fetal acidosis. *J Reprod Med* 1983;28:857–861.

[9]Blackwell SC, Sahai A, Hassan SS, Treadwell MC, Tomlinson MW, Jones TB, et al. Effects of intrapartum zidovudine therapy on fetal heart rate parameters in women with human immunodeficiency virus infection. *Fetal Diagn Ther* 2001;16:413–416.

*Source:* Reproduced with permission from ACOG Practice Bulletin, Number 70. Intrapartum Fetal Heart Rate Monitoring. *Obstet Gynecol* 2005;106(6):1453–1461.

# OBSTETRICS

## UMBILICAL CORD GAS VALUES

| Value | Yeomans (1985)[a] (n=146) | Ramin (1989)[a] (n=1292) | Riley (1993)[b] (n=3522) |
|---|---|---|---|
| **Arterial blood in term newborns (Mean ± one standard deviation)** | | | |
| pH | 7.28 ± 0.05 | 7.28 ± 0.07 | 7.27 ± 0.069 |
| $PCO_2$ (mm Hg) | 49.2 ± 8.4 | 49.9 ± 14.2 | 50.3 ± 11.1 |
| $HCO_3^-$ (meq/L) | 22.3 ± 2.5 | 23.1 ± 2.8 | 22.0 ± 3.6 |
| Base excess (meq/L) | —[c] | –3.6 ± 2.8 | –2.7 ± 2.8 |
| **Venous blood in term newborns (Mean ± one standard deviation)** | | | |
| pH | 7.35 ± 0.05 | — | 7.34 ± 0.063 |
| $PCO_2$ (mm Hg) | 38.2 ± 5.6 | — | 40.7 ± 7.9 |
| $HCO_3^-$ (meq/L) | 20.4 ± 4.1 | — | 21.4 ± 2.5 |
| Base excess (meq/L) | — | — | –2.4 ± 2.0 |

[a]Data are from infants of selected patients with uncomplicated vaginal deliveries.
[b]Data are from infants of unselected patients with vaginal deliveries.
[c]Data were not obtained.

Ramin SM, Gilstrap LC III, Leveno KJ, Burris J, Little BB. Umbilical artery acid-base status in the preterm infant. *Obstet Gynecol* 1989;74:256–258.
Riley RJ, Johnson JWC. Collecting and analyzing cord blood gases. *Clin Obstet Gynecol* 1993;36:13–23.
Yeomans ER, Hauth JC, Gilstrap LC III, Strickland DM. Umbilical cord pH, $PCO_2$, and bicarbonate following uncomplicated term deliveries. *Am J Obstet Gynecol* 1985;151:798–800.

| Value | Ramin (1989)[a] (n=77) | Dickinson (1992)[b] (n=949) | Riley (1993)[c] (n=11015) |
|---|---|---|---|
| **Arterial blood in preterm newborns (Mean ± one standard deviation)** | | | |
| pH | 7.29 ± 0.07 | 7.27 ± 0.07 | 7.28 ± 0.089 |
| $PCO_2$ (mm Hg) | 49.2 ± 9.0 | 51.6 ± 9.4 | 50.2 ± 12.3 |
| $HCO_3^-$ (meq/L) | 23.0 ± 3.5 | 23.9 ± 2.1 | 22.4 ± 3.5 |
| Base excess (meq/L) | –3.3 ± 2.4 | –3.0 ± 2.5 | –2.7 ± 3.0 |

[a]Data are from infants of selected patients with uncomplicated vaginal deliveries.
[b]Data are from infants of unselected patients with vaginal deliveries.

Dickinson JE, Eriksen NL, Meyer BA, Parisi VM. The effect of preterm birth on umbilical cord blood gases. *Obstet Gynecol* 1992;79:575-578.
Ramin SM, Gilstrap LC III, Leveno KJ, Burris J, Little BB. Umbilical artery acid-base status in the preterm infant. *Obstet Gynecol* 1989;74:256-258.
Riley RJ, Johnson JWC. Collecting and analyzing cord blood gases. *Clin Obstet Gynecol* 1993;36:13–23.

*Source:* American College of Obstetricians and Gynecologists: Umbilical Artery Blood Acid-Base Analysis. ACOG Technical Bulletin #216, November 1995. ACOG, Washington, DC © 2000.

# NEONATAL RESUSCITATION

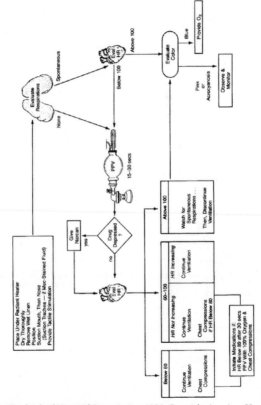

*Source: Textbook of Neonatal Resuscitation,* 1994. Copyright American Heart Association. Reproduced with permission.

# OBSTETRICS
## INFANT CPR

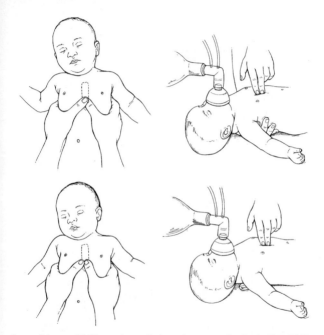

*Source:* Schuman AJ. Neonatal resuscitation: what you need to know. *Cont Ob/Gyn* 1992;37(12):96. Reproduced with the permission of the publisher, Medical Economics Publishing: Montvale, N.J.

## Apgar Score

| Feature | 0 | 1 | 2 |
| --- | --- | --- | --- |
| Appearance | Blue, pale | Body pink, extremities blue | Pink |
| Pulse | Absent | <100 beats/min | >100 beats/min |
| Grimace (tone) | None | Grimace | Cough, sneeze |
| Activity | Limp | Some tone | Active |
| Respirations | Absent | Crying | Good cry |

## Neonatal Drug Doses

| Drug | Dose |
| --- | --- |
| Epinephrine | (1:10,000) 0.2 mL/kg IV or ET. Give rapidly. Dilute 1:1 with saline for ET use. |
| Volume Expansion | (Whole blood, saline, 5% albumin, LR) 10 mL/kg, give over 5–10 mins. |
| $NaHCO_3$ | (0.5 meq/mL) 1–2 meq/kg IV. Give slowly, only if ventilation adequate. |
| Naloxone | (0.4 mg/mL) 0.1 mg/kg = 0.25 mL/kg IV, ET, IM, SQ. Give rapidly |
| Glucose | D10W 2 mL/kg IV. Give over 1–2 mins. |

*Source:* Baker ER, Shepard B. Neonatal resuscitation & care of the newborn at risk. In: DeCherney AH, Pernoll ML, ed. *Current Obstetric & Gynecologic Diagnosis & Treatment.* 8th ed. Norwalk, Conn.: Appleton & Lange, 1994.
Reproduced with the permission of the publisher.

# OBSTETRICS

## ANTEPARTUM TESTING

### Indications

Patients at high risk of uteroplacental insufficiency
  Prolonged pregnancy
  Diabetes mellitus (DM)
  Hypertension
  Previous stillbirth
  Suspected intrauterine growth restriction (IUGR)
  Advanced maternal age
  Multiple gestations with discordant growth
  Antiphospholipid syndrome
When other tests suggests fetal compromise
  Suspected IUGR
  Decreased fetal movement
  Oligohydramnios
Routine antepartum surveillance

### Non-Stress Test

- Can be used in an outpatient setting to assess fetal well-being.
- After 32-week gestation, a reactive non-stress test (NST) includes two 15-beat accelerations lasting 15 seconds during a 20-minute period.
- A non-reactive NST can be caused by a sleep cycle, maternal medications, smoking, an abnormal CNS, or fetal hypoxia.
- A reactive NST is associated with a perinatal mortality of 5/1000.
- A non-reactive NST is associated with a perinatal mortality of 30–40/1000, but has a 75–90% false positive rate.
- If the NST is non-reactive, vibroacoustic stimulation (VAS) can be applied to the fetal head for 3 seconds to wake the fetus from a sleep cycle. Reactivity after VAS is as reassuring as spontaneous reactive NST.
- Bradycardia (a FHR deceleration to 90 or 40 beats below baseline × 60 seconds or more) during an NST is associated with 25% perinatal mortality with expectant management.
- Twice weekly NSTs are recommended for DM, prolonged gestation, and IUGR.

## Contraction Stress Test

- The contraction stress test (CST) was the first test used to assess antepartum fetal well being.
- During the CST the FHR response to the stress of contractions (either spontaneous or induced with Pitocin) is assessed.
- CST are limited by a high (>30%) false positive rate, time required to perform the test, and need for access to labor and delivery if the induced contractions cause FHR abnormalies that necessitate delivery.
- A negative CST, however, has been shown to be more reassuring than a reactive NST.
- CST can be used to follow up non-reactive NST.

| Interpretation | Description | Incidence (%) |
|---|---|---|
| Negative | No late decelerations appearing anywhere on the tracing with adequate uterine contractions (three in 10 mins) | 80 |
| Positive | Late decelerations that are consistent and persistent, present with the majority (>50%) of contractions without excessive uterine activity; if persistent late decelerations seen before the frequency of contractions is adequate, test interpreted as positive | 3–5 |
| Suspicious | Inconsistent late decelerations | 5 |
| Hyperstimulation | Uterine contractions closer than every 2 mins or lasting >90 secs, or five uterine contractions in 10 mins; if no late decelerations, test interpreted as negative | 5 |
| Unsatisfactory | Quality of the tracing inadequate for interpretation or adequate uterine activity cannot be achieved | 5 |

# OBSTETRICS

## Biophysical Profile

| Biophysical Variable | Normal (Score = 2) | Abnormal (Score = 0) |
|---|---|---|
| Fetal breathing movements | At least one episode of >30 secs duration in 30 mins observation | Absent or no episode of ≥30 secs duration in 30 minutes |
| Gross body movement | At least three discrete body/limb movements in 30 mins (episodes of active continuous movement considered a single movement) | Up to two episodes of body/limb movements in 30 mins |
| Fetal tone | At least one episode of active extension with return to flexion of fetal limb(s) or trunk; opening and closing of hand considered normal tone | Either slow extension with return to partial flexion or movement of limb in full extension or absent fetal movement |
| Reactive fetal heart rate | At least two episodes of acceleration of ≥15 bpm and 15 secs duration associated with fetal movement in 30 mins | Fewer than two accelerations or acceleration <15 bpm in 30 mins |
| Qualitative amniotic fluid volume | At least one pocket of amniotic fluid measuring 2 cm in two perpendicular planes | Either no amniotic fluid pockets or a pocket <2 cm in two perpendicular planes |

bpm, beats per minute.
*Source:* Adapted from Manning FA: Biophysical profile scoring. In Nijhuis J, ed. *Fetal Behaviour.* New York: Oxford University Press, 1992, p 241.

## Management Based on Biophysical Profile

| Score | Interpretation | Management |
|---|---|---|
| 10 | Normal infant; low risk of chronic asphyxia | Repeat testing at weekly intervals; repeat twice weekly in diabetic patients and patients at ≥41 wks gestation |
| 8 | Normal infant; low risk of chronic asphyxia | Repeat testing at weekly intervals; repeat testing twice weekly in diabetics and patients at ≥41 wks gestation; oligohydramnios is an indication for delivery |
| 6 | Suspect chronic asphyxia | If ≥36 wks gestation and conditions are favorable, deliver; if at >36 wks and L/S <2.0, repeat test in 4–6 hrs; deliver if oligohydramnios is present |
| 4 | Suspect chronic asphyxia | If ≥36 wks gestation is present, deliver; if <32 wks gestation, repeat score |
| 0–2 | Strongly suspect chronic asphyxia | Extend testing time to 120 mins; if persistent score ≤4, deliver, regardless of gestational age |

*Source:* Adapted from Manning FA, Harman CR, Morrison I, et al. Fetal assessment based on fetal biophysical profile scoring. *Am J Obstet Gynecol* 1990;162:703, and Manning FA. Biophysical profile scoring. In Nijhuis J ed. *Fetal Behaviour.* New York: Oxford University Press, 1992, p 241.

- Biophysical profile (BPP) can be used for assessment as early as 26–28 weeks.
- If the BPP is <6, VAS can be applied and the BPP repeated.
- The risk of fetal death is increased by 14 × with absence of movement and by 18 × with absence of breathing.
- BPP may be artificially low within 24–96 hours of receiving steroids for fetal lung maturity.
- A lower BPP score is associated with a higher risk of cerebral palsy; increased risk of cerebral palsy with decreasing score.

## Umbilical Artery Dopplers

- During normal pregnancies there is increased blood flow during diastole as gestation progresses.
- The ratio of systolic to diastolic blood flow (S/D ratio) reflects placental resistance.
- Typically recommended when placental insufficiency is suspected.
- The S/D ratio is not affected by fetal hypoxia.
- Abnormally elevated S/D ratios are associated with IUGR and possibly chromosomal and fetal anomalies.
- Absent end-diastolic flow is associated with an increase in perinatal morbidity and mortality. Reverse end-diastolic flow is predictive of poor fetal outcome including a 36% mortality rate.
- If the S/D ratio shows absent or reverse end-diastolic flow, increased fetal monitoring is indicated. Delivery is not mandatory, but can be considered in the clinical context of the gestational age, fetal and maternal health, and results of other monitoring tests.

# OBSTETRICS

## Antenatal Testing Guidelines

| Condition | Timing of Testing | Test and Frequency |
|---|---|---|
| **Diabetes Mellitus** | | |
| Diet-controlled with no complications | 34 wks–delivery | NST qwk |
| Insulin-dependent in good control | 34 wks–delivery | NST qwk |
| Diet-controlled with previous IUFD and/or other medical problem | 26 wks–32 wks | NST qwk |
| Insulin-dependent with poor control | 32 wks–delivery | NST 2 × wk |
| Previous IUFD | at ≥40 wks | NST 2 × wk and BPP |
| *Good control = pregestational diabetic in good control prior to 12 wks, or GDM in good control before 32 wks.* | | |
| **Post dates / poor dates using earliest EDC** | | |
| | 40–40.6 wks | NST qwk |
| | 41–41.6 wks | NST 2 × wk and AFI |
| | | NST 3 × wk, BPP at 42 wks |
| *Delivery is often advocated at ≥42 wks, but if the delivery option is not chosen, observe the above protocol.* | | |
| *Normal NST, CST, BPP with low or very low AFI, → consider delivery.* | | |
| **Multiple mild variables (>3 in 5 min) or any lasting 30 secs** | | |
| | | Perform AFI → frequency of subsequent testing on case by case basis |
| **Assorted Clinical Problems** | | |
| Abnormal FHTs by auscultation | 26 wks or at onset of problem | NST qwk |
| Asthma (with hypoxia) | | |
| Cardiac disease | | |
| Cholestasis of pregnancy | | |
| Collagen vascular disease—in remission | | |
| Congenital anomalies | | |
| Decreased fetal movement | | |
| Late prenatal care (3rd trimester) 1 test only if normal | | |
| Multiple gestation | | |
| Oligohydramnios | | |
| Placenta previa—no bleeding | | |
| Polyhydramnios | | |
| Thyroid disease | | |

| Condition | Timing of Testing | Test and Frequency |
|---|---|---|
| Poor OB history | 26 wks or at onset of problem | NST q wk |
| Preterm labor | | |
| PUBS or IUT | | |
| Renal disease | | |
| Rh disease | | |
| Sickle cell disease (daily in crisis) | | |
| Previous IUFD | | |
| Third trimester bleeding | | |
| Chronic HTN | | NST 2× wk |
| Preeclampsia | | |
| IUGR | | |
| PROM | | |

AFI, amniotic fluid index; BPP, biophysical profile; CST, contraction stress test; EDC, expected day of confinement; FHT, fetal heart tracing; HTN, hypertension; IUFD, intrauterine fetal death; IUGR, intrauterine growth restriction; IUT, intrauterine transfusions; NST, nonstress test; OB, obstetric; PROM, premature rupture of the membranes; PUBS, percutaneous umbilical blood sampling.

# OBSTETRICS

## INTRAUTERINE GROWTH RESTRICTION

### Risk Factors Associated with Fetal Intrauterine Growth Restriction

| Fetal | Placental | Maternal |
|---|---|---|
| Chromosomal abnormalities | Small placenta | Extremes of under and/or malnutrition |
| Multifactorial congenital malformations | Circumvallate placenta | Vascular/renal disease |
| Multiple gestations | Chorioangiomata | Congenital or acquired thrombophylic disorder |
| Infection | | Drugs/lifestyle |
| | | High altitude or significant hypoxic disorder |

*Source:* Reproduced with permission from Resnick R. Intrauterine Growth Restriction. *Obstet Gynecol.* 2002;99(3):490–496.

### Evaluation and Management of the IUGR Fetus

| | Constitutionally Small Fetus | Fetus with Structural and/or Chromosome Abnormality; Fetal Infection | Substrate Deprivation; Uteroplacental Insufficiency |
|---|---|---|---|
| Growth rate and pattern | Usually below but parallel to normal; symmetric | Markedly below normal; symmetric | Variable; usually asymmetric |
| Anatomy | Normal | Usually abnormal | Normal |
| Amniotic fluid volume | Normal | Normal or hydramnios; decreased in the presence of renal agenesis or urethral obstruction | Low |
| Additional evaluation | None | Karyotype; specific testing for viral DNA in amniotic fluid as indicated | Fetal lung maturity testing as indicated |
| Additional laboratory evaluation of fetal well-being | Normal BPP/UAV | BPP variable; normal UAV | BPP score decreases; UAV evidence of vascular resistance |
| Continued surveillance and timing of delivery | None; anticipate term delivery | Dependent upon etiology | BPP and UAV; delivery timing requires balance of gestational age and BPP/UAV findings; fetal lung maturity testing often helpful |

IUGR, intrauterine growth restriction; BPP, biophysical profile; UAV, umbilical artery velocimetry.
*Source:* Reproduced with permission from Resnick R. Intrauterine Growth Restriction. *Obstet Gynecol.* 2002;99(3):490–496.

## ASTHMA IN PREGNANCY

### Fast Facts

- No predictable effect on asthma.
- $1/3$ improved, $1/3$ worsened, $1/3$ unchanged.
- Mild asthmatics at low risk.
- Severe asthmatics should have high-risk follow-up.
- Mortality of asthma is that of mechanical ventilatory fatigue.

### Medical Management of Asthma

| Type | Management | |
| --- | --- | --- |
| | Preferred | Alternative |
| Mild intermittent asthma | No daily medications; albuterol as needed | |
| Mild persistent asthma | Low-dose inhaled corticosteroid | Cromolyn, leukotriene receptor antagonist, or theophylline (serum level 5–12 mcg/mL) |
| Moderate persistent asthma | Low-dose inhaled corticosteroid and salmeterol or medium-dose inhaled corticosteroid or (if needed) medium-dose inhaled corticosteroid and salmeterol | Low-dose or (if needed) medium-dose inhaled corticosteroid and either leukotriene receptor antagonist or theophylline (serum level 5–12 mcg/mL) |
| Severe persistent asthma | High-dose inhaled corticosteroid and salmeterol and (if needed) oral corticosteroid | High-dose inhaled corticosteroid and theophylline (serum level 5–12 mcg/mL) and oral corticosteroid if needed |

Albuterol 2–4 puffs as needed for peak expiratory flow rate or forced expiratory volume in 1 sec less than 80%, asthma exacerbations, or exposure to exercise or allergens; oral corticosteroid burst if inadequate response to albuterol regardless of asthma severity.

Information adapted from National Institutes of Health, National Heart, Lung, and Blood Institute. National Asthma Education Program. Report of the Working Group on Asthma and Pregnancy: Management of asthma during pregnancy.

|  | Mild Intermittent | Mild Persistent | Moderate Persistent | Severe Persistent |
|---|---|---|---|---|
| **Symptoms** | $\leq 2$ times/wk<br>Asymptomatic between exacerbations | >2 times/wk but <1 time a day | Daily<br>Exacerbations occur $\geq 2$ times/wk | Continual<br>Frequent exacerbations |
| **Pulmonary function tests** | Normal PEFR between exacerbations<br>$FEV_1$ or PEFR >80% of predicted<br>PEFR variability <20% | $FEV_1$ or PEFR >80% of predicted<br>PEFR variability 20-30% | $FEV_1$ or PEFR 60-80% of predicted<br>PEFR variability >30% | $FEV_1$ or PEFR <60% of predicted<br>PEFR variability >30% |
| **Nocturnal awakening** | $\leq 2$ times/mo | >2 times/mo | >1 time/wk | Nightly awakenings |
| **Interference with daily activities** | None | Mild | Some interference with normal activities but rare severe exacerbation | Limitations of physical activity |
| **Treatment** | Inhaled short-acting $\beta_2$-agonist (albuterol) | Inhaled short-acting $\beta_2$-agonist + daily anti-inflammatory (low-dose inhaled corticosteroid or cromolyn) | Inhaled $\beta_2$-agonist + daily medication (medium-dose inhaled corticosteroid OR low-medium dose inhaled corticosteroid AND long-acting bronchodilator) | Inhaled short-acting $\beta_2$-agonist + daily medication (inhaled high-dose corticosteroid AND long-acting bronchodilator AND oral corticosteroid) |

NAEPP, National Asthma Education and Prevention Program; PEFR, peak expiratory flow rate; $FEV_1$, forced expiratory volume in 1 sec.

*Source:* Adapted from NIH publication 93-3279, 1993; Gardner MO, et al. NIH publication 97-4051, 1997, and NAEPP: Working Group on Managing Asthma during Pregnancy. Recommendations for Pharmacologic Treatment, Update 2004. NIH publication No. 05-5236, March 2005.

## Management of Chronic Asthma in Pregnancy

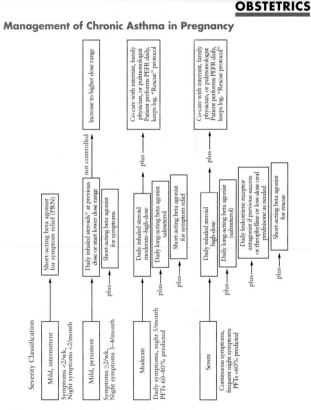

Severity Classification

**Mild, intermittent**
Symptoms <2/wk,
Night symptoms <2/month
→ Short-acting beta agonist for symptom relief (PRN)

**Mild, persistent**
Symptoms ≥2/wk,
Night symptoms 3–4/month
→ Daily inhaled steroids* at previous dose or start lower dose range
  plus→ Short-acting beta agonist for symptoms
  → not controlled → Increase to higher dose range

**Moderate**
Daily symptoms, night 5/month
PFTs 60–80% predicted
→ Daily inhaled steroid moderate–high-dose
  plus→ Daily long-acting beta agonist salmeterol
  plus→ Short-acting beta agonist for symptom relief
  → plus → Co-care with internist, family physician, or pulmonologist. Patient performs PEFR daily, keeps log. "Rescue" protocol

**Severe**
Continuous symptoms, frequent night symptoms
PFTs <60% predicted
→ Daily inhaled steroid high-dose
  plus→ Daily long-acting beta agonist (salmeterol)
  plus→ Daily leukotriene receptor antagonist of previous success or theophylline or low-dose oral prednisone as needed
  plus→ Short-acting beta agonist for rescue
  → plus → Co-care with internist, family physician, or pulmonologist. Patient performs PEFR daily, keeps log. "Rescue protocol"

*Alternatives: Cromolyn or nedocromil if previous good response.
PEFR, peak expiratory flow rate; PFT, pulmonary function test.
*Source:* Reproduced with permission from Sakornbut E. How to treat pregnant patients with asthma. *Cont Ob/Gyn.* 2003;April:26–43. *Cont OB/GYN* is a copyrighted publication of Advanstar Communications Inc. All rights reserved.

# OBSTETRICS

## Dosages of Commonly Used Asthma Medications

| Medication | Dosage Range | FDA Category[a] | Class of Asthma |
|---|---|---|---|
| Albuterol (Proventil, Ventolin) | 2 puffs q4–6hrs prn | B | All |
| Salmeterol (Serevent) | 2 puffs q12hrs or hs | C | Moderate to severe |
| Cromolyn (Intal) | 2 puffs qid | B | Mild persistent to severe |
| Beclomethasone (Beclovent, Vancenase, Qvar) | 2–4 puffs (42 mcg) tid or qid double strength (84 mcg) 2 puffs bid | C | Mild persistent to severe |
| Triamcinolone (Azmacort, Nasacort) | 2–4 puffs (100 mcg) tid or qid | C | Mild persistent to severe |
| Budesonide (Pulmicort, Rhinocort) | 200 or 400 pg/inhalation, 1–2 inhalations bid | C | Mild persistent to severe |
| Flunisolide (Aerobid) | 2–4 puffs (250 mcg) bid | C | Mild persistent to severe |
| Fluticasone (Flovent, Advair) | 44,110,220 mcg/puffs, 1 inhalation bid | C | Mild persistent to severe |
| Montelukast (Singular) | 10 mg hs | B | Severe, possibly moderate |
| Zafirlukast (Accolate) | 20 mg bid | B | Severe, possibly moderate |

[a]B no evidence to risk in humans; C risk cannot be ruled out.

*Source:* Reproduced with permission from Sakornbut E. How to treat pregnant patients with asthma. *Cont Ob/Gyn.* 2003;April:26–43. *Cont OB/GYN* is a copyrighted publication of Advanstar Communications Inc. All rights reserved.

## Drugs for Treating an Acute Severe Asthma Exacerbation

| Medication | Dosage |
|---|---|
| *Inhaled beta-agonists* | |
| Albuterol | Nebulizer: 2.5–5.0 mg (0.5–1.0 mL of a 0.5% solution, diluted with 2–3 mL normal saline) given every 20 mins for three doses MDI with a holding chamber: 90 mcg/puff given as 4–8 puffs every 20 mins up to 4 hrs |
| Metaproterenol | Nebulizer: 15 mg (0.3 mL of a 5% solution, diluted with 2–3 mL normal saline) |
| *Subcutaneous beta-agonists* | |
| Terbutaline | 0.25 mg every 20 mins for three doses |
| Epinephrine | 0.3 mg of 1:1000 solution every 20 mins for three doses |
| *Corticosteroids* | |
| Methylprednisolone | 60–80 mg IV every 6–8 hrs or 125 mg IV bolus followed by inhaled/subcutaneous beta-agonist or oral steroids, depending on initial response |
| Hydrocortisone | 2.0 mg/kg IV bolus every 4 hr or 2.0 mg/kg IV bolus followed by 0.5 mg/kg/hr continuous infusion |
| *Anticholinergics* | |
| Ipratropium bromide | Nebulizer: 0.5 mg (one vial 0.02% solution) every 30 mins for three doses |
| | MDI: 18 mcg/puff given as 4–8 puffs as needed |
| *Other* | |
| Magnesium sulfate | 2 g IV bolus over 2 min, followed immediately by inhaled beta-agonist |
| Heliox | 80% helium/20% oxygen mixture (or alternative ways to prepare heliox depending on a given hospital pharmacy of 70%/30% or 60%/40%) through a nonrebreather mask |

*Source:* Reproduced with permission from Sakornbut E. How to treat pregnant patients with asthma. *Cont Ob/Gyn.* 2003;April:26–43. *Cont OB/GYN* is a copyrighted publication of Advanstar Communications Inc. All rights reserved.

# OBSTETRICS

## Home Management of Acute Asthma Exacerbations[a]

Use albuterol metered-dose inhaler (MDI) 2–4 puffs and measure peak expiratory flow rate (PEFR).

**Poor response:**

PEFR less than 50% predicted, or severe wheezing and shortness of breath, or decreased fetal movement, repeat albuterol 2–4 puffs by MDI and obtain emergency care.

**Incomplete response:**

PEFR is 50–80% predicted or if persistent wheezing and shortness of breath, then repeat albuterol treatment 2–4 puffs MDI at 20-min intervals up to two more times. If repeat PEFR 50–80% predicted or if decreased fetal movement, contact caregiver or go for emergency care.

**Good response:**

PEFR more than 80% predicted, no wheezing or shortness of breath, and fetus is moving normally. May continue inhaled albuterol 2–4 puffs MDI every 3–4 hrs as needed.

[a]Information from National Institutes of Health, National Heart, Lung, and Blood Institute. National Asthma Education Program. Report of the Working Group on Asthma and Pregnancy, management of asthma during pregnancy, 1993.

## Emergency Department and Hospital-Based Management of Asthma Exacerbation

### Initial assessment and treatment

- History and examination (auscultation, use of accessory muscles, heart rate, respiratory rate), peak expiratory flow rate (PEFR) or forced expiratory volume in 1 second ($FEV_1$), oxygen saturation, and other tests as indicated.
- Initiate fetal assessment (consider fetal monitoring and/or biophysical profile if fetus is potentially viable).
- If severe exacerbation ($FEV_1$ or PEFR less than 50% with severe symptoms at rest), then high-dose albuterol by nebulization every 20 minutes or continuously for 1 hour and inhaled ipratropium bromide and systemic corticosteroid.
- Albuterol by metered-dose inhaler or nebulizer, up to three doses in first hour.
- Oral corticosteroid if no immediate response or if patient recently treated with systemic corticosteroid.
- Oxygen to maintain saturation more than 95%.
- Repeat assessment: symptoms, physical examination, PEFR, oxygen saturation.
- Continue albuterol every 60 minutes for 1–3 hours provided there is improvement.

### Repeat assessment

- Symptoms, physical examination, PEFR, oxygen saturation, other tests as needed.
- Continue fetal assessment.

### Good response

- $FEV_1$ or PEFR 70% or more.
- Response sustained 60 minutes after last treatment.
- No distress.

- Physical examination is normal.
- Reassuring fetal status.
- Discharge home.

**Incomplete response**
- $FEV_1$ or PEFR 50% or more but less than 70%.
- Mild or moderate symptoms.
- Continue fetal assessment until patient is stabilized.
- Monitor $FEV_1$ or PEFR, oxygen saturation, pulse.
- Continue inhaled albuterol and oxygen.
- Inhaled ipratropium bromide.
- Systemic (oral or intravenous) corticosteroid.
- Individualize decision for hospitalization.

**Poor response**
- $FEV_1$ or PEFR less than 50%.
- $PCO_2$ more than 42 mm Hg.
- Physical examination: symptoms severe, drowsiness, confusion.
- Continue fetal assessment.
- Admit to intensive care unit.
- Intravenous corticosteroid.

*Source:* Information from National Institutes of Health, National Heart, Lung, & Blood Institute. National Asthma Education Program. Report of the working group on asthma and pregnancy, management of asthma during pregnancy, 1993.

# OBSTETRICS

## MATERNAL VALVULAR HEART DISEASE

### Recommendations for the Evaluation and Care of Women of Childbearing Age with Mechanical Valve Prostheses Who Are Taking Anticoagulants

**Before conception**

Clinical evaluation of cardiac functional status and previous cardiac events

Echocardiographic assessment of ventricular and valvular function and pulmonary pressure

Discussion of risks associated with pregnancy

Discussion of risks and benefits associated with anticoagulant therapy

Family or pregnancy planning

**Conception**

Change to therapeutic, adjusted-dose unfractionated heparin (titrated to a mid-interval therapeutic activated partial-thromboplastin time or anti-factor Xa level) from time of confirmed pregnancy through wk 12

**Completion of first trimester**

Warfarin therapy, wk 12–36

**Week 36[a]**

Discontinue warfarin

Change to unfractionated heparin titrated to a therapeutic activated partial-thromboplastin time or anti-factor Xa level

**Delivery**

Restart heparin therapy 4–6 hr after delivery if no contraindications

Resume warfarin therapy the night after delivery if no bleeding complications

[a]If labor begins while the woman is receiving warfarin, anticoagulation should be reversed and cesarean delivery should be performed.

*Source:* Reproduced with permission from Reimold SC, Rutherford JD. Valvular heart disease in pregnancy. *N Engl J Med.* 2003;349(1):52–59. Copyright © 2003 Massachusetts Medical Society. All rights reserved.

## Classification of Valvular Heart Lesions According to Maternal, Fetal, and Neonatal Risk

| Low Maternal and Fetal Risk | High Maternal and Fetal Risk | High Maternal Risk | High Neonatal Risk |
|---|---|---|---|
| Asymptomatic aortic stenosis with a low mean outflow gradient (<50 mm Hg) in the presence of normal left ventricular systolic function | Severe aortic stenosis with or without symptoms | Reduced left ventricular systolic function (left ventricular ejection fraction <40%) | Maternal age <20 yrs or >35 yrs |
| Aortic regurgitation of NYHA class I or II with normal left ventricular systolic function | Aortic regurgitation with NYHA class III or IV symptoms | Previous heart failure | Use of anticoagulant therapy throughout pregnancy |
| Mitral regurgitation of NYHA class I or II with normal left ventricular systolic function | Mitral stenosis with NYHA class II, III, or IV symptoms | Previous stroke or transient ischemic attack | Smoking during pregnancy |
| Mitral-valve prolapse with no mitral regurgitation or with mild-to-moderate mitral regurgitation and with normal left ventricular systolic function | Mitral regurgitation with NYHA class III or IV symptoms | | Multiple gestations |
| Mild-to-moderate mitral stenosis (mitral-valve area >1.5 cm$^2$, gradient <5 mm Hg) without severe pulmonary hypertension | Aortic-valve disease, mitral-valve disease, or both, resulting in severe pulmonary hypertension (pulmonary pressure >75% of systemic pressures) | | |
| Mild-to-moderate pulmonary-valve stenosis | Aortic-valve disease, mitral-valve disease, or both, with left ventricular systolic dysfunction (ejection fraction <0.40) | | |
| | Maternal cyanosis | | |
| | Reduced functional status (NYHA class III or IV) | | |

# OBSTETRICS

**Fetal Effects of, Maternal Indications for, and Risks Associated with Drugs Used in the Treatment of Maternal Valvular Heart Disease[a]**

| Drug | Fetal Effects | Indications in Pregnant Patients with Valve Disease | Risk Category |
|------|---------------|----------------------------------------------------|---------------|
| **Diuretics** | | | |
| Furosemide | Increased urinary sodium and potassium levels | To decrease congestion associated with valvular heart disease | $C_m$ |
| **Antihypertensive agents** | | | |
| Beta-blockers | Possible decreased heart rate, possible lower birth weight | Hypertension, supraventricular arrhythmias, to control heart rate in women with clinically significant mitral stenosis | $D_m$ |
| Methyldopa | No major adverse effects | Hypertension | C |
| **Vasodilator agents** | | | |
| Angiotensin-converting–enzyme inhibitors | Urogenital defects, death, intrauterine growth retardation | Not indicated during pregnancy and should be discontinued | $D_m$ |
| Hydralazine | No major adverse effects | For vasodilation in cases of aortic regurgitation and ventricular dysfunction | $C_m$ |
| Nitrates | Possible bradycardia | Rarely used to decrease venous congestion | $B–C_m$ |
| **Anticoagulant and antithrombotic agents** | | | |
| Warfarin | Hemorrhage, developmental abnormalities when used between wk 6–12 of gestation | For anticoagulation of mechanical heart valves, valvular heart disease with associated atrial fibrillation during wk 12–36 of pregnancy | $D_m$ |
| Unfractionated heparin | Hemorrhage, no congenital defects | For anticoagulation of mechanical heart valves, valvular heart disease with associated atrial fibrillation during wk 6–12 and after wk 36 of pregnancy | $C_m$ |
| Low-molecular-weight heparin | Hemorrhage | Not currently indicated during pregnancy | $D_m$ |
| Aspirin | Hemorrhage, prolongation of labor, low birth weight (when taken in high doses) | Low-dose aspirin (81 mg/day) occasionally used as an adjunct in patients with previous embolic events or prosthetic-valve thrombosis | C |

| Drug | Fetal Effects | Indications in Pregnant Patients with Valve Disease | Risk Category |
|------|---------------|----------------------------------------------------|---------------|
| **Antiarrhythmic agents** | | | |
| Digoxin | No major adverse effects | For suppression of supraventricular arrhythmias | C |
| Adenosine | No major adverse effects | For immediate conversion of supraventricular arrhythmias | $C_m$ |
| Quinidine | High doses may be oxytocic | Occasionally used for suppression of atrial or ventricular arrhythmias | $C_m$ |
| Procainamide | No major adverse effects | Occasionally used for suppression of atrial or ventricular arrhythmias | $C_m$ |
| Amiodarone | Hypothyroidism, intrauterine growth retardation, premature birth | Rarely used during pregnancy because of side effects; may be used to suppress atrial or ventricular arrhythmias in high-risk patients | $C_m$ |
| **Antibiotics for prophylaxis against endocarditis[b]** | | | |
| Ampicillin | No major adverse effects | Given along with gentamicin to high-risk patients to prevent endocarditis | B |
| Vancomycin | No major adverse effects | Given along with gentamicin to high-risk patients with allergy to penicillin to prevent endocarditis | $C_m$ |
| Gentamicin | No major adverse effects | Given along with ampicillin or vancomycin to high-risk patients to prevent endocarditis | C |

[a]The risk categories are defined as follows. For drugs in category B, either studies of animal reproduction have not demonstrated a fetal risk but there have been no controlled studies in pregnant women or studies of animal reproduction have shown an adverse effect (other than a decrease in fertility) that was not confirmed in controlled studies in women in the first trimester of pregnancy (and there is no evidence of a risk in later trimesters). For drugs in category C, either studies in animals have revealed adverse effects on the fetus and there have been no controlled studies in pregnant women or no studies in women or animals are available; these drugs should be given only if the potential benefit justifies the potential risk to the fetus. For drugs in category D, there is evidence of risk to the human fetus, but the benefits from use in pregnant women may be acceptable despite the risk. A subscript m indicates that the manufacturer has rated the risk.

[b]Antibiotic prophylaxis against endocarditis may be used at the discretion of the treating physician at the time of delivery in high-risk patients. High-risk patients include those with prosthetic cardiac valves, previous bacterial endocarditis, surgically constructed systemic pulmonary shunts or conduits, or complex cyanotic congenital heart disease. Ampicillin should be given intramuscularly or intravenously in a dose of 2.0 g within 30 mins before delivery; 1 g should be given orally, intramuscularly, or intravenously 6 hrs later. Vancomycin should be given intravenously in a dose of 1 g over a period of 1 to 2 hrs, beginning 30 mins before delivery. Gentamicin should be given in a dose of 1.5 mg per kilogram of body weight (not to exceed 120 mg) within 30 mins before delivery.

*Source:* Reproduced with permission from Reimold SC, Rutherford JD. Valvular heart disease in pregnancy. *N Engl J Med.* 2003;349(1):52–59. Copyright © 2003 Massachusetts Medical Society. All rights reserved.

# OBSTETRICS

## GESTATIONAL DIABETES

### Screening for Gestational Diabetes
- Use either a two-step screening with initial 50 g GCT followed by a diagnostic OGTT or eliminate the GCT and screen all appropriate patients with OGTT.
- GCT = non-fasting 50 g oral glucose challenge test.
  - Venous plasma glucose measured one hour later.
  - Value of ≥140 mg/dL indicates need for 3 hour OGTT (~80% sensitivity).
  - Value of ≥130 mg/dL will improve sensitivity to 90% but will necessitate OGTT on 25% of women.

### Testing Recommendations from the Major Professional Organizations

| Issue Being Debated | North American Diabetes and Pregnancy Study Group[a] | American Diabetes Association[b] | American College of Obstetricians and Gynecologists[c] |
|---|---|---|---|
| Universal versus selective screening | Universal | Selective | No recommendation |
| Types of procedures | | One or two step | Two step |
| | | | One step for certain Native American populations only |
| Screening threshold | | 130-140 mg/dL | 130–140 mg/dL |
| Diagnostic criteria | | Carpenter-Coustan | Carpenter-Coustan or NDDG |

NDDG, National Diabetes Data Group.

[a]Reece EA, Homko C, Miodovnik M, Langer O. A consensus report of the Diabetes in Pregnancy Study Group of North America Conference, Little Rock, Ark., May 2002, *J Maternal-Fetal Neonatal Med.* 2002;12:362–364.

[b]American Diabetes Association. Gestational diabetes mellitus: clinical practice recommendations. *Diabetes Care.* 2003;26(suppl 1):S103–S105.

[c]ACOG Practice Bulletin, No. 30. Gestational Diabetes. *Obstet Gynecol.* 2001;98:525–538.

Adapted from Expert Committee on the Diagnosis and Classification of Diabetes Mellitus. Report of the Expert Committee on the Diagnosis and Classification of Diabetes Mellitus. *Diab Care.* 2000;23 (suppl 1):S4–S19.

## Screening Options for Gestational Diabetes

| Status | Plasma or Serum Glucose Level Carpenter/Coustan Conversion | | Plasma Level National Diabetes Data Group Conversion | |
|--------|--------|--------|--------|--------|
| | mg/dL | mmol/L | mg/dL | mmol/L |
| Fasting | 95 | 5.3 | 105 | 5.8 |
| One hour | 180 | 10.0 | 190 | 10.6 |
| Two hours | 155 | 8.6 | 165 | 9.2 |
| Three hours | 140 | 7.8 | 145 | 8.0 |

| Risk Category | Recommendations for Screening |
|---------------|-------------------------------|
| **High risk (one or more of the following)** | |
| Advanced maternal age (Stanford Protocol) | Screen at initial antepartum visit or as soon as possible; repeat at 24–28 wks gestation if initial screening negative for gestational diabetes |
| Prior pregnancy with gestational diabetes (ACOG) | |
| Marked obesity | |
| Diabetes in first degree relative | |
| History of glucose intolerance | |
| Previous infant with macrosomia | |
| Current glycosuria | |
| **Average risk** | |
| Patient fits neither the high-risk nor low-risk profile | Screen between 24–28 wks gestation |
| **Low risk (all of the following)** | |
| Age <25 yrs | Not required |
| Belongs to a low-risk race or ethnic group[a] | |
| No diabetes in first degree relative | |
| Normal prepregnancy weight and weight gain during pregnancy | |
| No history of abnormal blood glucose levels | |
| No prior poor obstetrical outcomes | |

[a]Low-risk races and ethnic groups are those other than Hispanic, black, Native American, South or East Asian, Pacific Islander or Indigenous Australian.
*Source:* Kjos SL and Buchanan TA. Gestational Diabetes Mellitus. *N Engl J Med* 1999;341(23):1749–1756. Copyright © 1999 Massachusetts Medical Society. All rights reserved.

# OBSTETRICS

## Management

For an excellent review, see Metzger BE, Coustan DR et al. Summary and Recommendations of the Fourth International Workshop-Conference on Gestational Diabetes Mellitus. *Diabetes Care* 1998;21 Supp 2, B161–B168.

### Diet (Body Mass Index)

- Ideal body weight (IBW) = 100 lb @ 5 feet, plus 5 lb/inch >5 feet
- Daily kcal: 36 kcal/kg or 15 kcal/lb of IBW + 100 kcal/trimester
- Nutrients
  - 40–50% carbohydrate
  - 12–20% protein
  - 30–35% fat

### Glucose Monitoring

- Desired ranges
*California Diabetes in Pregnancy Program "Sweet Success"*
  Fasting 70–105 mg/dL
  2 hour post-prandial 100–140 mg/dL

### Insulin

- Usually begun for fasting >105 mg/dL consistently
- Anticipated eventual insulin requirements for gestational diabetic listed below
- Distribution
  A.M. $^2/_3$ Total: $^2/_3$ NPH, $^1/_3$ Reg
  P.M. $^1/_3$ Total: $^1/_2$ NPH, $^1/_2$ Reg
- Insulin dependent diabetes mellitus requires individualization (see following page)

### Action Profile of Commonly Used Insulins

| Type | Onset of Action | Peak of Action (hrs) | Duration of Action (hrs) |
|---|---|---|---|
| Insulin lispro | 1–15 mins | 1–2 | 4–5 |
| Insulin aspart | 1–15 mins | 1–2 | 4–5 |
| Regular insulin | 30–60 mins | 2–4 | 6–8 |
| Isophane insulin suspension | 1–3 hrs | 5–7 | 13–18 |
| Insulin zinc suspension | 1–3 hrs | 4–8 | 13–20 |
| Extended insulin zinc suspension | 2–4 hrs | 8–14 | 18–30 |
| Insulin glargine | 1 hr | No peak | 24 |

*Source:* Modified from Gabbe SG, Graves CR. Mangagement of diabetes mellitus complicating pregnancy. *Obstet Gynecol.* 2003;102:857–868.

## Anticipated Insulin Dosage

| Gestational Age (wks) | Anticipated Insulin Dose |
|---|---|
| 6–18 | 0.7 Units/kg |
| 18–26 | 0.8 Units/kg |
| 26–36 | 0.9 Units/kg |
| 36–40 | 1.0 Units/kg |

## Oral Hypoglycemics

- Glyburide does not cross into placenta.
- Glyburide is pregnancy category B.
- If elevated values, start with glyburide 2.5 mg PO with morning meal. Add 2.5 mg increments every week if level not achieved.
- If 10 mg is exceeded, change to twice daily dosing.
- If 20 mg is reached, change to insulin.
- Up to 85% will be well controlled on Gyburide.

*Source: Am J Obstet Gynecol. 2005;193:118–124.*

## Insulin Management during Labor and Delivery

- Usual dose of intermediate-acting insulin is given at bedtime.
- Morning dose of insulin is withheld.
- Intravenous infusion of normal saline is begun.
- Once active labor begins or glucose levels decrease to less than 70 mg/dL, the infusion is changed from saline to 5% dextrose and delivered at a rate of 100–150 cc/hr (2.5 mg/kg/min) to achieve a glucose level of approximately 100 mg/dL.
- Glucose levels are checked hourly using a bedside meter allowing for adjustment in the insulin or glucose infusion rate.
- Regular (short-acting) insulin is administered by intravenous infusion at a rate of 1.25 U/hr if glucose levels exceed 100 mg/dL.

*Source:* Data from Coustan DR. Delivery: timing, mode, and management. In: Reece EA, Coustan DR, Gabbe SG, editors. Diabetes in women: adolescence, pregnancy, and menopause. 3rd ed. Philadelphia (PA): Lippincott Williams & Wilkins; 2004; and Jovanovic L, Peterson CM. Management of the pregnant, insulin-dependent diabetic woman. Diabetes Care 1980;3:63–68.

# OBSTETRICS

## Management of Diabetes in Active Labor

- Check ketones Q void.
- Use the following insulin scale to ensure normoglycemia at delivery.

| FSBG | Insulin Drip |
|------|-------------|
| <70 | 0 |
| 70–90 | 0.5 Units/hr for DM I |
| 91–110 | 1 Units/hr for DM I |
| 111–130 | 2 Units/hr for DM I/DM II/GDM |
| 131–150 | 3 Units/hr |
| 151–170 | 4 Units/hr |
| 171–200 | 5 Units/hr |
| >200 | Check urine ketones and call physician |

DM I, type 1 diabetes; DM II, type II diabetes; GDM, gestational diabetes.
*Source:* Personal communication Dr. Jeffery Faig.

## INSULIN DEPENDENT DIABETES AND PREGNANCY

### Management of Insulin Dependent Diabetics in Pregnancy

- √ HgB$_{A1C}$ preconception and during 1st trimester.
  - Rate of malformations 22% for HgB$_{A1C}$ >8.5.
- Fetal cardiac echocardiogram at 22 weeks.
- Ophthalmology evaluation during 1st and 3rd trimesters.
- 24 hour urine for creatinine clearance, total protein.
- Ultrasound at 18, 22, 26, 38 weeks; consider amniocentesis for maturity at 38 weeks.

### DKA during Pregnancy

| Evaluation | Therapy |
|---|---|
| Laboratory assessment | Arterial blood gas, then glucose, ketones, electrolytes q2hr |
| Insulin | Low dose, intravenous regular insulin |
| | Loading dose: 0.2–0.4 Units/kg |
| | Maintenance 2.0–10 Units/hr |
| Fluids | Isotonic NaCl |
| | Total replacement in first 12 hr = 4–6 L |
| | 500–1000 mL/hr for 2–4 hrs |
| | 250 mL/hr until 80% replaced |
| Glucose | Begin D5-NS when plasma glucose reaches 250 mg/dL |
| Potassium | If initially normal or reduced then add 40–60 mEq/L |
| | If initially elevated then give 20–30 mEq/L once levels begin to decline |
| Bicarbonate | Add one amp (44 mEq) to 1 L of 0.45 NS if pH is <7.10 |

*Source:* Landon MB. Diabetes mellitus and other endocrine diseases. In: Gabbe SG, Niebyl JR, Simpson JL, ed. *Obstetrics: Normal and Problem Pregnancies.* 2nd ed. New York: Churchill Livingstone, 1991. Reproduced with the permission of the publisher.

### White Classification

| Class | Onset | Duration | Vascular Disease |
|---|---|---|---|
| A | Any | Any | None |
| B | >20 yrs old | <10 yrs | None |
| C | 10–19 yrs old | 10–19 yrs | None |
| D | ≤10 yrs old | ≥20 yrs | Benign retinopathy |
| EF | Any | Any | Nephropathy |
| R | Any | Any | Proliferative retinopathy |
| 14 | Any | An | Heart disease |
| RT | Any | Any | Renal transplant |

# OBSTETRICS

## CLASSIFICATION OF HYPERTENSIVE DISORDERS OF PREGNANCY

### Chronic Hypertension

- Hypertension present and observable before pregnancy or prior to 20th week of gestation.
- Hypertension defined as blood pressure >140 mm Hg systolic or 90 mm Hg diastolic.
  - Persistence of hypertension beyond the usual post partum period
  - Use of antihypertensive medications before pregnancy (*Source:* ACOG bulletin. Chronic hypertention in pregnancy. Number 29, 2001.)

### Preeclampsia–Eclampsia

- Preeclampsia is defined as
1. Blood pressure of 140 mm Hg systolic or higher or 90 mm Hg diastolic or higher that occurs after 20 weeks of gestation in a woman with previously normal blood pressure AND
2. Protenuria, defined as urinary excretion of 0.3 g protein or higher in a 2-hour urine specimen
- Severe preeclampsia is diagnosed if one or more of the following is present:
1. Blood pressure of 160 mm Hg systolic or higher or 110 mm Hg diastolic or higher on two occasions at least 6 hours apart while the patient is on bed rest
2. Proteinuria of 5 g or higher in a 24-hour urine specimen or 3+ or greater on two random urine samples collected at least 4 hours apart
3. Oliguria of less than 500 mL in 24 hours
4. Cerebral or visual disturbances
5. Pulmonary edema or cyanosis
6. Epigastric or right upper-quadrant pain
7. Impaired liver function
8. Thrombocytopenia
9. Fetal growth restriction

*Source:* ACOG practice bulletin. Diagnosis and management of preeclampsia and eclampsia. Number 33, January 2002.

Note: Previous incremental rise in blood pressure has not been included but rise in blood pressure of 30 mm Hg systolic or 15 mm Hg diastolic warrants close observation.

Edema has been abandoned as a marker.

Eclampsia is the occurrence of seizures in a woman with preeclampsia (unattributed to other causes).

## Preconception Risk Factors for Preeclampsia

| | |
|---|---|
| 20–30% | Previous preeclampsia |
| 50% | Previous preeclampsia at 28 wks |
| 15–25% | Chronic hypertension |
| 40% | Severe hypertension |
| 25% | Renal disease |
| 20% | Pregestational diabetes mellitus |
| 10–15% | Class B/C diabetes |
| 35% | Class F/R diabetes |
| 10–40% | Thrombophilia |
| 10–15% | Obesity/insulin resistance |
| 10–20% | Age >35 years |
| 10–15% | Family history of preeclampsia |
| 6–7% | Nulliparity/primipaternity |

## Pregnancy-Related Risk Factors for Preeclampsia

| Magnitude of risk depends on the number of factors | |
|---|---|
| 2-fold normal | Unexplained midtrimester elevations of serum AFP, HCG, inhibin-A |
| 10–30% | Abnormal uterine artery Doppler velocimetry |
| 0–30% | Hydrops/hydropic degeneration of placenta |
| 10–20% | Multifetal gestation (depends on number of fetuses and maternal age) |
| 10% | Partner who fathered preeclampsia in another woman |
| 8–10% | Gestational diabetes mellitus |
| 8–10% | Limited sperm exposure (teenage pregnancy) |
| 6–7% | Nulliparity/primipaternity |
| Limited data | Donor insemination, oocyte donation |
| Limited data | Unexplained persistent proteinuria or hematuria |
| Unknown | Unexplained fetal growth restriction |

*Source:* Reproduced with permission from Sibai BM. Preeclampsia: 3 preemptive tactics. *OBG Management.* 2005;20–32.

# OBSTETRICS

## Preeclampsia Superimposed upon Chronic Hypertension

- Prognosis worse than in either condition alone.
- Overdiagnosis is appropriate and unavoidable.
- Consider this diagnosis in following findings:
  - New onset proteinuria (300 mg/24 hour) in a hypertensive woman without previous proteinuria
  - Hypertension and proteinuria prior to 20 weeks gestation
  - Sudden increase in proteinuria
  - Sudden increase in blood pressure in a previously well-controlled patient
  - Platelet count <100,000 cells/mm$^3$
  - Elevated hepatic enzymes (AST and ALT)

## Complication Rates in Women with Superimposed Preeclampsia vs. Women without Hypertension[a]

| Complication | Without Hypertension (per 1000 Cases) | Preeclampsia Superimposed on Chronic Hypertension (per 1000 Cases) |
|---|---|---|
| Abruptio placentae | 9.6 | 30.6 |
| Thrombocytopenia | 1.6 | 11.5 |
| Disseminated intravascular coagulation | 2.9 | 17.4 |
| Pulmonary edema | 0.2 | 6.4 |
| Blood transfusion | 1.5 | 16.3 |
| Mechanical ventilation | 0.2 | 17.0 |

[a]US women, 1988–1997.
*Source:* Reproduced with permission from Sibai BM. Preeclampsia: 3 preemptive tactics. *OBG Management.* 2005;20–32.

## Mild Preeclampsia

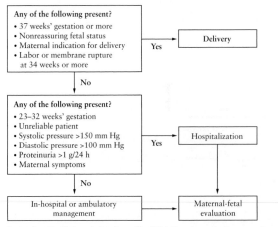

*Source:* Reproduced with permission from Sibai BM. Preeclampsia: 3 preemptive tactics. *OBG Management.* 2005;20–32.

# OBSTETRICS

## Management of Mild Preeclampsia

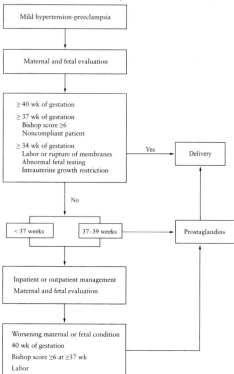

```
        ┌─────────────────────────────────────┐
        │   Mild hypertension-preeclampsia    │
        └─────────────────────────────────────┘
                          │
        ┌─────────────────────────────────────┐
        │    Maternal and fetal evaluation    │
        └─────────────────────────────────────┘
                          │
        ┌─────────────────────────────────────┐
        │  ≥ 40 wk of gestation               │
        │                                     │
        │  ≥ 37 wk of gestation               │        ┌──────────┐
        │  Bishop score ≥6                    │        │          │
        │  Noncompliant patient               │──Yes──▶│ Delivery │
        │                                     │        │          │
        │  ≥ 34 wk of gestation               │        └──────────┘
        │  Labor or rupture of membranes      │
        │  Abnormal fetal testing             │
        │  Intrauterine growth restriction    │
        └─────────────────────────────────────┘
                          │ No
         ┌────────────┐  ┌────────────┐                 ┌───────────────┐
         │ < 37 weeks │  │ 37–39 weeks│────────────────▶│ Prostaglandins│
         └────────────┘  └────────────┘                 └───────────────┘
                          │
        ┌─────────────────────────────────────┐
        │ Inpatient or outpatient management  │
        │ Maternal and fetal evaluation       │
        └─────────────────────────────────────┘
                          │
        ┌─────────────────────────────────────┐
        │ Worsening maternal or fetal condition│
        │ 40 wk of gestation                  │
        │ Bishop score ≥6 at ≥37 wk           │
        │ Labor                               │
        └─────────────────────────────────────┘
```

*Source:* Adapted from Sibai BM. Gestational Hypertension-Preeclampsia. *Obstet Gynecol.* 2003.

## Management of Severe Preeclampsia

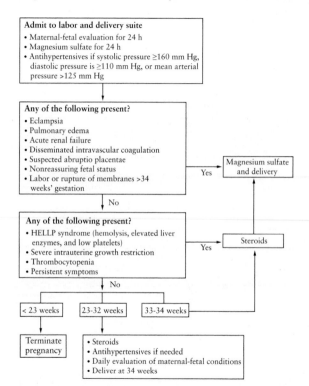

*Source:* Reproduced with permission from Sibai BM. Preeclampsia: 3 preemptive tactics. *OBG Management.* 2005;20–32.

# OBSTETRICS

## Magnesium Sulfate Toxicity

| $MgSO_4$ Overdose | |
|---|---|
| **Toxicity** | |
| EKG changes | 5–10 mEq/L |
| Loss of deep tendon reflexes | 10 mEq/L |
| Respiratory suppression | 15 mEq/L |
| Cardiovascular collapse | >25 mEq/L |

Treatment of toxicity is: 1 gm $Ca^{+2}$ gluconate IV push.

## Laboratory Evaluation of PIH

| Test | Rationale |
|---|---|
| Hemoglobin and hematocrit | Hemoconcentration supports the diagnosis of preeclampsia and is an indicator of severity. Values may be decreased, however, if hemolysis accompanies the disease. |
| Platelet count | Thrombocytopenia suggests preeclampsia. |
| Quantification of protein excretion | Pregnancy hypertension with proteinuria should be considered preeclampsia (pure or superimposed) until it is proven otherwise. |
| Serum creatinine level | Abnormal or rising creatinine levels, especially in association with oliguria, suggest severe preeclampsia. |
| Serum uric acid level | Increased uric acid levels suggest the diagnosis of preeclampsia. |
| Serum transaminase levels | Rising serum transaminase levels suggest severe preeclampsia with hepatic involvement. |
| Serum albumin, lactic acid dehydrogenase, blood smear and coagulation profile | For women with severe disease, these values indicate the extent of endothelial leak (hypoalbuminemia), presence of hemolysis (LDH level, peripheral smear), and possible coagulopathy including thrombocytopenia. |

LDH, lactate dehydrogenase.
*Source:* National High Blood Pressure Education Program Working Group Report on High Blood Pressure in Pregnancy, NIH Publication No. 00-3029, July 2000.

## Hypertensive Emergency

| Drug | Administration |
| --- | --- |
| Hydralazine | Start with 5 mg IV or 10 mg IM. If blood pressure is not controlled, repeat at 20-min intervals (5–10 mg depending on response). Once blood pressure is controlled repeat as needed (usually about 3 hrs). If no success by 20 mg IV or 30 mg IM total, consider another drug. |
| Labetalol | Start with 20 mg IV as a bolus; if effect is suboptimal, then give 40 mg 10 mins later and 80 mg every 10 mins for two additional doses. Use a maximum of 220 mg. If desired blood pressure levels are not achieved, switch to another drug. Do not give labetalol to women with asthma or congestive heart failure. |
| Nifedipine | Start with 10 mg orally and repeat in 30 mins if necessary. Short acting nifedipine is NOT approved by the FDA for managing hypertension. Refer to the Working Group Report for details. |
| Sodium nitro-prusside | Rarely needed for hypertension not responding to the drugs listed above and/or if there are clinical findings of hypertensive encephalopathy. Start at a rate of 0.25 mcg/kg/min to a maximum of 5 mcg/kg/min. Fetal cyanide poisoning may occur if used for more than 4 hrs. |

Caution: Sudden and severe hypotension can result from the administration of any of these agents, especially short-acting oral nifedipine. The goal of blood pressure reduction in emergency situations should be a gradual reduction of blood pressure to the normal range.

*Source:* National High Blood Pressure Education Program Working Group Report on High Blood Pressure in Pregnancy, NIH Publication No. 00-3029, July 2000.

# OBSTETRICS

## Acute and Long-Term Drug Treatment

| Drug | Starting Dose | Maximum Dose | Comments |
|------|---------------|--------------|----------|
| **Acute Treatment of Severe Hypertension** | | | |
| Hydralazine | 5–10 mg IV every 20 mins | 30 mg[a] | |
| Labetalol | 20–40 mg IV every 10–15 mins | 220 mg[a] | Avoid in women with asthma or congestive heart failure |
| Nifedipine | 10–20 mg orally every 30 mins | 50 mg[a] | |
| **Long-Term Treatment of Hypertension** | | | |
| Methyldopa | 250 mg bid | 4 g/day | Rarely indicated |
| Labetalol | 100 mg bid | 2400 mg/day | First choice |
| Atenolol | 50 mg/day | 100 mg/day | Associated with intrauterine growth restriction |
| Propanolol | 40 mg bid | 640 mg/day | Use with associated thyroid disease |
| Hydralazine | 10 mg tid | 100 mg/day | Use in cases of left ventricular hypertrophy |
| Nifedipine | 10 mg bid | 120 mg /day | Use in women with diabetes |
| Diltiazem | 120–180 mg/day | 540 mg/day | |
| Thiazide diuretic | 12.5 mg bid | 50 mg/day | Use in salt-sensitive hypertension and/or congestive heart failure |
| | | | May be added as second agent |
| | | | Avoid if preeclampsia develops or intrauterine growth restriction is present |
| Angiotensin-converting enzyme inhibitors and angiotensin receptor blockers | — | — | Do not use after 16–18 wks |

[a]If desired blood pressure levels are not achieved, switch to another drug.

*Source:* Reproduced with permission from Sibai BM, Ghulmiyyah LM. Controlling chronic hypertension in pregnancy. *OBG Management.* 2006;41–55.

## ECLAMPSIA

### Signs and Symptoms of Eclampsia[a]

| Condition | Frequency (%) in Women with Eclampsia | Remarks |
|---|---|---|
| **Signs** | | |
| Hypertension | 85 | Should be documented on at least 2 occasions more than 6 hrs apart |
| Severe: 160/110 mm Hg or more | 20–54 | |
| Mild: 140–160/90–110 mm Hg | 30–60 | |
| No hypertension | 16 | |
| Proteinuria | 85 | |
| At least 1+ on dipstick | 48 | |
| At least 3+ on dipstick | 14 | |
| No proteinuria | 15 | |
| **Symptoms** | | |
| At least 1 of the following: | 33–75 | Clinical symptoms may occur before or after a convulsion |
| Headache | 30–70 | Persistent, occipital, or frontal |
| Right upper quadrant or epigastric pain | 12–20 | |
| Visual changes | 19–32 | Blurred vision, photophobia |
| Altered mental changes | 4–5 | |

[a]Summary of 5 series.
*Source:* Reproduced with permission from Sibai BM. Managing an eclamptic patient. *OBG Management.* 2005:37–50.

### Usual Times of Onset[a]

| Onset | Frequency (%) | Remarks |
|---|---|---|
| Antepartum | 38–53 | Maternal and perinatal mortality, and the incidence of complications and underlying disease, are higher in antepartum eclampsia, especially in early cases |
| ≤20 wks | 1.5 | |
| 21 to 27 wks | 7.5 | |
| ≥28 wks | 91 | |
| Intrapartum | 18–36 | Intrapartum eclampsia more closely resembles postpartum disease than antepartum cases |
| Postpartum | 11–44 | Late postpartum eclampsia occurs more than 48 hrs but less than 4 wks after delivery |
| ≤48 hrs | 7–39 | |
| >48 hrs | 5–26 | |

[a]Summary of 5 series.
*Source:* Reproduced with permission from Sibai BM. Managing an eclamptic patient. *OBG Management.* 2005:37–50.

# OBSTETRICS

## Maternal Complications

| Complication | Rate (%) | Remarks |
|---|---|---|
| Death | 0.5–2.0 | Risk of death is higher: <br> Older than 30 yrs of age <br> No prenatal care <br> African Americans <br> Onset of preeclampsia or eclampsia before 28 wks gestation |
| Intracerebral hemorrhage | <1 | Usually related to several risk factors |
| Aspiration pneumonia | 2–3 | Heightened risk of maternal hypoxemia and acidosis |
| Disseminated coagulopathy | 3–5 | Regional anesthesia is contraindicated in these patients, and there is a heightened risk of hemorrhagic shock |
| Pulmonary edema | 3–5 | Heightened risk of maternal hypoxemia and acidosis |
| Acute renal failure | 5–9 | Usually seen in association with abruptio placentae, maternal hemorrhage, and prolonged maternal hypotension |
| Abruptio placentae | 7–10 | Can occur after a convulsion; suspect it if fetal bradycardia or late decelerations persist |
| HELLP syndrome | 10–15 | |

HELLP, hemolysis, elevated liver enzymes and low platelets.

## Management of Eclamptic Seizure

| **Avoid Maternal Injury** |
|---|
| Insert padded tongue blade |
| Avoid inducing gag reflex |
| Elevate padded bedside rails |
| Use physical restraints as needed |
| **Maintain Oxygenation to Mother and Fetus** |
| Apply face mask with or without oxygen reservoir at 8–10 L/min |
| Monitor oxygenation and metabolic status via <br> Transcutaneous pulse oximetry <br> Arterial blood gases (sodium bicarbonate administered accordingly) |
| Correct oxygenation and metabolic status before administering anesthetics that may depress myocardial function |
| **Minimize Aspiration** |
| Place patient in lateral decubitus position (which also maximizes uterine blood flow and venous return) |
| Suction vomitus and oral secretions |
| Obtain chest x-ray after the convulsion is controlled to rule out aspiration |

*Source:* Reproduced with permission from Sibai BM. Managing an eclamptic patient. *OBG Management.* 2005:37–50.

## ACUTE FATTY LIVER, HELLP, HEPATITIS, ETC.

### Frequency of Various Signs and Symptoms among Imitators of Preeclampsia–Eclampsia

| Signs and Symptoms | HELLP Syndrome | AFLP | TTP | HUS | Exacerbation of SLE |
|---|---|---|---|---|---|
| Hypertension | 85 | 50 | 20–75 | 80–90 | 80 with APA, nephritis |
| Proteinuria | 90–95 | 30–50 | With hematuria | 80–90 | 100 with nephritis |
| Fever | Absent | 25–32 | 20–50 | NR | Common during flare |
| Jaundice | 5–10 | 40–90 | Rare | Rare | Absent |
| Nausea and vomiting | 40 | 50–80 | Common | Common | Only with APA |
| Abdominal pain | 60–80 | 35–50 | Common | Common | Only with APA |
| Central nervous system | 40–60 | 30–40 | 60–70 | NR | 50 with APA |

AFLP, acute fatty liver of pregnancy; APA, antiphospholipid antibodies with or without catastrophic antiphospholipid syndrome; Common, reported as the most common presentation; HELLP, hemolysis, elevated liver enzymes, low platelets; HUS, hemolytic uremic syndrome; NR, values are not reported; SLE, systemic lupus erythematosus; TTP, thrombotic thrombocytopenic purpura.

Data are %.

*Source:* Reproduced with permission from Sibai BM. Imitators of Preeclampsia. *Obstet Gynecol.* 2007 Apr;109(4):956–66.

# OBSTETRICS

## Frequency and Severity of Laboratory Findings among Imitators of Preeclampsia–Eclampsia

| Laboratory Findings | HELLP Syndrome | AFLP | TTP | HUS | Exacerbation of SLE |
|---|---|---|---|---|---|
| Thrombocytopenia (less than 100,000/mm³) | More than 20,000 | More than 50,000 | 20,000 or less | More than 20,000 | More than 20,000 |
| Hemolysis (%) | 50–100 | 15–20 | 100 | 100 | 14–23 with APA |
| Anemia (%) | Less than 50% | Absent | 100 | 100 | 14–23 with APA |
| DIC (%) | Less than 20 | 50–100 | Rare | Rare | Rare |
| Hypoglycemia (%) | Absent | 50–100 | Absent | Absent | Absent |
| VW factor multimers (%) | Absent | Absent | 80–90 | 80 | Less than 10 |
| ADAMTS13 less than 5% (%) | Absent | Absent | 33–100 | Rare | Rare |
| Impaired renal function (%) | 50 | 90–100 | 30 | 100 | 40–80 |
| LDH (IU/L) | 600 or more | Variable | More than 1000 | More than 1000 | With APA |
| Elevated ammonia (%) | Rare | 50 | Absent | Absent | Absent |
| Elevated bilirubin (%) | 50–60 | 100 | 100 | NA | Less than 10 |
| Elevated transaminases (%) | 100 | 100 | Usually mild* | Usually mild* | With APA |

AFLP, acute fatty liver of pregnancy; ADAMTS, von Willebrand factor-cleaving metalloprotease; APA, antiphospholipid antibodies; DIC, disseminated intravascular coagulopathy; HELLP, hemolysis, elevated liver enzymes, low platelets; HUS, hemolytic uremic syndrome; LDH, lactic dehydrogenase; NA, values are not available; SLE, systemic lupus erythematosus; TTP, thrombotic thrombocytopenic purpura; VW, von Willebrand.

*Levels less than 100 IU/L.

*Source:* Reproduced with permission from Sibai BM. Imitators of Preeclampsia. *Obstet Gynecol.* 2007 Apr;109(4):956–66.

# INTRAUTERINE FETAL DEMISE

## Recommended Evaluation

| Recommended in most cases: |
| --- |
| Perinatal autopsy |
| Placental evaluation |
| Karyotype |
| Antibody screen[a] |
| Serologic test for syphilis[b] |
| Screen for fetal–maternal hemorrhage (Kleihauer-Betke or other) |
| Urine toxicology screen |
| Parvovirus serology |

| Recommended if clinical suspicion: |
| --- |
| Lupus anticoagulant screen[c] |
| Anticardiolipin antibodies[c] |
| Factor V Leiden mutation[c] |
| Prothrombin G20210A mutations |
| Screen for protein C, protein S, and antithrombin III deficiency[d] |
| Uterine imaging study[e] |
| MTHFR mutation screening[f] |

| Not recommended at present: |
| --- |
| Thyroid-stimulating hormone |
| Glycohemoglobin |
| TORCH titers[g] |
| Placental cultures |
| Testing for other thrombophilias |

[a]Negative first-trimester screen does not require repeat testing.
[b]Repeat testing in cases of negative first trimester screen if high-risk population.
[c]Test in cases of thrombosis, placental insufficiency, and recurrent fetal death.
[d]These thrombophilias are rare in the absence of personal or family history of thrombosis.
[e]Test in cases of unexplained recurrent loss, preterm premature rupture of membranes, and preterm labor.
[f]MTHFR, methylenetetrahydrofolate reductase.
[g]TORCH titers, serology for toxoplasmosis, rubella, cytomegalovirus, and herpes simplex.
*Source:* Reproduced with permission from Silver RM. Fetal Death. *Obstet Gynecol.* 2007:109;153–167.

# OBSTETRICS

## NON-IMMUNE HYDROPS EVALUATION

| Ultrasound | Maternal Blood |
|---|---|
| **Placenta** | 3 hr OGTT |
| Hemangioma | Type and screen |
| Thickened | Kleihauer-betke |
| Triploidy syndromes | AFP |
| Maternal diabetes | G-6-PD |
| Fetal anemia | CMV, toxo, parvovirus B19 titers |
| Thin (dysmaturity) | VDRL |
| **Umbilical cord** | Rheumatoid factor, anti-nuclear antibody (ANA) |
| Thrombus | BUN creatinine, uric acid |
| **Amniotic fluid** | Mirror syndrome |
| Polyhydramnios (usual) |    Preeclampsia type maternal illness associated |
| Oligohydramnios (with triploidy) |      with fetal hydrops |
| **Fetus** | Thrombophilia screen |
| Ascites, pleural effusion, pericardial effusion | |
| Edema | |
| Twin-twin transfusion | |
| Fetal sex (G-6-PD deficiency) | |
| Enlarged heart, cardiac tumor | |
| Fetal bradycardia (heart block) | |
| Pulmonary hypoplasia | |
| Cystic adenomatoid malformation of lung | |
| Diaphragmatic hernia | |
| Sacrococcygeal teratoma | |
| Short-limbed dwarfism | |
| Cystic hygroma | |
| Alpha thalassemia | |

### ISOIMMUNIZATION
**Evaluation of Obstetric Patients with a Positive Indirect Coombs' Test Result**

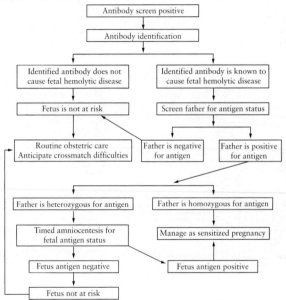

*Source:* American College of Obstetricians and Gynecologists. PROLOG: Obstetrics. 5th ed. Washington, DC: ACOG; 2003.

### Middle Cerebral Artery Doppler Evaluation
- Ultrasound measurement of the MCA peak systolic blood flow velocity can be used to predict fetal anemia instead of the DOD-450.
- MCA Dopplers are 88% sensitive and 82% specific for fetal anemia whereas DOD-450 was 76% sensitive 77% specific for fetal anemia.

*Source:* Oepkes D, et al. Doppler ultrasonography versus amniocentesis to predict fetal anemia. *N Engl J Med.* 2006;355(2):156–164.

# OBSTETRICS

## Managing the Sensitized Pregnancy

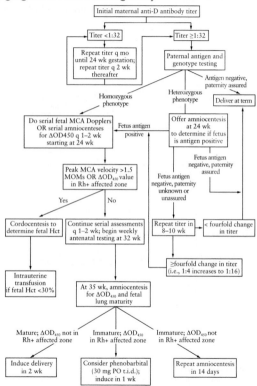

## Managing Patients with a Previously Affected Fetus

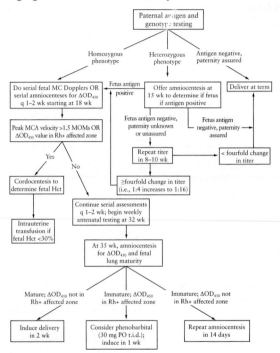

# OBSTETRICS

## MULTIPLE GESTATION

### Fast Facts
- Dizygotic: fertilization of 2 separate ova by 2 sperm
- Monozygotic: division of single ovum fertilized by single sperm
- Since 1980, 65% increase in the number of twin, and 500% increase in the number of triplet pregnancies

### Placentation
- Dizygotic twins ($^2/_3$ of U.S. twins) have separate chorion/amnion.
- Type of Monozygotic twins ($^1/_3$ of U.S. twins) dependent on timing of embryonic division.

| | |
|---|---|
| 0–72 hrs | diamniotic, dichorionic (30%) |
| 4–8 days | monochorionic, diamniotic (68%) |
| 8–13 days | monochorionic, monoamniotic (2%) |
| >13 days | conjoined twins |

### Maternal Complications of Twin Gestation
- 6× more likely to be hospitalized with pregnancy complications
- Hyperemesis
- Pregnancy-induced hypertension (PIH)
- Pyelonephritis
- Postpartum hemorrhage
- Preterm labor
- Acute fatty liver
- Thromboembolism

### Antepartum Management
- High risk for preterm labor
- Serial sonogram for growth
- NST as indicated
  - May be useful in multiple gestations to assess fetal well-being and predict cord compression

## Morbidity and Mortality in Multiple Gestation

| Characteristic | Twins | Triplets | Quadruplets |
|---|---|---|---|
| Average birth weight[a] | 2347 g | 1687 g | 1309 g |
| Average gestational age at delivery[a] | 35.3 wks | 32.2 wks | 29.9 wks |
| Percentage with growth restriction[b] | 14–25 | 50–60 | 50–60 |
| Percentage requiring admission to neonatal intensive care unit | 25 | 75 | 100 |
| Average length of stay in neonatal intensive care unit[c–i] | 18 days | 30 days | 58 days |
| Percentage with major handicap[i,j] | — | 20 | 50 |
| Risk of cerebral palsy[i,j] | 4 times more than singletons | 17 times more than singletons | — |
| Risk of death by age 1 year[k–m] | 7 times higher than singletons | 20 times higher than singletons | — |

[a]Martin JA, Hamilton BE, Sutton PD, Ventura SJ, Menacker F, Munson ML. Births: final data for 2002. *Natl Vital Stat Rep* 2003;52(10):1–102.

[b]Mauldin JG, Newman RB. Neurologic morbidity associated with multiple gestation. *Female Pat* 1998;23(4):27–28, 30, 35–36, passim.

[c]Ettner SL, Christiansen CL, Callahan TL, Hall JE. How low birthweight and gestational age contribute to increased inpatient costs for multiple births. *Inquiry* 1997–1998;34:325–339.

[d]McCormick MD, Brooks-Gunn J, Workman-Daniels K, Turner J, Peckham GI. The health and developmental status of very low-birth-weight children at school age. *JAMA* 1992;267:2204–2208.

[e]Luke B, Bigger HR, Leurgans S, Sietsema D. The cost of prematurity: a case-control study of twins vs singletons. *Am J Public Health* 1996;86:809–814.

[f]Albrecht IL, Tomich PG. The maternal and neonatal outcome of triplet gestations. *Am J Obstet Gynecol* 1996;174:1551–1556.

[g]Newman RB, Hamer C, Miller MC. Outpatient triplet management: a contemporary review. *Am J Obstet Gynecol* 1989;161:547–553; discussion 553–555.

[h]Seoud MA, Toner JP, Kruithoff C, Muasher SJ. Outcome of twin, triplet, and quadruplet in vitro fertilization pregnancies: the Norfolk experience. *Fertil Steril* 1992;57:825–834.

[i]Elliott JP, Radin TG. Quadruplet pregnancy: contemporary management and outcome. *Obstet Gynecol* 1992;80:421–424.

[j]Grether JK, Nelson KB, Cummins SK. Twinning and cerebral palsy: experience in four northern California counties, births 1983 through 1985. *Pediatrics* 1993;92:854–858.

[k]Luke B, Minogue J. The contribution of gestational age and birth weight to perinatal viability in singletons versus twins. *J Mat-Fetal Med* 1994;3:263–274.

[l]Kiely JL, Kleinman JC, Kiely M. Triplets and higher order multiple births: time trends and infant mortality. *Am J Dis Child* 1992;146:862–868.

[m]Luke B, Keith LG. The contribution of singletons, twins, and triplets to low birth weight, infant mortality, and handicap in the United States. *J Reprod Med* 1992;37:661–666.

*Source:* Reproduced with permission from ACOG Committee on Practice Bulletins: Multiple Gestation: Complicated Twin, Triplet, and High-Order Multifetal Pregnancy. ACOG Practice Bulletin 2004;104(4):869–882.

## OBSTETRICS

**Presentation of Twins**

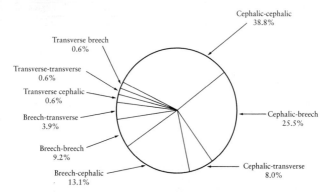

*Source:* Thompson SA, Lyons TL, Makowski EL. Outcomes of twin gestations at the University of Colorado Health Sciences Center, 1973–1983. *J Reprod Med* 1987;32 (5):328–339. Reproduced with the permission of the publisher, the Journal of Reproductive Medicine.

## Management of Multiple Gestation Delivery

Delivery method is controversial

| Presentation | Birth Wt | Number of Cesarean Sections Needed to Prevent One Instance of Composite Morbidity and Mortality |
|---|---|---|
| Vtx/Non-vtx | 500–1499 g | 7 |
| Vtx/Non-vtx | 1500–4000 g | 25 |

*Source:* Meyer, MC. Translating data to dialogue: How to discuss mode of delivery with you patient with twins. American Journal of Obstetrics and Gynecology 2006;195(4):899–906.

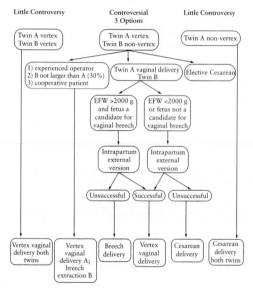

*Source:* Chervenak FA, Johnson RE, Youcha S, et al. Intrapartum management of twin gestation. *Obstet Gynecol* 1985;65(1):119–24. Reproduced with the permission of the publisher, the American College of Obstetricians and Gynecologists.

# OBSTETRICS

## PRETERM LABOR

### Fast Facts

- Preterm birth causes 85% of all perinatal morbidity and mortality
- 12.5% of all pregnancies (National vital statistics report 2004)
  - Spontaneous preterm labor (70–80%)
  - Indicated preterm delivery (20–30%)

### Diagnosis

1. Estimated gestational age <37 completed weeks
2. Uterine activity
3. Cervical dilation >2 cm or 80% effaced
4. Documented cervical change from single examiner

### Principles of Management (Outpatient)

- Weekly cervical exams (20–37 wks)
- Home self-monitoring
- Pelvic rest
- Bedrest
- Early intervention for cervical change
- Education
- Identification of high risk patients

### Prevention

17-Alpha-hydroxyprogesterone caproate 250 mg IM weekly, starting between 16 and 20 weeks until 36 weeks, reduces the risk of delivery before 37 weeks in patients with a history of preterm delivery.

*Source:* Meis et al. *N Engl J Med.* 2003;348:2379–2385. Copyright © 2003 Massachusetts Medical Society. All rights reserved.

### Gestational Age at Delivery, Fetal and Neonatal Outcome of Women Treated with Either 17P or Placebo in NICHD Trial

|  | 17P | Placebo | RR | CL |
|---|---|---|---|---|
| N | 306 | 153 |  |  |
| Gestational age at delivery |  |  |  |  |
| <37 wks | 36.3% | 54.9 | 0.66 | 0.54–0.81 |
| <35 wks | 20.6% | 30.7% | 0.67 | 0.48–0.93 |
| <32 wks | 11.4% | 19.6% | 0.58 | 0.37–0.91 |
| BW < 2,500 g | 27.2% | 41.1% | 0.66 | 0.51–0.87 |
| BW < 1,500 g | 8.6% | 13.9% | 0.62 | 0.36–1.07 |
| Neonatal death | 2.6% | 5.9% | 0.44 | 0.17–1.13 |
| Necrotizing enterocolitis | 1.3% | 5.2% | 0.25 | 0.8–0.82 |
| Intraventricular hemorrhage | 0 | 2.6% | NA | NA |
| Supplemental $O_2$ | 14.9% | 23.8% | 0.62 | 0.42–0.92 |
| Respiratory distress syndrome | 9.5% | 15.1% | 0.63 | 0.38–1.05 |

*Source:* Reproduced with permission from Armstrong JA, Nageotte M: Can progesterone prevent preterm birth? *Cont Ob/Gyn.* 2005;Oct:30–35. *Cont OB/GYN* is a copyrighted publication of Advanstar Communications Inc. All rights reserved.

## The Four Major Pathways to Preterm Delivery

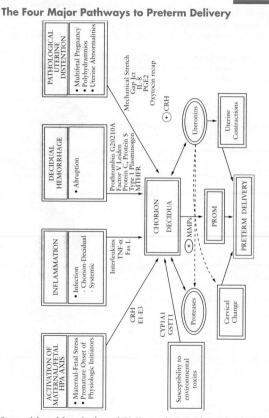

*Source:* Adapted from Lockwood CJ, Kvczynski E. *Paediatr Edimol.* 2001;15:78, and Wang X et al. *Paediatr Perinat Epidemol.* 2001;15:63.

# OBSTETRICS

## Predicting Preterm Delivery

- Home uterine activity monitoring of unproven benefit.
- Fetal fibronectin screening has a strong negative predictive value between 24 and 34 weeks.
- Cervical length on sonogram may be predictive of preterm delivery.
- Prophylactic treatment of mother for Group B *streptococcus* is appropriate pending culture results to prevent neonatal infection, but not to prevent preterm delivery.
- Tocolytic therapy may at least provide for administration of corticosteroids or transport to tertiary center for delivery.

## Determining Risk of Preterm Delivery in Parous Women at 24 Weeks of Gestation

| Technique for Determining Risk | % Risk Based on History of Delivery | | | |
|---|---|---|---|---|
| | 18–26 wks | 27–31 wks | 32–36 wks | 37 wks |
| | *Risk of delivery at <35 wks* | | | |
| By obstetric history | 15 | 15 | 14 | 3 |
| FFN (+) | 49 | 48 | 46 | 13 |
| FFN (−) | 13 | 13 | 12 | 2 |
| CL (cm) at 24 wks | | | | |
| ≤2.5 | 31 | 32 | 31 | 8 |
| 26–3.5 | 16 | 16 | 16 | 4 |
| >3.5 | 8 | 8 | 8 | 2 |
| | *Risk of spontaneous preterm delivery at <35 wks* | | | |
| FFN (−) by CL (cm) | | | | |
| ≤2.5 | 25 | 25 | 25 | 6 |
| 2.6–3.5 | 14 | 14 | 13 | 3 |
| >3.5 | 7 | 7 | 7 | 1 |
| FFN (+) by CL (cm) | | | | |
| ≤2.5 | 64 | 64 | 63 | 25 |
| 2.6–3.5 | 64 | 45 | 45 | 14 |
| >3.5 | 28 | 28 | 27 | 7 |

FNN, fetal fibronectin; CL, cervical length.
*Source:* Modified from Iams JD, Goldberg RL, Mercer BM, Moawad A, Thom E, Meis PJ, et al. The Preterm Prediciton Study: recurrence risk of spontaneous preterm birth. *Am J Obstet Gynecol* 1998;178:1038–1039.

# FETAL FIBRONECTIN TESTING

## Women with Signs & Symptoms of Preterm Labor[a]

| | | |
|---|---|---|
| Negative predictive value | 99.2% | 124 out of 125 women with a normal (negative) fetal fibronectin test result **will not** deliver within the next 14 days. |
| Positive predictive value | 16.7% | 1 out of 6 women with an elevated (positive) fetal fibronectin test result **will** deliver preterm within 14 days. However, almost 1 out of 2 women with an elevated (positive) fetal fibronectin test result **will** spontaneously give birth before 37 wks. |

## Women with Risk Factors but No Symptoms[b]

| | | |
|---|---|---|
| Negative predictive value | 93.9% | 15 out of 16 women with a normal (negative) fetal fibronectin test result **will not** spontaneously give birth before 37 wks. |
| Positive predictive value | 46.3% | Almost 1 out of 2 women with an elevated (positive) fetal fibronectin test result **will** spontaneously give birth before 37 wks. |

[a]*Source*: Peaceman AM, Andrews WW, Thorp JM, et al. Fetal fibronectin as a predictor of preterm birth in patients with symptoms: a multicenter trial. *Am J of Obstet Gynecol* 1997 Jul;177(1):13–18.
[b]*Source*: Nageotte MP, Casal D, Senyei AE. Fetal fibronectin in patients at increased risk for premature birth. *Am J Obstet Gynecol.* 1994;170(1 Pt 1):20–25.

## Predicting Recurrent Preterm Birth

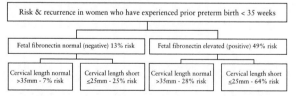

*Source:* Reproduced with permission from Iams JD, Goldenberg RL, Mercer BM. The preterm prediction study: recurrence risk of spontaneous preterm birth. *Am J of Obstet Gynecol* 1998;178:1035–1040.

# OBSTETRICS

## Evaluation of Patient with PTL Risk Factors

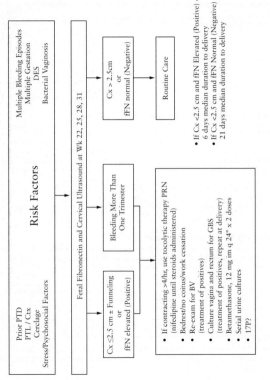

**Risk Factors**

Prior PTD
PTL / Ctx
Cerclage
Stress/Psychosocial Factors

Multiple Bleeding Episodes
Multiple Gestation
DES
Bacterial Vaginosis

Fetal Fibronectin and Cervical Ultrasound at Wk 22, 25, 28, 31

Cx > 2.5cm
or
fFN normal (Negative)

Routine Care

Bleeding More Than
One Trimester

Cx ≤2.5 cm ± Funneling
or
fFN elevated (Positive)

- If contracting >4/hr, use tocolytic therapy PRN
  (nifedipine until steroids administered)
- Bedrest/no coitus/work cessation
- Re-exam for BV
  (treatment of positives)
- Culture vagina and rectum for GBS
  (treatment of positives, repeat at delivery)
- Betamethasone, 12 mg im q 24" x 2 doses
- Serial urine cultures
- 17P?

- If Cx <2.5 cm and fFN Elevated (Positive) =
  6 days median duration to delivery
- If Cx <2.5 cm and fFN Normal (Negative) =
  21 days median duration to delivery

*Source:* Reproduced, courtesy of Cytyc Corporation and affiliates. Adapted from algorithm by Charles J. Lockwood, MD, Chair, Department of Obstetrics and Gynecology, Yale University.

## Triage Protocol for PTL Symptoms

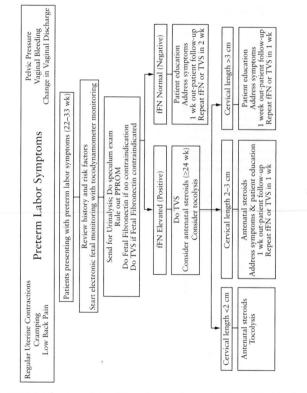

*Source:* Reproduced, courtesy of Cytyc Corporation and affiliates. Algorithm by Herman L. Hedriana, M.D., Sutter Medical Center Sacramento.

# OBSTETRICS

## Maternal Characteristics Associated with Increased Risk

- History of previous preterm birth
- Maternal race (more black than nonblack)
- Poor nutrition/low body mass index
- Low socioeconomic status
- Absent or inadequate prenatal care
- Age <18 or >40 yrs
- Strenuous work
- High personal stress
- Cigarette smoking
- Anemia (hemoglobin <10 g/dL)
- Bacteriuria
- Genital colonization or infection (e.g., bacterial vaginosis, *Neisseria gonorrhea*, *Chlamydia trachomatis*, *Mycoplasma*, and *Ureaplasma*)
- Cervical injury or abnormality (e.g., in utero exposure to diethylstilbesterol, history of cervical conization, second trimester induced abortion)
- Uterine anomaly or fibroids
- Excessive uterine contractility
- Premature cervical dilation (>1 cm) or effacement (~80%)

*Source:* APGO Educational Series on Women's Health Issues: *Prevention and Management of Preterm Birth.* © 1998 Association of Professors of Gynecology and Obstetrics. Washington, DC.

## Antenatal Steroids

## National Institutes of Health Consensus Panel Recommendations for Antenatal Steroid Use

- The benefits of antenatal administration of corticosteroids to fetuses at risk of preterm delivery vastly outweigh the risks. The benefits include not only a reduction in the risk of respiratory distress syndrome but also a substantial decrease in mortality and intraventricular hemorrhage.
- All women who are between 24 and 34 wks of pregnancy and who are at risk for preterm delivery are candidates for antenatal corticosteroid therapy.
- Fetal race, gender, and availability of surfactant therapy should not influence the decision to use antenatal corticosteroid therapy.
- A patient eligible for therapy with tocolytic agents also should be eligible for treatment with antenatal corticosteroids when she requires repetitive intravenous tocolytics.
- Treatment should consist of either two doses of 12 mg betamethasone, intramuscularly, given 24 hrs apart, or four doses of 6 mg dexamethasone, intramuscularly, given 12 hrs apart. Optimal benefits begin 24 hrs after initiation of therapy and last 7 days.
- Because treatment for less than 24 hrs still can result in significant reductions in neonatal mortality, antenatal corticosteroids should be given unless immediate delivery is anticipated.
- Antenatal corticosteroid use is recommended in women with preterm premature rupture of membranes at less than 30–32 wks of gestation in the absence of clinical chorioamnionitis because of the high risk of intraventricular hemorrhage at those early gestational ages.
- In women with complicated pregnancies for whom delivery before 34 wks of gestation is likely, antenatal corticosteroid use is recommended unless there is evidence that corticosteroids will have an adverse effect on the mother or delivery is imminent.

*Source:* Adapted from Effect of antenatal steroids for fetal maturation on perinatal outcomes. NIH Consens Statement 1994 Feb 28–Mar 2;12(2):1–24.

## Dose

β-Methasone
- 12 mg IM given in 2 doses 24 hours apart

Dexamethasone
- 6 mg IM given in 4 doses, one every 12 hours

Use of repeated courses of steroids is controversial as it may lead to decreased birth weight and head circumference and generally should be limited to women enrolled in study protocols.

*Source:* ACOG Committee Opinion No. 273, May 2002.

# OBSTETRICS

## Tocolytics for Preterm Labor

| Tocolytic Agent | Dosage and Administration | Contraindications |
|---|---|---|
| Beta-mimetic | Terbutaline, 0.25 mg subcutaneously every 20 min to 3 hrs (hold or pulse >120 beats per min) | Cardiac arrhythmias |
| | Ritodrine initial dose of 50–100 mcg/min, increase 50 mcg/min every 10 mins until contractions cease or side effects develop | Poorly controlled thyroid disease |
| | Maximum dose = 350 mcg/min | Poorly controlled diabetes mellitus |
| Magnesium sulfate | 4–6 g bolus for 20 mins, then 2–3 g/hr | Myasthenia gravis |
| Calcium channel blockers | 30 mg loading dose, then 10–20 mg every 4–6 hrs | Cardiac disease, use caution with renal disease, maternal hypotension (<90/50 mm Hg), avoid concomitant use with magnesium sulfate |
| Prostaglandin synthetase inhibitors | Indomethacin loading dose of 50 mg rectally or 50–100 mg orally, then 25–50 mg orally every 6 hrs × 48 hrs | Significant renal or hepatic impairment |
| | Ketorolac loading dose of 60 mg intramuscularly, then 30 mg intramuscularly every 6 hrs × 48 hrs | Active peptic ulcer disease |
| | Sulindac, 200 mg orally every 12 hrs × 48 hrs | Coagulation disorders or thrombocytopenia, NSAID-sensitive asthma, other sensitivity to NSAIDs |

| Maternal Side Effects | Fetal and Neonatal Side Effects |
|---|---|
| Cardiac or cardiopulmonary arrhythmias, pulmonary edema, myocardial ischemia, hypotension, tachycardia | Fetal tachycardia, hyperinsulinemia, hyperglycemia, myocardial and septal hypertrophy, myocardial ischemia |
| Metabolic hyperglycemia, hyperinsulinemia, hypokalemia, antidiuresis, altered thyroid function | Neonatal tachycardia, hypoglycemia, hypocalcemia, hyperbilirubinemia, hypotension, intraventricular hemorrhage |
| Physiologic tremor, palpitations, nervousness, nausea or vomiting, fever, hallucinations | — |
| Flushing, lethargy, headache, muscle weakness, diplopia, dry mouth, pulmonary edema, cardiac arrest | Lethargy, hypotonia, respiratory depression, demineralization with prolonged use |
| Flushing, headache, dizziness, nausea, transient hypotension | None noted as yet |
| Nausea, heartburn | Constriction of ductus arteriosus, pulmonary hypertension, reversible decrease in renal function with oligohydramnios, intraventricular hemorrhage, hyperbilirubinemia, necrotizing enterocolitis |
| — | — |
| — | — |

NSAIDs, nonsteroidal antiinflammatory drugs.

*Source:* Reproduced with permission from ACOG Practice Bulletin. Clinical management guidelines for obstetrician-gynecologist. Number 43, May 2003. Management of preterm labor. *Obstet Gynecol.* 2003;101(5):1039–1047.

# OBSTETRICS

## Cochrane Reviews of Tocolytic Therapy

| Agent (Cochrane Reference) | Trials and Subjects | Is the Agent an Effective Tocolytic? | Cochrane Review Advice or Conclusion |
|---|---|---|---|
| **Ineffective** | | | |
| Hydration | 2 trials, 228 subjects | Not superior to bed rest alone | No advantage over bed rest unless the woman is dehydrated |
| Magnesium | 23 trials, 2036 subjects | Not superior to control treatments | Magnesium is ineffective at delaying birth or preventing preterm birth, compared with control treatments; its use is associated with increased morbidity for the infant |
| Atosiban | 11 trials, 1695 subjects | Not superior to placebo | Caution against use |
| Antibiotics with intact membranes | 11 trials, 7428 subjects | Reduced maternal infection, but no improvement in newborn outcomes; may increase complexity of neonatal infections | Not recommended for routine practice |
| **May be Ineffective** | | | |
| Nitric oxide donors (nitroglycerine) | 5 trials, 466 subjects | Reduced risk of delivery before 37 wks, but not 32 or 34 wks; headache is a common side effect | Insufficient evidence to support use |
| Cyclooxygenase inhibitors (indomethacin) | 13 trials, 713 subjects | Reduction in delivery before 37 wks compared with controls | Estimates are imprecise and should be interpreted with caution |
| **Effective Compared with Controls** | | | |
| Calcium-channel blockers | 12 trials, 1029 subjects | Reduction in birth within 7 days of treatment and prior to 34 wks gestation; reduced likelihood of termination of therapy because of adverse effects compared with betamimetics | Calcium-channel blockers are preferable to other tocolytic agents; nifedipine[a] not evaluated against placebo; control groups typically received a betamimetic |
| Betamimetics | 17 trials, 1320 subjects | Reduced risk of delivery within 48 hrs; many adverse effects reported | Betamimetics delay delivery, allowing for completion of a course of glucocorticoids; multiple adverse effects occur |

[a]Nifedipine is not approved by the FDA for treating preterm labor.

*Source:* Reproduced with permission from Barbieri RL. Is the end of an era here for magnesium sulfate tocolysis? *OBG Management.* 2007;January:6–10.

## PRETERM PREMATURE RUPTURE OF MEMBRANES (PPROM)

### Fast Facts

- Associated with 25–33% of preterm deliveries.
- 90% of term and 50% of preterm patients will enter labor within 24 hours.
- 85% of preterm patients will be in labor within 1 week.
- Clinically evident intraamniotic infection present in 13–60% of preterm PROM patients.
- Rate of fetal malpresentation increased.
- Abruptio placentae occurs in 4–12%.
- Risk of antenatal fetal demise 1–2%.
- Risk of pulmonary hypoplasia variable.
  - Rarely occurs if PROM after 26 weeks.
- PPROM associated with amniocentesis has better outcome than spontaneous PPROM.

### Risk Factors

- Intraamniotic infection
- Lower socioeconomic classes, teenagers, smokers, single mothers, previous STD in pregnancy
- 2nd and 3rd trimester bleeding, cervical cerclage, prior cervical conization
- Low BMI, nutritional deficiencies (copper, ascorbic acid)
- Connective tissue disorders (Ehlers-Danlos Syndrome)
- Pulmonary disease
- Uterine overdistention
- Prior PROM (16–32% recurrence risk)

### Diagnosis/Evaluation

- History
- Sterile speculum exam (SSE)
  - Pooling
  - Ferning
  - Nitrazine positive (this may be falsely positive with blood, semen, alkaline antiseptic, BV, or anything the elevates the vaginal pH >6)
  - Vaginal/cervical cultures
  - Vaginal pool for L/S, PG
- For definitive diagnosis, one can use the "tampon test" and inject indigo carmine into the amnion via amniocentesis. If a vaginal tampon turns blue, rupture can be confirmed.
- Ultrasound for presentation, careful monitoring for cord prolapse if the infant is non-vertex
- Evaluate for chorioamnionitis

# OBSTETRICS

## Management of PROM

| Gestational Age | Management |
| --- | --- |
| Term (37 wks or more) | Proceed to delivery, usually by induction of labor |
| | Group B streptococcal prophylaxis recommended |
| Near term (34 wks to 36 completed wks) | Same as for term |
| Preterm (32 wks to 33 completed wks) | Expectant management, unless fetal pulmonary maturity is documented |
| | Group B streptococcal prophylaxis recommended |
| | Corticosteroid—no consensus, but some experts recommend |
| | Antibiotics recommended to prolong latency if there are no contraindications |
| Preterm (24 wks to 31 completed wks) | Expectant management |
| | Group B streptococcal prophylaxis recommended |
| | Single-course corticosteroid use recommended |
| | Tocolytics—no consensus |
| | Antibiotics recommended to prolong latency if there are no contraindications |
| Less than 24 wks[a] | Patient counseling |
| | Expectant management |
| | Group B streptococcal prophylaxis is not recommended |
| | Corticosteroids are not recommended |
| | Antibiotics—there are incomplete data on use in prolonging latency |

[a]The combination of birthweight, gestational age, and sex provide the best estimate of chances of survival and should be considered in individual cases.

- Monitor CBC and vitals for evidence of changing status.
  - Antibiotics can prolong latency.
    Ampicillin, 2 gm IV q6hrs, and erythromycin, 250 mg IV q6hrs × 48 hours *then*
    Amoxicillin, 250 mg PO q8hrs, and erythromycin, 333 mg PO q8hrs × 5 days

## Summary of Recommendations and Conclusions

*The following recommendations and conclusions are based on good and consistent scientific evidence (Level A):*

- For women with PROM at term, labor should be induced at the time of presentation, generally with oxytocin infusion, to reduce the risk chorioamnionitis.
- Patients with PROM before 32 weeks of gestation should be cared for expectantly until 33 completed weeks of gestation if no maternal or fetal contraindications exist.
- A 48-hour course of intravenous ampicillin and erythromycin followed by 5 days of amoxicillin and erythromycin is recommended during expectant management of preterm PROM remote from term to prolong pregnancy and to reduce infectious and gestational age–dependent neonatal morbidity.
- All women with PROM, including those known to be carriers of group B streptococci and those who give birth before carrier status can be delineated, should receive intrapartum chemoprophylaxis to prevent vertical transmission of group B streptococci regardless of earlier treatments.
- A single course of antenatal corticosteroids should be administered to women with PROM before 32 weeks of gestation to reduce the risks of RDS, perinatal mortality, and other morbidities.

*The following recommendations and conclusions are based on limited and inconsistent scientific evidence (Level B):*

- Delivery is recommended when PROM occurs at or beyond 34 weeks of gestation.
- With PROM at 32–33 completed weeks of gestation, labor induction may be considered if fetal pulmonary maturity has been documented.
- Digital cervical examinations should be avoided in patients with PROM unless they are in active labor or imminent delivery is anticipated.

*The following recommendations and conclusions are based primarily on consensus and expert opinion (Level C):*

- A specific recommendation for or against tocolysis administration cannot be made.
- The efficacy of corticosteroid use at 32–33 completed weeks is unclear based on available evidence, but treatment may be beneficial particularly if pulmonary immaturity is documented.
- For a woman with preterm PROM and a viable fetus, the safety of expectant management at home has not been established.

*Source:* ACOG Practice Bulletin, Number 80, April 2007). Premature rupture of membranes. Clinical management guidelines for obstetricians-gynecologist. *Obstet Gynecol.* 2007;109(4):1007–1019.

# OBSTETRICS

## SYSTEMIC LUPUS ERYTHEMATOSUS
### Diagnosis

| | |
|---|---|
| Must have 4 of 11 criteria of American College of Rheumatologists. | |
| Malar rash | Arthritis |
| Discoid lesions | Pleuritis or pericarditis |
| Photosensitivity | Oral ulcers |
| Proteinuria >0.5 g/day or cellular cast | Neurologic disorder - seizure, psychosis |
| Hematologic | Immunologic |
|    Anemia |    (+) LE prep |
|    Leukopenia |    Anti double-stranded DNA |
|    Thrombocytopenia |    Anti-Sm |
|    Anemia |    False positive VDRL |
| |    Positive FANA |

DNA, deoxyribonucleic acid; FANA, fluorescent antinuclear antibody test; LE, lupus erythematosus; VDRL, Venereal Disease Research Laboratory test for syphilis.

### Common Complaints of Lupus Patients
- Arthritis or rheumatism for >3 months
- Fingers that become cold, pale, numb, or uncomfortable in the cold
- Mouth sores for ≥2 weeks
- Prominent facial rash for >1 month
- Photosensitivity
- Pleurisy
- Rapid hair loss
- Seizures or convulsions

### Initial Labs in Pregnancy
- Antinuclear antibody screen and titer
- Anti-double-stranded DNA
- Anti-Ro, La
- Lupus anticoagulant
- Anticardiolipin antibodies (see below)
- C3, C4
- CH50
- Chemistry panel, electrolytes
- Thyroid function tests (as indicated)
- Anti-platelet antibodies
- 24-hour urine for creatinine clearance, total protein

## Common Lab Abnormalities

| | |
|---|---|
| (+) ANA | >90% |
| Anti-DNA (DS) | >80% |
| Anti-DNA (SS) | 50% |
| Anti-SM | 30% |
| Anti-Ro (SSA)[a] | 25% |

[a]Associated with neonatal lupus-rash, thrombocytopenia, and heart block.

## Pregnancy

- Studies are inconsistent, but as a rule of thumb $1/3$ get better, $1/3$ get worse, and $1/3$ remain stable.
- Patients should be counseled to get pregnant when their disease is in remission.
- Monitor for disease flare and hypertensive complications of pregnancy (especially in women with a history of lupus nephritis).
- Patients are best managed in collaboration with a rheumatology.

## Revised Classification Criteria for the Antiphospholipid Syndrome

Antiphospholipid antibody syndrome is present if at least one of the clinical criteria and one of the laboratory criteria that follow are met.[a]

Clinical criteria

1. Vascular thrombosis[b]

One or more clinical episodes[c] of arterial, venous, or small vessel thrombosis,[d] in any tissue or organ. Thrombosis must be confirmed by objective validated criteria (i.e., unequivocal findings of appropriate imaging studies or histopathology). For histopathologic confirmation, thrombosis should be present without significant evidence of inflammation in the vessel wall.

2. Pregnancy morbidity

   (a) One or more unexplained deaths of a morphologically normal fetus at or beyond the 10th wk of gestation, with normal fetal morphology documented by ultrasound or by direct examination of the fetus, or

   (b) One or more premature births of a morphologically normal neonate before the 34th wk of gestation because of: (i) eclampsia or severe preeclampsia defined according to standard definitions, or (ii) recognized features of placental insufficiency,[e] or

   (c) Three or more unexplained consecutive spontaneous abortions before the 10th wk of gestation, with maternal anatomic or hormonal abnormalities and paternal and maternal chromosomal causes excluded.

In studies of populations of patients who have more than one type of pregnancy morbidity, investigators are strongly encouraged to stratify groups of subjects according to a, b, or c above.

*(continued)*

# OBSTETRICS

## Revised Classification Criteria for the Antiphospholipid Syndrome *(continued)*

Laboratory criteria[f]

1. Lupus anticoagulant present in plasma, on two or more occasions at least 12 wks apart, detected according to the guidelines of the International Society on Thrombosis and Haemostasis (Scientific Subcommittee on LAs/phospholipid-dependent antibodies).

2. Anticardiolipin antibody of IgG and/or IgM isotype in serum or plasma, present in medium or high titer (i.e. >40 IgG antiphospholipid or IgM antiphospholipid, or > the 99th percentile), on two or more occasions, at least 12 wks apart, measured by a standardized enzyme-linked immunosorbent assay.

3. Anti-$\beta_2$ glycoprotein-I antibody of IgG and/or IgM isotype in serum or plasma (in titer > the 99th percentile), present on two or more occasions, at least 12 wks apart, measured by a standardized enzyme-linked immunosorbent assay, according to recommended procedures.

[a]Classification of antiphospholipid antibody syndrome should be avoided if less than 12 wks or more than 5 yrs separate the positive antiphospholipid test and the clinical manifestation.

[b]Coexisting inherited or acquired factors for thrombosis are not reasons for excluding patients from APS trials. However, two subgroups of APS patients should be recognized, according to: (a) the presence, and (b) the absence of additional risk factors for thrombosis. Indicative (but not exhaustive) such cases include: age (>55 in men. and >65 in women), and the presence of any of the established risk factors for cardiovascular disease (hypertension, diabetes mellitus, elevated LDL or low HDL cholesterol, cigarette smoking, family history of premature cardiovascular disease, body mass index ≥30 kg m$^{-2}$, microalbuminuria, estimated glomerular filtration rate <60 mL min$^{-1}$), inherited thrombophilias, oral contraceptives, nephrotic syndrome, malignancy, immobilization, and surgery. Thus, patients who fulfil criteria should be stratified according to contributing causes of thrombosis.

[c]A thrombotic episode in the past could be considered as a clinical criterion, provided that thrombosis is proved by appropriate diagnostic means and that no alternative diagnosis or cause of thrombosis is found.

[d]Superficial venous thrombosis is not included in the clinical criteria.

[e]Generally accepted features of placental insufficiency include: (i) abnormal or non-reassuring fetal surveillance test(s), e.g. a non-reactive non-stress test, suggestive of fetal hypoxemia, (ii) abnormal Doppler flow velocimetry waveform analysis suggestive of fetal hypoxemia, e.g., absent end-diastolic flow in the umbilical artery, (iii) oligohydramnios, e.g., an amniotic fluid index of 5 cm or less, or (iv) a postnatal birth weight less than the 10th percentile for the gestational age.

[f]Investigators are strongly advised to classify APS patients in studies into one of the following categories: I, more than one laboratory criteria present (any combination):IIa. LA present alone; IIb, aCL antibody present alone; IIc, anti-$\beta_2$ glycoprotein-I antibody present alone.

*Source:* Reproduced with permission from Miyakis S, Lockshin MD, Atsumi T et al. International consensus statement on an update of the classification criteria for definite antiphospholipid syndrome (APS). *J Throm Haemost.* 2006;4:295–306.

## Management of Women with Antiphospholipid Antibodies

| Feature | Pregnant[a] | Nonpregnant |
|---|---|---|
| **Antiphospholipid Syndrome (APS)** | | |
| APS without prior fetal death or recurrent pregnancy loss | Heparin in prophylactic doses (15,000–20,000 U of unfractionated heparin or equivalent per day) administered subcutaneously in divided doses and low-dose aspirin daily<br><br>Calcium and vitamin D supplementation | Optimal management uncertain; options include no treatment or daily treatment with low-dose aspirin |
| APS with prior thrombosis or stroke | Heparin to achieve full anticoagulation<br>**or**<br>Heparin in prophylactic doses (15,000–20,000 U of unfractionated heparin or equivalent per day) administered subcutaneously in divided doses *plus* low-dose aspirin daily and calcium and vitamin D supplementation | Warfarin administered daily in doses to maintain international normalized ratio >3.0 |
| APS without prior pregnancy loss or thrombosis | Optimal management uncertain; options include no treatment, daily treatment with low-dose aspirin, daily treatment with prophylactic doses of heparin and low-dose aspirin | Optimal management uncertain; options include no treatment or daily treatment with low-dose aspirin |
| **Antiphospholipid Antibodies without APS** | | |
| Lupus anticoagulant (LA) or medium-to-high positive IgG anticardiolipin antibodies (aCL) | Optimal management uncertain; options include no treatment, daily treatment with low-dose aspirin, daily treatment with prophylactic doses of heparin and low-dose aspirin | Optimal management uncertain; options include no treatment or daily treatment with low-dose aspirin |
| Low levels of IgG aCL, only IgM aCL, only IgA aCL without LA, antiphospholipid antibodies other than LA or aCL | Optimal management uncertain; options include no treatment or daily treatment with low-dose aspirin | Optimal management uncertain; options include no treatment or daily treatment with low-dose aspirin |

The medications shown should not be used in the presence of contraindications.
[a]Close observation of mother and fetus is necessary in all cases.
The patient should be counseled in all cases regarding symptoms of thrombosis and thromboembolism.
*Source:* ACOG Educational Bulletin Number 244. February 1998. Antiphospholipid Syndrome.

# OBSTETRICS

## ABRUPTIO PLACENTAE

### Fast Facts

- Premature separation of the normally-implanted placenta.
- Abruption represents 30% of third trimester bleeding, seen in 1% of all births.
- Occurs most often between 24–26 weeks.

### Evidence and Strength of Association Linking Major Risk Factors with Placental Abruption Based on Published Studies

| Risk Factors | Strength | RR or OR |
| --- | --- | --- |
| Maternal age and parity | + | 1.1–3.7 |
| Cigarette smoking | + + | 1.4–2.5 |
| Cocaine and drug use | + + + | 5.0–10.0 |
| Multiple gestations | + + | 1.5–3.0 |
| Chronic hypertension | + + | 1.8–5.1 |
| Mild and severe preeclampsia | + + | 0.4–4.5 |
| Chronic hypertension with preeclampsia | + + + | 7.8 |
| Premature rupture of membranes | + + | 1.8–5.1 |
| Oligohydramnios | + | 2.5–10.0 |
| Chorioamnionitis | + + | 2.0–2.5 |
| Dietary or nutritional deficiency | +/– | 0.9–2.0 |
| Male fetus | +/– | 0.9–1.3 |

RR, relative risk; OR, odds ratio.
These estimates are the ranges of RR or OR found in independent studies.
*Source:* Reproduced with permission from Yeo, Ananth CV, Vintzileos AM. Placental abruption. In: Sciarra J, editor. *Gynecology and Obstetrics.* Vol 2. Hagerstown (MD). Lippincott Williams & Wilkins.

- Recurrence risk
  - 5–16%
  - Increases to 25% after 2 previous abruptions
- Classic signs and symptoms
  - Painful vaginal bleeding
  - Abdominal pain
  - Uterine hypertonicity and tenderness
  - Fetal distress or fetal death (usually with at least a 50% abruption)

## Management

- Consider expectant management or tocolytic with mild abruption and premature fetus.
- Moderate to severe abruptions indicate need for delivery.
- Amniotomy useful in augmenting labor in anticipation of vaginal delivery.
- Close fetal monitoring.
- Perinatal mortality has been reduced by appropriate intervention with C/S.
- Lab studies: CBC, type and cross, prothrombin time/partial thromboplastin time, and fibrinogen.
- Replace blood products and coagulation factors aggressively.

## Ultrasonographic Criteria for Diagnosis of Placental Abruption

24% sensitive, 96% specific, 88% positive predictive value, 53% negative predictive value

| |
|---|
| 1. Preplacental collection under the chorionic plate (between the placenta and amniotic fluid) |
| 2. Jello-like movement of the chorionic plate with fetal activity |
| 3. Retroplacental collection |
| 4. Marginal hematoma |
| 5. Subchorionic hematoma |
| 6. Increased heterogeneous placental thickness (more than 5 cm in a perpendicular plane) |
| 7. Intra-amniotic hematoma |

*Source:* Reproduced with permission from Yeo, Ananth CV, Vintzileos AM. Placental abruption. In: Sciarra J, editor. *Gynecology and Obstetrics.* Vol 2. Hagerstown (MD): Lippincott Williams & Wilkins.

# OBSTETRICS

## Management of Abruption

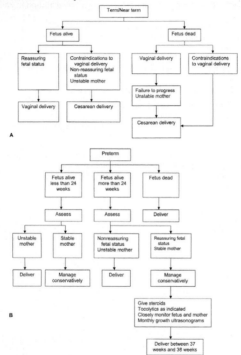

Algorithm for the management of placental abruption in term or near term (**A**) and preterm births (**B**). In all cases, complete blood count and coagulation indices should be checked; blood or blood volume should be replaced; coagulopathy should be corrected; and intake, output, and renal function should be monitored.

*Source:* Reproduced with permission from Oyelese Y, Ananth CV: Placental Abruption. *ObstetGynecol.* 2006;108(4):1005–1016.

## PLACENTA PREVIA
### Fast Facts

- Definitions:
  - Complete—placenta completely covers the internal os
  - Partial—when the os is partially dilated, the placenta only partially covers the os
  - Marginal—the placenta just reaches, but does not cover the os
  - Low-lying—placenta extends into the lower uterine segment, but does not reach the os
- Placenta previa represents 20% of third trimester bleeding
- In the United States, 0.03% maternal mortality
- Incidence 1/250 live births
- Bleeding is maternal
- Often presents as painless, bright-red bleeding
- May be associated with contractions

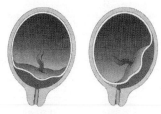

Complete          Partial

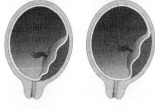

Marginal          Low lying

Types of placenta previa. Illustration: John Yanson.
*Source:* Reproduced with permission from Oyelese Y, Smulian JC: Placenta Privia, Placenta Accreta, and Vasa Previa. *ObstetGynecol.* 2006;107(4):927–941.

- Risk factors
  - Previous C/S (RR 4.5 with one prior c/s, 44.9 with 4 prior C/D)

# OBSTETRICS

- Grand multiparity
- Intrauterine surgery, smoking, multifetal gestation, maternal age

## Management
- Transvaginal ultrasound for accurate diagnosis

## Studies of Second Trimester Transvaginal Sonography in the Prediction of Placenta Previa at Delivery
- Tocolytic of choice is MgSO$_4$.
- No vaginal exams.
- Serial ultrasound for interval growth, resolution of partial previa.
- Delivery by cesarean; if placenta is >2 cm from the os, vaginal delivery is okay, but monitor closely for postpartum hemorrhage.
- Hospitalization usually after first bleed, but depends on clinical situation.
- Consider delivery as soon as lung maturity documented.
- β-Methasone if bleeding and or contractions occur between 24 and 34 weeks.
- High risk for accreta, hemorrhage (especially if previous C/S).
- Discuss blood products, risk of hysterectomy.
- See section on uterine packing (page 78).

| Author | Gestational Age at Sonogram (wk) | Number of Women | Incidence of Placenta Previa at First- or Second-Trimester Sonography [n (%)] | Incidence at Delivery [n (%)] |
|---|---|---|---|---|
| Becker[a] | 20–23 | 8650 | 99 (1.1) | 28 (0.32) |
| Taipale[b] | 18–23 | 3969 | 57 (1.5) | 5 (0.14) |
| HIV[c] | 9–13 | 1252 | 77 (6.2) | 4 (0.31) |
| Mustafa[d] | 20–24 | 203 | 8 (3.9) | 4 (1.9) |
| Lauria[e] | 15–20 | 2910 | 36 (1.2) | 5 (0.17) |
| Rosati[f] | 10–16 | 2158 | 105 (4.9) | 8 (0.37) |

[a]Becker RH, Vonk R, Mende BC, et al. The relevance of placental location at 20–23 gestational weeks for prediction of placenta previa at delivery: evaluation of 8650 cases. *Ultrasound Obstet Gynecol.* 2001 Jun;17(6):496–501.

[b]Taipale P, Hiilesmaa V, Ylostalo P. Transvaginal ultrasonography at 18–23 weeks in predicting placenta previa at delivery. *Ultrasound Obstet Gynecol.* 1998 Dec;12(6):422–425.

[c]Hill LM, DiNofrio DM, Chenevey P. Transvaginal sonographic evaluation of first-trimester placenta previa. *Ultrasound Obstet Gynecol.* 1995 May;5(5):301–303.

[d]Mustafa SA, Brizot ML, Carvalho MH, et al. Transvaginal ultrasonography in predicting placenta previa at delivery: a longitudinal study. *Ultrasound Obstet Gynecol.* 2002 Oct;20(4):356–359.

[e]Lauria MR, Smith RS, Treadwell MC, et al. The use of second-trimester transvaginal sonography to predict placenta previa. *Ultrasound Obstet Gynecol.* 1996 Nov;8(5):337–340.

[f]Rosati P, Guariglia L. Clinical significance of placenta previa detected at early routine transvaginal scan. *J Ultrasound Med.* 2000 Aug;19(8):581–585.

*Source:* Oyelese Y, Sumulian, JC. Placenta Previa, Plancenta Accreta, and VasaPrevia. *Obstetrics and Gynecology.* 2006;107:927–941.

## Evaluation

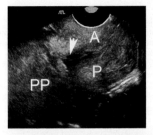

Transvaginal sonogram of a complete placenta previa *(PP)*. Note that both the placenta and the internal cervical os *(arrow)* are clearly depicted. *A,* anterior lip of cervix; *P,* posterior lip of cervix. The placenta just overlaps the internal os. One can see how this could become a partial placenta previa covering just the anterior lip of the cervix if cervical dilation were to occur.

*Source:* Reproduced with permission from Oyelese Y, Smulian JC: Placenta Privia, Placenta Accreta, and Vasa Previa. *ObstetGynecol.* 2006;107(4):927–941.

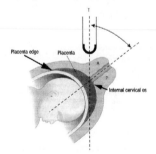

Diagram demonstrating the technique for transvaginal sonography of placenta previa. *T,* transvaginal transducer; *A,* anterior lip of cervix; *P,* posterior lip of cervix. Complete placenta previa is shown completely covering the internal os *(arrow).* The transvaginal transducer lies within the vagina, about 2 cm from the anterior lip of the cervix. The angle between the transducer and the cervical canal is 32 degrees, demonstrating why the probe does not enter the cervix. Illustration: John Yanson.

*Source:* Reproduced with permission from Oyelese Y, Smulian JC: Placenta Privia, Placenta Accreta, and Vasa Previa. *ObstetGynecol.* 2006;107(4):927–941.

# OBSTETRICS

## THROMBOEMBOLIC DISORDERS

### Fast Facts

Venous thromboembolism (VTE) occurs in 0.05–0.3% of pregnancies.

Risk of deep vein thrombosis (DVT) is equal across trimesters and postpartum, but pulmonary embolism (PE) is more common post-partum (*Source:* ACOG Bulletin #19, 2000).

Monthly rates of DVT: 0.001% antepartum, 0.06% postpartum.

- 3–16× more common after C/S.

PE occurs in 15–24% of untreated DVT cases with mortality rate of 15%.

- PE occurs in 4.5% treated cases with mortality rate of 1%.

### Risk Factors for Thromboembolism

| |
| --- |
| Hereditary thrombophilia (prevalence in general population) |
| Factor V Leiden mutation (5–9%)[a] |
| AT-III deficiency (0.02–0.2%) |
| Protein C deficiency (0.2–0.5%) |
| Protein S deficiency (0.08%) |
| Hyperhomocysteinemia (1–11%) |
| Prothrombin gene mutation G20210A (2–4%) |
| Prior history of deep vein thrombosis |
| Mechanical heart valve |
| Atrial fibrillation |
| Trauma/prolonged immobilization/major surgery |
| Other familial hypercoagulable states |
| Antiphospholipid syndrome |

[a]For African-Americans, about 1%; for Caucasians 6–11%.

Data from Lockwood CJ. Heritable coagulopathies in pregnancy. *Obstet Gynecol Surv* 1999;54:754–765.

**Estimated Prevalence (%) of Inherited Risk Factors for VTE and Risk of VTE**

| Genetic Risk Factor | Prevalence in the General Population | Prevalence in Patients with First VTE | Risk of VTE (OR) |
|---|---|---|---|
| Antithrombin deficiency | 0.07% | 1% | 10–20 |
| Protein C deficiency | 0.3% | 3% | 6–8 |
| Protein S deficiency | 0.2% | 3% | 2–6 |
| Factor V Leiden (heterozygous) | 5–8% | 20% | 4–8 |
| Factor V Leiden (homozygous) | 0.06% | 1.5% | 80 |
| Prothrombin gene mutation | 3% | 6% | 2–4 |
| Hyperhomocystinemia | 5% | 10% | 2–3 |
| Antiphospholipid antibodies | 2% | 10–15% | 9 |

VTE, venous thromboembolism; OR, odds ratio.
*Source:* Reproduced with permission from Kujovich JL. Thrombophilia and pregnancy complications. Am J Obstet Gynecol. 2004;191:412–424.

## Pregnancy Associated Changes in Coagulation

- Increases in clotting factors (I, VII, VIII, IX, X)
- Decreases in protein S
- Decreases in fibrinolytic activity
- Increased venous stasis
- Vascular injury associated with delivery
- Increased activation of platelets
- Resistance to activated protein C

*Source:* American College of Obstetricians and Gynecologists: *Thromboembolism in Pregnancy.* ACOG Practice Bulletin #19, August 2000. ACOG, Washington, DC © 2000. Reproduced with the permission of the publisher.

## Diagnosis

- Doppler ultrasound diagnostic study of choice in proximal DVT.
- Ventilation-perfusion scan or CT angiogram needed in cases of suspected pulmonary embolism.

# OBSTETRICS

## Common Hypercoagulable States

| Abnormality | Prevalence in Patients with Thrombosis | Testing Methods | Can Patients Be Tested during Pregnancy? | Is the Test Reliable during Acute Thrombosis? | Is the Test Reliable while on Anticoagulation? |
|---|---|---|---|---|---|
| Factor V Leiden | 40–70%[a] | APC resistance assay | No | Yes | Yes |
| Prothrombin gene mutation G20210A | 8–30%[b] | DNA analysis | Yes | Yes | Yes |
| Antiphospholipid antibody | 10–15%[c] | Functional assay (e.g., dilute Russell viper venom time) | Yes | Yes | Yes |
| | | Anticardiolipin antibodies | Yes | Yes | Yes |
| | | β2 Glycoprotein-1 antibodies | Yes | Yes | Yes |
| Protein C deficiency | — | Protein C activity | Yes | No | No |
| Protein S deficiency | 10–15%[d] | Protein S total and free antigen | Yes | No | No |
| AT-III deficiency | — | AT-III activity | Yes | No | No |
| Hyperhomocysteinemia | 8–25% | Fasting plasma homocystine | Yes | Unclear | Yes |

[a]Bokarewa MI, Bremme K, Blombäck M. Arg506-Gln mutation in factor V and risk of thrombosis during pregnancy, Br J Haematol. 1996;92:473–478; Hellgren M, Svensson PJ, Dahlbäck B. Resistance to activated protein C as a basis for venous thromboembolism associated with pregnancy and oral contraceptives. Am J Obstet Gynecol. 1995;173:210–213; Faioni EM, Razzari C, Martinelli I, Panzeri D: Franchi F, Mannucci PM. Resistance to activated protein C in unselected patients with arterial and venous thromboembolism. Am J Hematol. 1997;55:59–64.

[b]Grandone E, Margaglione M, Colaizzo D, D'Andrea G, Cappucci G, Brancaccio V, et al, Genetic susceptibility to pregnancy-related venous thromboembolism: roles of factor V Leiden, prothrombin G20210A, and methylenetetrahydrofolate reductase C677T mutations, Am J Obstet Gynecol. 1998;179:1324–1328; Martinelli I, Taioli E, Bucciarelli P, Akhavan S, Mannucci PM. Interaction between the G20210A mutation of the prothrombin gene and oral contraceptive use in deep vein thrombosis. Arterioscler Thromb Vasc Biol 1999;19:700–703; Salomon O, Steinberg DM, Zivelin A, Gitel S, Dardik R, Rosenberg N, et al. Single and combined prothrombotic factors in patients with idiopathic venous thromboembolism prevalence and risk assessment. Arterioscler Thromb Vasc Biol. 1999;19:511–518.

[c]Ginsberg JS, Wells PS, Brill-Edwards P, Donovan D, Moffatt K, Johnston M, et al. Antiphospholipid antibodies and venous thromboembolism, Blood. 1995;86:3685–3691.

[d]Auch M, Borgel D, Gaussem P, Emmerich J, Alhenc-Gelas M, Gandrille S, Protein C and protein S deficiencies. Semin Hematol 1997;34:205–216; De Stefano V Leone G, Mastrangelo S, Tripodi A, Rodeghiero F, Castaman G, et al. Clinical manifestations and management of inherited thrombophilia: retrospective analysis and follow-up after diagnosis of 238 patients with congenital deficiency of antithrombin III, protein C, or protein S deficiency. A cooperative, retrospective study, Gesellschaft fur Thrombose- und Hamostaseforschung (GTH) Study Group on Natural Inhibitors, Arterioscler Thromb Vasc Biol. 1996;16:742–748.

Source: American College of Obstetricians and Gynecologists. PROLOG: Obstetrics. 5th ed. Washington, DC: ACOG; 2003.

## Heparin Therapy

### Unfractionated Heparin

| Low-Dose Prophylaxis | Adjusted-Dose Prophylaxis |
| --- | --- |
| 5000–7500 U every 12 hrs during the first trimester | 10,000 U twice to three times daily to achieve APTT of 1.5–2.5 |
| 7500–10,000 U every 12 hrs during the second trimester | |
| 10,000 U every 12 hrs during the third trimester unless the APTT is elevated. The APTT may be checked near term and the heparin dose reduced if prolonged. | |
| OR | |
| 5000–10,000 U every 12 hrs during the entire pregnancy | |

### Low-Molecular-Weight Heparin

| Low-Dose Prophylaxis | Adjusted-Dose Prophylaxis |
| --- | --- |
| Dalteparin 5000 U once or twice daily | Dalteparin 5000–10,000 U every 12 hrs |
| Enoxapin 40 mg once or twice daily | Enoxapin 30–80 mg every 12 hrs |

*Source:* American College of Obstetricians and Gynecologists: *Thromboembolism in Pregnancy.* ACOG Practice Bulletin #19, August 2000. ACOG, Washington, DC © 2000. Reproduced with the permission of the publisher.

# OBSTETRICS

## ACCP and ACOG Guidelines Overview

| ACCP (2004) | ACOG (2000) |
|---|---|

### VTE Prophylaxis

**Women receiving long-term VKA therapy who are considering pregnancy:** For women on long-term VKA therapy who are attempting pregnancy, it is suggested to perform frequent pregnancy tests and substitute UFH or LMWH for warfarin when pregnancy is achieved (Grade 2C).

**Women with prior VTE:**

(1) In patients with a history of a single episode of VTE associated with a transient risk factor that is no longer present, clinical surveillance and postpartum anticoagulants are recommended (Grade 1C). If the previous event was pregnancy or estrogen related or there are additional risk factors (such as obesity), antenatal anticoagulant prophylaxis is suggested.

(2) In patients with a history of a single idiopathic episode of VTE who are not receiving long-term anticoagulants, prophylactic LMWH, mini-dose UFH, moderate-dose UFH, or clinical surveillance plus postpartum anticoagulants is suggested (Grade 2C).

(3) In patients with a history of a single episode of VTE and thrombophilia (confirmed laboratory abnormality) or strong family history of thrombosis and not receiving long-term anticoagulants, prophylactic or intermediate-dose LMWH, or mini-dose or moderate-dose UFH, plus postpartum anticoagulants is suggested (Grade 2C).

(4) In antithrombin-deficient women, compound heterozygous for prothrombin G20210A and factor V Leiden, and homozygotes for these conditions with a history of VTE, intermediate-dose LMWH prophylaxis or moderate-dose UFH is suggested (Grade 2C).

(5) In patients with multiple (≥2) episodes of VTE and/or women receiving long-term anticoagulants (e.g., single episode of VTE—either idiopathic or associated with thrombophilia), adjusted-dose UFH or adjusted-dose LMWH followed by resumption of long-term anticoagulants postpartum is suggested (Grade 2C).

(6) In all women with previous DVT, antenatally and postpartum, use of graduated elastic compression stockings is suggested (Grade 2C).

(1) History of isolated VTE associated with a transient thrombogenic event (no underlying thrombophilia); heparin or no prophylaxis antepartum. Warfarin for 6 wks postpartum.

(2) History of any of the following: idiopathic thrombosis; thrombosis related to pregnancy or oral contraceptive use; thrombosis accompanied by thrombophilia (other than homozygous for factor V Leiden mutation, heterozygous for both factor V Leiden and prothrombin G20210A mutation, or antithrombin III deficiency); low-dose heparin antepartum and postpartum.

(3) Thrombophilia and strong family history of thrombosis, but no personal history of thrombosis; candidate for antepartum and postpartum prophylaxis. At minimum, postpartum prophylaxis should be offered.

(4) Any of the following: artificial heart valve; history of life-threatening thrombosis; recent thrombosis; recurrent thrombosis; receiving chronic anticoagulation; history of rheumatic heart disease with current atrial fibrillation; antithrombin III deficiency; antiphospholipid syndrome; thrombosis accompanied by any of the following: homozygous for factor V Leiden mutation or G20210A mutation or heterozygous for both factor V Leiden mutation and G20210A mutations; adjusted-dose heparin every 8 hrs; LMWH BID is an alternative.

(5) Antiphospholipid syndrome and a history of thrombosis: adjusted-dose prophylactic anticoagulation.

(6) Withhold heparin injections at onset of labor. High-risk patients can resume injections 4–8 hrs after an uncomplicated delivery and warfarin can be given the following morning.

| ACCP (2004) | ACOG (2000) |
|---|---|
| **Women with thrombophilia:** | |
| (1) In antithrombin-deficient women, compound heterozygotes for prothrombin G20210A and factor V Leiden, and homozygotes for these conditions with no prior VTE, active prophylaxis is suggested (Grade 2C). | LEVEL C *(Based primarily on consensus and expert opinion)* |
| (2) In all other patients with prior VTE and thrombophilia (confirmed laboratory abnormality), surveillance or prophylactic LMWH or mini-dose UFH, plus postpartum anticoagulants, is suggested (Grade 2C). | |

### VTE Treatment

| | |
|---|---|
| (1) In women with acute VTE, either adjusted-dose LMWH throughout pregnancy or IV UFH (bolus followed by a continuous infusion to maintain aPTT in therapeutic range) for at least 5 days, followed by adjusted-dose UFH or LMWH for the remainder of the pregnancy, is recommended. Anticoagulants should be administered for at least 6 wks postpartum (Grade 1C+). | (1) During pregnancy: heparin (IV bolus + infusion for 5–7 days) followed by SC adjusted-dose heparin every 8 hrs; continue every 8–12 hrs ≥ 3 months after acute event. Some experts recommend continuing therapeutic dose for remainder of pregnancy; others recommend a lower dose. LMWH may be an alternative; dosing should achieve peak anti-factor Xa level of 0.5–1.2 U/mL. |
| (2) In women receiving adjusted-dose LMWH or UFH therapy, discontinuation of heparin 24 hrs prior to elective induction of labor is recommended (Grade 1C). | (2) During delivery: may switch to IV heparin (short half-life). |
| | (3) Postpartum: switch to warfarin (overlap with heparin for first 5–7 days until international normalized ratio = 2.0–3.0). |

*Source:* Reproduced with permission from Duhl AJ: Update on the use of antithrombotic agents in pregnancy. *Excerpta Medica.* 2006:3–12.

# OBSTETRICS

## HEPARIN-INDUCED THROMBOCYTOPENIA
### Diagnostic algorithm to confirm or rule out heparin-induced thrombocytopenia (HIT)

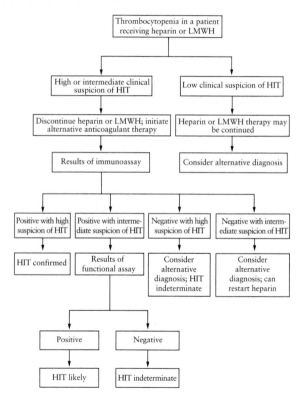

Diagnostic algorithm to confirm or rule out heparin-induced thrombocytopenia (HIT) in patients who have not undergone bypass surgery. Thrombocytopenia can be absolute (platelet count, <150,000 per cubic millimeter) or relative (defined as a decrease in the platelet count of >50 percent from the highest level before the initiation of heparin therapy). The clinical index of suspicion should be based on a temporal association between the start of heparin therapy and the development of thrombocytopenia (typically beginning 5–10 days after the start of heparin) or a new thrombosis; the exclusion of other causes of thrombocytopenia (e.g., drugs other than heparin, disseminated intravascular coagulopathy or other consumptive processes, post-transfusion purpura); rebound in the platelet count on discontinuation of heparin; or some combination of these criteria. On the bases of the criteria, the suspicion could be assessed as high when all three criteria are met, intermediate when one or two are met, and low when none are met. Alternatively, the clinical risk can be assessed according to score based on other criteria. The decision to initiate alternatively, the clinical risk can be assessed according to scores based on other criteria. The decision to initiate alternative anticoagulant therapy should be guided by assessment of the patient's bleeding risk and coexisting conditions. The decision to continue unfractionated heparin or low-molecular-weight heparin (LMWH) should be tailored to the patient. A functioning assay is recommended, where clinically available. Antibodies not specific to PF4–heparin may cause HIT. The decision to continue alternative anticoagulant therapy should be individualized.

# OBSTETRICS

**Incidence of Heparin-Induced Thrombocytopenia, According to Population at Risk, and Recommendations for Monitoring of Platelet Count**

| Therapy | Risk | Clinical Population at Risk |
|---------|------|----------------------------|
| Heparin (new or remote [>100 days] exposure) | High | Patients undergoing orthopedic surgery |
| | Intermediate | Adults undergoing cardiac surgery |
| | | Children undergoing cardiac surgery |
| | Intermediate | General medical patents |
| | | Patients with neurologic conditions |
| | | Patients undergoing percutaneous coronary intervention for acute coronary syndrome |
| | | Patients undergoing acute hemodialysis |
| | Low to rare | General pediatric patients |
| | | Pregnant women |
| | | Patients undergoing chronic hemodialysis |
| Low-molecular-weight heparin (new or remote [>100 days] exposure) | Intermediate | Medical patients |
| | | Patients with neurologic conditions |
| | | Patients undergoing surgical or orthopedic procedures[a] |
| | Rare | Pregnant women |
| | | General pediatric patients |
| Heparin or low-molecular-weight heparin (exposure within 100 days) | Unknown | All clinical populations |

| Incidence of PF4-Heparin Antibodies[a] (%) | Incidence of HIT (%) | Platelet-Count Monitoring |
|---|---|---|
| 14 | 3–5 | At baseline and at least every other day from days 4–14 of heparin therapy or until heparin discontinued[b,c] |
| 25–50 | 1–2 | |
| 8–20 | 0.8–3.0 | |
| 0–2.3 | 0–0.1 | Not essential[b] |
| 2–8 | 0–0.9 | At baseline and every 2–4 days after days 4–14 of low-molecular weight heparin therapy or until therapy discontinued[c] |
| Unknown | 0–0.1 | Routine monitoring not recommended[b] |
| Unknown | Unknown | At baseline, within 24 hrs, and every other day from days 4–14 until heparin is discontinued[b,c] |

[a]Rates of seropositivity were determined by antigen or serologic enzyme-linked immunosorbent assays.
[b]Recommendations for monitoring platelets are those of the American College of Chest Physicians.
[c]Recommendations for monitoring platelets are those of the British Committee for Standards in Haematology.

*Source:* Reproduced with permission from Arepally GM, Ortel TL: Heparin-Induced Thrombocytopenia. *N Engl J Med.* 2006;355:807–817. Copyright © 2006 Massachusetts Medical Society. All rights reserved.

# OBSTETRICS

## THROMBOCYTOPENIA IN PREGNANCY

### Fast Facts
- Defined as platelet count <150,000/ mL.
  - Repeat platelet count and obtain a CBC to exclude pancytopenia and lab artifact.
- Occurs in 8% of pregnancies.
- Obtaining antiplatelet antibodies is not recommended (does not help with the Dx or Rx).
- Epidural anesthesia should not be given if maternal platelets are <50 k.

### Gestational Thrombocytopenia
- Most common cause of thrombocytopenia in pregnancy ($^2/_3$ of cases).
- Manifests itself usually in the third trimester and is usually mild (rarely <70 k).
- Usually not associated with fetal thrombocytopenia, thus there is no risk for fetal hemorrhage.
- Does not require any other testing than routine antepartum platelet count every 1–2 months.
- Can be difficult to distinguish from immune thrombocytopenic purpura since antibodies can also be present.
  - Usually milder, occurs later in gestation, with no maternal history of thrombocytopenia.
- Women are asymptomatic.
- No history of thrombocytopenia except in prior pregnancies.
- Resolves 2–12 weeks postpartum.

### Neonatal Alloimmune Thrombocytopenia
- Occurs in 1:1–2000 pregnancies.
- Caused by maternal antibodies to paternal originating platelet antigens (HPA-1 and -2).
- Similar to Rh disease but can occur during a first pregnancy.
- Maternal platelet count is usually normal.
- 10–20% of neonates will develop intracranial hemorrhage which often occurs *in utero*.
- Treatment is intravenous immunoglobulin (± steroids, fetal transfusion) to increase fetal platelet count.
- Assessment of fetal platelet count prior to treatment is one approach.
  - Fetal blood sampling at 22–24 weeks gestation may optimize medical treatment.
- Most investigators suggest delivery at 37 weeks.
  - Assessing fetal platelet count to determine mode of delivery is one possible approach (<50 k, cesarean recommended).

- Recurrence rate is extremely high; consider testing parents for platelet incompatibility.
- Usually diagnosed postpartum with neonate with symptomatic thrombocytopenia.

## Immune Thrombocytopenia Purpura

- Occurs in 1:1000 to 1:10,000 pregnancies.
- Caused by maternal IgG antiplatelet antibodies destroying maternal and fetal platelets.
- Maternal platelet count usually <100 k; maternal count correlates poorly with fetal count.
- 15% of infants to mothers with immune thrombocytopenia purpura will have counts <50 k, 5% with counts <20 k.
- Rate of intracranial hemorrhage is extremely low (<1%) as compared to neonatal alloimmune Tc.
- Maternal treatment for fetal indications is not recommended.
- Obtain platelet counts frequently.
  - Maternal therapy indicated for platelet count <50 k.
    ⇨ Prednisone 1–2 mg/kg/d, PRN intravenous immunoglobulin and platelet transfusion.
- Obtaining fetal platelet count is probably not warranted.
  - Mode of delivery should be based upon obstetric considerations only.
    ⇨ C/S does not seem to decrease risk of intracranial hemorrhage.
- Diagnosis of exclusion.

## Pregnancy-Induced Hypertension

- Etiology in 20% of cases.
- Cause is unknown but platelet count rarely <20 k.
- Primary treatment in the setting of PIH or HELLP syndrome is delivery.
- Consider increasing the platelet count to >50 k if considering C/S and/or epidural.

# OBSTETRICS

## Characteristics of Maternal Thrombocytopenia

| | Timing of Diagnosis | Clinical Features |
|---|---|---|
| Gestational thrombocytopenia | Third trimester | Typically asymptomatic |
| Preeclampsia | Second to third trimester | Hypertension, renal dysfunction, and proteinuria |
| | | May have hematologic and liver dysfunction |
| | | May have headaches, changes in vision, epigastric discomfort |
| HELLP syndrome | Second to third trimester | Hepatic dysfunction and hemolysis |
| | | May have features of preeclampsia |
| Idiopathic thrombocytopenia | Variable | Often asymptomatic |
| | | Patient commonly has a history of ITP |
| | | May present with abnormal bruising |
| Thrombotic thrombocytopenic purpura (UP) | Second to third trimester | Neurologic dysfunction, fever, hemolytic anemia |
| | | May have hypertension and renal dysfunction |
| Hemolytic uremic syndrome | Second to third trimester | Hypertension, renal dysfunction, hemolytic anemia |
| | | May have neurologic findings, fevers |
| | | Preceded by gastrointestinal infection |
| Human immunodeficiency virus infection (HIV) | Variable | May be asymptomatic, though many patients complain of malaise and low-grade fever |
| | | May be associated with mild anemia and neutropenia |
| Heparin-induced thrombocytopenia | Variable | Typically occurs within 2 wks of heparin use |
| | | Venous and arterial thromboses |

| Severity of Thrombocytopenia | Treatment |
|---|---|
| Mild | Expectant |
| Mild to severe | Terminate pregnancy |
| Mild to severe | Terminate pregnancy |
| Severe | Corticosteroids |
| | Intravenous IgG |
| | Splenectomy |
| Severe | Plasmapheresis |
| Severe | Plasmapheresis |
| Typically mild | Expectant |
| | Anti-retroviral therapy |
| Mild to moderate | Discontinue heparin |
| | Alternative anticoagulation for thrombotic disease |

*Source:* Reproduced with permission from Paidas MJ, Thung SF, Beardsley DS: Unmasking the many faces of maternal and fetal thrombocytopenia. *Cont OB/GYN.* 2006;Sept:42–52. *Cont OB/GYN* is a copyrighted publication of Advanstar Communications Inc. All rights reserved.

# OBSTETRICS

## MANAGEMENT OF ADULT THROMBOCYTOPENIC PURPURA

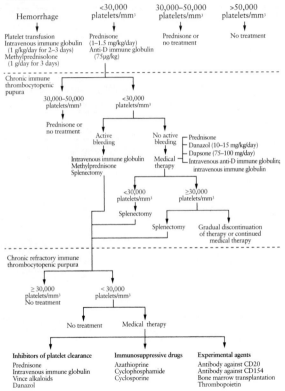

Management of adult-onset thrombocytopenic purpura. Some specialists advocate the use of 20,000 rather than 30,000 platelets per cubic millimeter as the threshold for therapy in patients who present with immune thrombocytopenic purpura. There is no consensus as to the appropriate duration of corticosteroid therapy. The use of anti-D immune globulin as initial therapy depends on the severity of thrombocytopenia and the extent of mucocutaneous bleeding. The decision whether to treat patients who present with a platelet count of 30,000 to 50,000 per cubic millimeter depends on whether there are coexisting risk factors for bleeding and whether there is a high risk of trauma. A platelet count of more than 50,000 per cubic millimeter may be appropriate before surgery or after trauma in some patients. In patients with chronic immune thrombocytopenic purpura and a platelet count of less than 30,000 per cubic millimeter, intravenous immune globulin or methylprednisolone may help to increase the platelet count immediately before splenectomy. The medications listed for the treatment of chronic immune thrombocytopenic purpura in patients with less than 30,000 platelets per cubic millimeter can be used individually, but either danazol or dapsone is often combined with the lowest dose of prednisone required to attain a hemostatic platelet count. Intravenous immune globulin and anti-D immune globulin are generally reserved for severe thrombocytopenia that is unresponsive to oral agents. The decision whether to perform a splenectomy, to continue medical therapy, or to taper doses and eventually discontinue therapy in patients with chronic immune thrombocytopenic purpura and a platelet count of 30,000 per cubic millimeter of higher depends on the intensity of therapy that is required, tolerance of side effects, the risk associated with surgery, and the preference of the patient. The decision whether to treat patients with chronic, refractory immune thrombocytopenic purpura involves weighing the risk of hemorrhage against the side effects of each form of therapy. Drugs are often used in combination. Patients who are receiving protracted courses of corticosteroids should be monitored for osteopenia and cataracts. This algorithm represents a synthesis of the published literature, expert opinion, American Society of Hematology guidelines, and the author's experience.

# OBSTETRICS

## EPILEPSY IN PREGNANCY

### Fast Facts

- Epilepsy prevalence rate 6.8 per 1000 population.
- In the United States, 1.1 million women with epilepsy are in their active reproductive years.
- Epilepsy affects 0.5–1% of pregnant women.
- Most frequently encountered neurologic condition in obstetric practice after migraine.
- 80% of pregnant women with epilepsy use antiepileptic drugs.

### Seizure Classification

Generalized seizures
    Absence
    Tonic
    Clonic
    Tonic-clonic
    Myoclonic
    Atonic
Focal seizures
    Simple partial
    Complex partial
    Secondary generalized

### Antiepileptic Drugs

| Traditional | Newer |
| --- | --- |
| Ethosuximide | Gabapentin |
| Valproate | Lamotrigine |
| Phenobarbitol | Topiramate |
| Carbamazepine | Tiagabine |
| Mysoline | Levetiracetam |
| Phenytoin | Oxcarbazepine |
| | Zonisamide |

*Source:* LaRoche SM, Helmers SL. The new antiepileptic drugs. *JAMA* 2004;291:605–620.

### Pregnancy and Epilepsy

Older reports indicate 8–75% of women experience increased seizure frequency. More recent reports indicate 15–33% of women experience reduced seizure control.

High seizure frequency antedating pregnancy possibly a predictor of increased seizures in pregnancy.

## Factors Contributing to Increased Seizures in Pregnancy

- High levels of estrogen
- Increased nausea and vomiting
- Changes in plasma volume
- Altered gastric motility
- Altered protein binding
- Increased metabolic capacity of the maternal liver
- Placental/fetal metabolism
- Poor compliance
- Increased life stressors

## Seizures in Pregnancy

- Profound alterations in maternal acid-base equilibrium with grand mal seizure.
- Maternal serum lactate concentration has been reported to rise 10-fold, and pH drop as low as 6.9.
- Changes in maternal acid-base equilibrium can be rapidly mediated through the placenta to the fetus.

## Epilepsy: Maternal-Fetal Complications

- Perinatal deaths not significantly different in epileptic mothers as compared to background.
- 5.3% had congenital malformations compared to 1.5% in controls (*Source: Sabers A et al. Acta Neurol Scand* 1998).
- No difference in pregnancy complications except for higher C/S rate.
- 2.7-fold increased risk of congenital malformations (*Source: Olafsson E et al. Epilepsia* 1998).

## Congenital Malformations

- 6–8% risk of birth defects in infants born to women taking antiepileptic drugs (AEDs)
- 2–3 times the risk of the general population
- Increased risk associated with
  - Polytherapy—malformation incidence 25% with four or more AEDs
  - High peak drug levels
- Not clearly associated with seizure frequency

# OBSTETRICS

## Management of Antiepileptic Drugs in Pregnancy

- Withdrawal of antiepileptic drug therapy
  - No seizure activity during the past 2–5 years
  - A single type of seizure
  - A normal EEG with treatment
  - A normal neurologic exam
  - Completed 6 months prior to planned conception
- Recurrence risk
  - 25% if no risk factors
  - 50% if risk factors
  - 90% of recurrences occur first year

## Monotherapy

- Single most effective drug at minimum effective dose
- Successful control in one third of patients undergoing planned polytherapy withdrawal

## Avoid Arbitrary Increases in Drug Doses for a Decreased Serum Level

- Free fraction if marked decline in total level
- Increase dose if more seizures or marked decline in free fraction
- Avoid high peak levels (3 or 4 divided doses)

## Antiepileptic Drug Monitoring in Pregnancy

- Levels before conception
- Beginning of each trimester
- During last month of pregnancy
- Through eighth postpartum week
- Monitoring schedule may need to be individualized

## Quality Standards Subcommittee of the American Academy of Neurology 1998

### Folate Supplementation

- Deficiency strongly associated with increased risk of neural tube defects.
- Supplementation provides risk reduction ranging from 60–100%.
- Supplementation studies not conducted on women taking AEDs, and efficacy unclear.
- Amount of folic acid supplementation extrapolated from general population.

### Folate Supplementation: Current Recommendations

- U.S. Public Health Service
  - 0.4 mg/day for all women in United States capable of becoming pregnant
- 1996 American College of Obstetricians and Gynecologists
  - 4 mg/day would "seem appropriate" for patients taking AEDs

### Vitamin K Supplementation

- Vitamin K deficiency described in neonates born to women using AEDs
- Neonatal administration of 1 mg vitamin K

### Antenatal Oral Supplementation

- Vitamin K 10 mg/day in last month of pregnancy
- Reduction in protein induced by vitamin K absence—decarboxylated forms of vitamin K dependant coagulation factors
- Reduction in neonatal hemorrhage?

### Intrapartum Administration

- Parenteral vitamin K 10 mg if antenatal oral supplementation not administered

# GUIDELINES FOR DIAGNOSTIC IMAGING IN PREGNANCY

## Fast Facts

- Diagnostic x-ray is a frequent source of patient anxiety.
- No single diagnostic x-ray procedure is enough to threaten the well-being of the embryo or fetus.
- Risk of fetal anomalies, growth restriction, or spontaneous abortion not increased at exposure level of <5 rad.

## Some Measures of Ionizing Radiation

| Measure | Definition | Unit | Unit |
|---|---|---|---|
| Exposure | Number of ions produced by x-rays per kilogram of air | Roentgen (R) | Roentgen (R) |
| Dose | Amount of energy deposited per kilogram of tissue | Rad (rad)[a] | Gray (Gy) 1 Gy =100 rad |
| Relative effective dose | Amount of energy deposited per kilogram of tissue normalized for biological effectiveness | Roentgen equivalents man (rem)[a] | Sievert (Sv) 1 Sv = 100 rem |

[a]For diagnostic x-rays, 1 rad = 1 rem.

## Estimated Fetal Exposure from Some Common Radiologic Procedures

| Procedure | Fetal Exposure |
|---|---|
| Chest x-ray (2 views) | 0.02–0.07 mrad |
| Abdominal film (single view) | 100 mrad |
| Intravenous pyelography | ≥1 rad[a] |
| Hip film (single view) | 200 mrad |
| Mammography | 7–20 mrad |
| Barium enema or small bowel series | 2–4 rad |
| CT[b] scan of head or chest | <1 rad |
| CT scan of abdomen and lumbar spine | 3.5 rad |
| CT pelvimetry | 250 mrad |

[a]Exposure depends on the number of films.
[b]CT, computed tomography.
*Source:* Reproduced with permission from Cunningham FG, Gant NF, Leveno KJ, et al. General considerations and maternal evaluation. In: *Williams' Obstetrics.* 21st ed. New York (NY): McGraw-Hill; 2001. 1143–1158.

# OBSTETRICS

## Guidelines from American College of Obstetricians and Gynecologists

1. X-ray exposure from a single diagnostic procedure does not result in harmful fetal effects.
   - Exposure to <5 rad not associated with adverse outcome
2. Concern about possible fetal effects should not prevent indicated diagnostic testing, but consider use of nonionizing radiation when possible.
3. MRI and ultrasound are not associated with known adverse fetal effects.
4. Consultation with an expert in dosimetry calculation may be helpful in estimating fetal dose when multiple studies are needed.
5. Radiopaque and paramagnetic contrast agents are unlikely to cause harm, but should only be used if the benefit justifies the potential risk to the fetus.
6. Use of radioactive isotopes of iodine is contraindicated.

*Source:* ACOG Committee on Obstetric Practice. Guidelines for diagnostic imaging during pregnancy. ACOG Committee Opinion. Number 299. Obstet Gynecol. 2004 Sep;104 (3):647–651.

## THYROID DISEASE IN PREGNANCY

### Fast Facts

- Thyroid disease is the second most common endocrine disease in reproductive age women.
- The American College of Obstetricians and Gynecologists does not recommend routine screening of asymptomatic pregnant patients.

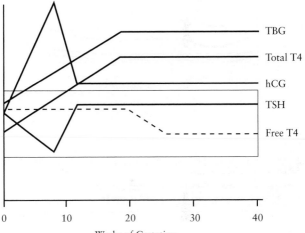

Weeks of Gestation

The pattern of changes in serum concentrations of thyroid function studies and hCG according to gestational age. The shading area represents the normal range of thyroid-binding globulin, total thyroxine, thyroid-stimulating hormone, or free T in the non-pregnant woman. TBG, thyroid-binding globulin; $T_4$, thyroxine; TSH, thyroid-stimulating hormone. Modified from Brent GA. Maternal thyroid function: interpretation of thyroid function tests in pregnancy.

*Source:* Reproduced with permission from American College of Obstetricians and Gynecologists, Thyroid Disease in Pregnancy. Practice Bulletin No. 2. August 2002. ACOG, Washington, D.C., 2002.387–396.

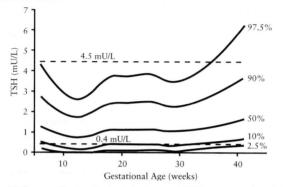

Gestational age-specific thyroid stimulating hormone (TSH) nomogram derived from 13,599 and 132 twin pregnancies as reported by Dashe and colleagues. Modified from Dashe JS, Casey BM, Wells CE, McIntire DD, Byrd EW, Leveno KJ, Cunningham FG. Thyroid-stimulating hormone in singleton and twin pregnancy: importance of gestational age–specific reference ranges.

*Source:* Reproduced with permission from American College of Obstetricians and Gynecologists, Thyroid Disease in Pregnancy. Practice Bulletin No. 2. August 2002. ACOG, Washington, D.C., 2002.387–396.

### Changes in Thyroid Function Test Results in Normal Pregnancy and in Thyroid Disease

| Maternal Status | TSH | FT$_4$ | FTI | TT$_4$ | TT$_3$ | RT$_3$U |
|---|---|---|---|---|---|---|
| Pregnancy | No change | No change | No change | Increase | Increase | Decrease |
| Hyperthyroidism | Decrease | Increase | Increase | Increase | Increase or no change | Increase |
| Hypothyroidism | Increase | Decrease | Decrease | Decrease | Decrease or no change | Decrease |

FT$_4$, free thyroxine; FTI, free thyroxine index; RT$_3$U, resin T3 uptake; TSH, thyroid-stimulating hormone; TT$_3$, total triiodothyronine; TT$_4$, total thyroxine.
*Source:* Reproduced with permission from American College of Obstetricians and Gynecologists, Thyroid Disease in Pregnancy. Practice Bulletin No. 2. August 2002. ACOG, Washington, D.C., 2002.387–396.

## Hyperthyroidism

- Signs and symptoms of hyperthyroidism
    - Nervousness
    - Tremors
    - Tachycardia
    - Excessive sweating
    - Heat intolerance
    - Weight loss
    - Goiter
    - Insomnia
    - Palpitations
    - Hypertension
- Graves' disease causes 95% of hyperthyroidism in pregnancy
    - Autoantibodies, thyroid-stimulating immunoglobulin and thyroid-stimulating hormone-binding inhibitory immunoglobulin, act on the thyroid-stimulating hormone receptor to cause thyroid stimulation or inhibition.
    - Thyroid-stimulating immunoglobulin and thyroid-stimulating hormone-binding inhibitory immunoglobulin can affect the fetal thyroid and cause fetal thyrotoxicosis or transient hypothyroidism in neonates of any woman with Graves' disease.
- Inadequately treated maternal thyrotoxicosis can lead to
    - Preterm delivery
    - Low birth weight
    - Fetal loss
    - Severe preeclampsia
    - Heart failure

## Management

- Measure free thyroxine or free thyroxine index (FTI) every 2–4 weeks.
- Keep free thyroxine or FTI in the high normal range using the lowest does of medication.
- Treat with either propylthiouracil (PTU) or methimazole.
- Both medications decrease thyroid hormone synthesis. PTU also reduces peripheral conversion of thyroxine to triiodothyronine.
- PTU and methimazole both enter breast milk, but are "compatible" with breastfeeding according to the American Academy of Pediatrics.
- β-blockers may be used to ameliorate the symptoms of thyrotoxicosis.

# OBSTETRICS

## Management of Hyperthyroidism in Pregnancy

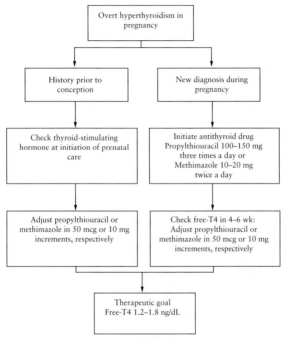

Source: Reproduced with permission from Casey BM, Leveno KJ: Thyroid Disease in Pregnancy. *Obstet Gynecol.* 2006;108(5):1283–1292.

## Treatment of Thyroid Storm in Pregnant Women

## Signs and Symptoms of Thyroid Storm

| |
|---|
| Hypermetabolism |
|     Fever above 4°C |
|     Perspiration |
|     Warm, flushed skin |
| Cardiovascular |
|     Tachycardia |
|     Atrial fibrillation |
|     Congestive heart failure |
| Central nervous system |
|     Irritability |
|     Agitation |
|     Tremor |
|     Mental status change (delirium, psychosis, coma) |
| Gastrointestinal |
|     Nausea, vomiting |
|     Diarrhea |
|     Jaundice |
| Supporting laboratory evidence |
|     Leukocytosis |
|     Elevated liver function values |
|     Hypercalcemia |
|     Low TSH, high $FT_4$ and/or $FT_3$ |

$FT_3$, free triiodothyronine; $FT_4$, free thyroxine; TSH, thyroid-stimulating hormone.
*Source:* Reproduced with permission from American College of Obstetricians and Gynecologists, Thyroid Disease in Pregnancy. Practice Bulletin No. 2. August 2002. ACOG, Washington, D.C., 2002.387–396.

# OBSTETRICS

## Management of Thyroid Storm

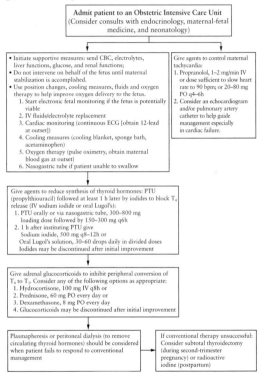

**Admit patient to an Obstetric Intensive Care Unit**
(Consider consults with endocrinology, maternal-fetal medicine, and neonatology)

- Initiate supportive measures: send CBC, electrolytes, liver functions, glucose, and renal functions;
- Do not intervene on behalf of the fetus until maternal stabilization is accomplished.
- Use position changes, cooling measures, fluids and oxygen therapy to help improve oxygen delivery to the fetus.
  1. Start electronic fetal monitoring if the fetus is potentially viable
  2. IV fluids/electrolyte replacement
  3. Cardiac monitoring (continuous ECG [obtain 12-lead at outset])
  4. Cooling measures (cooling blanket, sponge bath, acetaminophen)
  5. Oxygen therapy (pulse oximetry, obtain maternal blood gas at outset)
  6. Nasogastric tube if patient unable to swallow

Give agents to control maternal tachycardia:
1. Propranolol, 1–2 mg/min IV or dose sufficient to slow heart rate to 90 bpm; or 20–80 mg PO q4–6h
2. Consider an echocardiogram and/or pulmonary artery catheter to help guide management especially in cardiac failure.

Give agents to reduce synthesis of thyroid hormones: PTU (propylthiouracil) followed at least 1 h later by iodides to block T$_4$ release (IV sodium iodide or oral Lugol's):
1. PTU orally or via nasogastric tube, 300–800 mg loading dose followed by 150–300 mg q6h
2. 1 h after instituting PTU give
   Sodium iodide, 500 mg q8–12h or
   Oral Lugol's solution, 30–60 drops daily in divided doses
   Iodides may be discontinued after initial improvement

Give adrenal glucocorticoids to inhibit peripheral conversion of T$_4$ to T$_3$. Consider any of the following options as appropriate:
1. Hydrocortisone, 100 mg IV q8h or
2. Prednisone, 60 mg PO every day or
3. Dexamethasone, 8 mg PO every day
4. Glucocorticoids may be discontinued after initial improvement

Plasmapheresis or peritoneal dialysis (to remove circulating thyroid hormones) should be considered when patient fails to respond to conventional management

If conventional therapy unsuccessful: Consider subtotal thyroidectomy (during second-trimester pregnancy) or radioactive iodine (postpartum)

*Source:* Reproduced with permission from Belfort, MA Critical care in OB: part 4 navigating a thyroid storm. *Cont OB/GYN.* 2006;51(10):38-47. *Cont OB/GYN* is a copyrighted publication of Advanstar Communications Inc. All rights reserved.

# HYPOTHYROIDISM

## Signs and symptoms
Fatigue
Constipation
Intolerance to cold
Muscle cramps
Hair loss
Dry skin

## Etiology
Hashimoto's disease (chronic thyroiditis or chronic autoimmune thyroiditis)
Subacute thyroiditis
History of thyroidectomy
History of radioactive iodine treatment
Iodine deficiency
Postpartum thyroiditis (autoimmune inflammation of the thyroid gland causing thyrotoxicosis followed by hypothyroidism within 1 year postpartum)
Subclinical hypothyroidism (elevated TSH with normal FTI, asymptomatic)

## Inadequately treated hypothyroidism can lead to
Increased risk of preeclampsia
Placental abruption
Low birth weight
Congenital cretinism (growth failure, mental retardation, other neuropsychologic defects)

# OBSTETRICS

## Management of Hypothyroidism

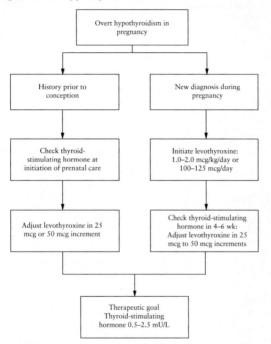

Overt hypothyroidism in pregnancy

History prior to conception → Check thyroid-stimulating hormone at initiation of prenatal care → Adjust levothyroxine in 25 mcg or 50 mcg increment

New diagnosis during pregnancy → Initiate levothyroxine: 1.0–2.0 mcg/kg/day or 100–125 mcg/day → Check thyroid-stimulating hormone in 4–6 wk: Adjust levothyroxine in 25 mcg to 50 mcg increments

Therapeutic goal
Thyroid-stimulating hormone 0.5–2.5 mU/L

*Source:* Reproduced with permission from Casey BM, Leveno KJ: Thyroid Disease in Pregnancy. *Obstet Gynecol.* 2006;108(5):1283–1292.

## METRIC/ENGLISH WEIGHT CONVERSION

| | | | | | | | | Ounces | | | | | | | | |
|---|---|---|---|---|---|---|---|---|---|---|---|---|---|---|---|---|
| **Pounds** | 0 | 1 | 2 | 3 | 4 | 5 | 6 | 7 | 8 | 9 | 10 | 11 | 12 | 13 | 14 | 15 |
| 0 | | 28 | 57 | 85 | 113 | 142 | 170 | 198 | 227 | 255 | 283 | 312 | 341 | 369 | 397 | 425 |
| 1 | 454 | 482 | 510 | 539 | 567 | 595 | 624 | 652 | 680 | 709 | 737 | 765 | 794 | 822 | 850 | 879 |
| 2 | 907 | 936 | 964 | 992 | 1021 | 1049 | 1077 | 1106 | 1134 | 1162 | 1191 | 1219 | 1247 | 1276 | 1304 | 1332 |
| 3 | 1361 | 1389 | 1417 | 1446 | 1474 | 1503 | 1531 | 1559 | 1588 | 1616 | 1644 | 1673 | 1701 | 1729 | 1758 | 1786 |
| 4 | 1814 | 1843 | 1871 | 1899 | 1928 | 1956 | 1984 | 2013 | 2041 | 2070 | 2098 | 2126 | 2155 | 2183 | 2211 | 2240 |
| 5 | 2268 | 2296 | 2325 | 2353 | 2381 | 2410 | 2438 | 2466 | 2495 | 2523 | 2551 | 2580 | 2608 | 2637 | 2665 | 1786 |
| 6 | 2722 | 2750 | 2778 | 2807 | 2835 | 2863 | 2892 | 2920 | 2948 | 2977 | 3005 | 3033 | 3062 | 3090 | 3118 | 3147 |
| 7 | 3175 | 3203 | 3232 | 3250 | 3289 | 3317 | 3345 | 3374 | 3402 | 3430 | 3459 | 3487 | 3515 | 3544 | 3572 | 3600 |
| 8 | 3629 | 3657 | 3685 | 3714 | 3742 | 3770 | 3799 | 3827 | 3856 | 3884 | 3912 | 3941 | 3969 | 3997 | 4026 | 4054 |
| 9 | 4082 | 4111 | 4139 | 4167 | 4196 | 4224 | 4252 | 4281 | 4309 | 4337 | 4366 | 4394 | 4423 | 4451 | 4479 | 4508 |
| 10 | 4536 | 4564 | 4593 | 4621 | 4649 | 4678 | 4706 | 4734 | 4763 | 4791 | 4819 | 4848 | 4876 | 4904 | 4933 | 4961 |
| 11 | 4990 | 5018 | 5046 | 5075 | 5103 | 5131 | 5160 | 5188 | 5216 | 5245 | 5273 | 5301 | 5330 | 5358 | 5386 | 5415 |
| 12 | 5443 | 5471 | 5500 | 5528 | 5557 | 5585 | 5613 | 5542 | 5670 | 5698 | 5727 | 5755 | 5783 | 5812 | 5840 | 5868 |
| 13 | 5897 | 5925 | 5953 | 5982 | 6010 | 6038 | 6067 | 6095 | 6123 | 6152 | 6180 | 6209 | 6237 | 6265 | 6294 | 6322 |
| 14 | 6350 | 6379 | 6407 | 6435 | 6464 | 6492 | 6520 | 6549 | 6577 | 6605 | 6634 | 6662 | 6690 | 6719 | 6747 | 6775 |

All converted English weights are in grams.

# GENETICS

## CARRIER TESTING FOR COMMON GENETIC DISEASES BASED UPON ETHNICITY

| Ethnic Groups | Common Diseases | Carrier Frequency | Testing Methodology |
|---|---|---|---|
| African Americans | Sickle cell anemia | 1 in 10 | CBC and quantitative hemoglobin electrophoresis |
| | Sickle C disease | 1 in 50 | |
| | α-Thalassemia | 1 in 30 | |
| | β-Thalassemia | 1 in 75 | |
| Ashkenazi Jews | Tay-Sachs disease | 1 in 30 | Biochemical testing |
| | Canavan disease | 1 in 40 | Molecular testing |
| | Cystic fibrosis | 1 in 29 | Molecular testing |
| | Gaucher disease | 1 in 15 | Molecular testing |
| | Dysautonomia | 1 in 32 | Molecular testing |
| Asians | α-Thalassemia | 1 in 20 | CBC and quantitative hemoglobin electrophoresis |
| | β-Thalassemia | 1 in 50 | |
| Caribbean | Sickle cell anemia | 1 in 12 to 1 in 30 | CBC and quantitative hemoglobin electrophoresis |
| | α-Thalassemia | 1 in 30 | |
| | β-Thalassemia | 1 in 50 to 1 in 75 | |
| Whites (non-Jewish) | Cystic fibrosis | 1 in 29 | Molecular testing |
| French Canadian | Tay-Sachs disease | 1 in 30 | Molecular testing |
| Hispanics | Sickle cell anemia | 1 in 30 to 1 in 200 | CBC and quantitative hemoglobin electrophoresis |
| | α-Thalassemia | Variable | |
| | β-Thalassemia | 1 in 30 to 1 in 75 | |
| Indian/Pakistani | Sickle cell anemia | 1 in 50 to 1 in 100 | CBC and quantitative hemoglobin electrophoresis |
| | α-Thalassemia | Variable | |
| | β-Thalassemia | 1 in 30 to 1 in 50 | |
| Mediterranean (Italian/Greek) | Sickle cell anemia | 1 in 30 to 1 in 50 | CBC and quantitative hemoglobin electrophoresis |
| | α-Thalassemia | 1 in 30 to 1 in 50 | |
| | β-Thalassemia | 1 in 20 to 1 in 30 | |
| Middle-Eastern (Arabic) | Sickle cell anemia | 1 in 50 to 1 in 100 | CBC and quantitative hemoglobin electrophoresis |
| | α-Thalassemia | Variable | |
| | β-Thalassemia | 1 in 50 | |
| South-East Asians | α-Thalassemia | 1 in 20 | CBC and quantitative hemoglobin electrophoresis |
| | β-Thalassemia | 1 in 30 | |

CBC, complete blood cell count.
*Note:* Numbers may not be exact and are estimates only.
*Source:* Adapted from March of Dimes.

## CYSTIC FIBROSIS

### Fast Facts

- Autosomal-recessive disorder; gene (cystic fibrosis transmembrane regulator) located on chromosome 7q.
- >1200 mutations reported; current recommendation is to screen individuals of European white and Ashkenazi Jewish descent for 25 common mutations.
- Clinical symptoms of cystic fibrosis (CF) include (but are not limited to):
  - Chronic sinopulmonary disease
    ⇨ Chronic cough and sputum production, chronic wheeze and air trapping, obstructive lung disease on lung function tests, persistent colonization with CF pathogens, chronic chest radiograph abnormalities, digital clubbing
  - Gastrointestinal/nutritional abnormalities
    ⇨ Malabsorption/pancreatic insufficiency, distal intestinal obstructive syndrome, rectal prolapse, recurrent pancreatitis, meconium ileus, chronic hepatobiliary disease, failure to thrive, hypoproteinemia, fat-soluble vitamin deficiencies
  - Obstructive azoospermia
  - Salt-loss syndromes
    ⇨ Acute salt depletion, chronic metabolic alkalosis
- Key points while screening for CF:
  - Two carriers have 25% chance of an affected child with each pregnancy.
  - Severity, age of onset, and organs affected not predictable.

| Ethnicity | Detection Rate (%) |
|-----------|--------------------|
| European white | 90 |
| African American | 69 |
| Hispanic | 72 |
| Asian American | Not available |

### Genetic Testing

- Preimplantation and prenatal genetic testing available for pregnancies at risk.
- The 5T allele reduces amount of cystic fibrosis transmembrane regulator protein produced (quantitative alteration).
- Implications of large size of gene and number of mutations:
  - Detection is not 100%.
  - Negative test does not rule out CF/carrier status but reduces likelihood.
  - Possibility of an unidentified mutation exists even after extensive testing.
  - Identification of one mutation does not rule out possibility of second unidentified mutation.

# GENETICS

## CF and Congenital Bilateral Absence of the Vas Deferens

- 19% of men with congenital bilateral absence of the vas deferens have two CF mutations.
- 33% have one identified CF mutation and one 5T allele.
- 20% have one identified CF mutation.
- 1% have two 5T alleles.
- 27% have no identified CF mutation with/without one 5T allele.

*Source:* Chillon et al., 1995.

## Cystic Fibrosis Carrier Rate before and after Screening in Different Racial and Ethnic Groups[a]

| Racial or Ethnic Group | Detection Rate | Estimated Carrier Risk | |
|---|---|---|---|
| | | Before Test | After Negative Test Result |
| Ashkenazi Jewish | 97% | 1/29 | ~ 1 in 930 |
| European Caucasian | 80% | 1/29 | ~ 1 in 140 |
| Hispanic American[b] | 57% | 1/46 | ~ 1 in 105 |
| African American | 69% | 1/65 | ~ 1 in 207 |
| Asian American | c | 1/90 | c |

[a]Presented in descending order of level of risk before testing. Assumes recommended panel of mutations tested and family history is negative for cystic fibrosis.
[b]Represents pooled data. Information for subgroups in this population may differ.
[c]Information not available.
*Source:* Adapted from the American College of Obstetricians and Gynecologists. Preconception and prenatal carrier screening for cystic fibrosis: clinical and laboratory guidelines. Washington, DC: ACOG, 2001.

## Risk of Offspring with Cystic Fibrosis[a]

| Racial or Ethnic Group Partners of Both Partners[b] | No Test | One Partner Negative, One Partner Untested | One Partner Positive, One Partner Negative | One Partner Positive, One Partner Untested | Both Negative |
|---|---|---|---|---|---|
| Ashkenazi Jewish | 1/3300 | 1/107,880 | 1/3720 | 1/116 | 1/3,459,600 |
| European Caucasian | 1/3300 | 1/16,240 | 1/560 | 1/116 | 1/78,400 |
| Hispanic American | 1/8464 | 1/19,320 | 1/420 | 1/184 | 1/44,100 |
| African American | 1/16,900 | 1/53,820 | 1/828 | 1/260 | 1/171,396 |
| Asian American | 1/32,400 | c | c | 1/360 | c |

[a]Estimates based on sensitivity of carrier test and frequency of carriers reported. If both partners are positive, risk is $^1/_4$ (25%) irrespective of ethnic or racial group.
[b]Calculation of risk for couples of different racial or ethnic background can be based on data in the above table, "Cystis Fibrosis Carrier Rate before and after Screening in Different Racial and Ethnic Groups" as follows:
No test: Carrier risk of one partner carrier of other partner × $^1/_4$.
One partner negative, one partner untested: Carrier risk after negative test of one partner × carrier risk of other partner without test × $^1/_4$.
One partner positive, one partner negative: Carrier risk of negative partner after testing × $^1/_4$.
One partner positive, one partner untested: Carrier risk of untested partner × $^1/_4$.
Both partners negative: Carrier risk of one partner after negative test × carrier risk of other partner after negative test × $^1/_4$.
[c]Information not available.
*Source:* Adapted from the American College of Obstetricians and Gynecologists. Preconception and prenatal carrier screening for cystic fibrosis: clinical and laboratory guidelines. Washington, DC: ACOG, 2001.

## Screening Recommendations

- Individuals with a family history of CF
- Reproductive partners of individuals who have CF
- Couples in whom one or both partners are Caucasian and are planning a pregnancy or seeking prenatal care

For couples planning pregnancy or seeking prenatal care, it is recommended that screening should be offered to those at higher risk of having children with CF (Caucasians, including Ashkenazi Jews) and in whom the testing is most sensitive in identifying carriers of a CF mutation. It is further recommended that screening should be made available to couples in other racial and ethnic groups who are at lower risk and in whom the test may be less sensitive. For those couples to whom screening will be offered, it is recommended that this be done when they seek preconception counseling or infertility care, or during the first and early second trimester of pregnancy.

*Source:* From the American College of Obstetricians and Gynecologists. Preconception and prenatal carrier screening for cystic fibrosis: clinical and laboratory guidelines. Washington, DC: ACOG, 2001.

# GENETICS

## ANEUPLOIDY SCREENING

### First Trimester Nuchal Translucency Screening
- Screening tests combine an ultrasound measurement of nuchal translucency, free β-hcG, pregnancy associated plasma protein A, and maternal age.
- Screening is done between 11–13$^{+6}$ weeks gestation.
- This screening method has an 87% detection rate with 5% false positive rate.

*Source:* Nicholaides KH. Nuchal translucency and other first-trimester sonographic markers of chromosomal abnormalities. *Am J Obstet Gynecol.* 2004;191(1):45–67.

### Second Trimester Triple Marker and Quad Screen
- California still uses a combination of alpha-fetoprotein (AFP), human chorionic gonadotropin, and unconjugated estriol to provide a second trimester risk of Down syndrome, trisomy 13, trisomy 18.
- Most states use the quadruple test, which uses AFP, unconjugated estriol, β-human chorionic gonadotropin, and inhibin-A.

| Genetic Disorder | AFP | uE3 | hCG | Inh A | PAPP-A |
|---|---|---|---|---|---|
| Down syndrome | ↓ | ↓ | ↑ | ↑ | ↓ |
| Trisomy 18 | ↓ | ↓↓ | ↓↓ | ↔ | ↓ |
| Trisomy 13 | ↔ | ↔ | ↔ | ↔ | |
| Turner syndrome with hydrops | ↓ | ↓ | ↑ | ↑ | |
| Turner syndrome without hydrops | ↓ | ↓ | ↓ | ↓ | |
| Triploidy (paternal) | ↔ | ↓ | ↑ | ? | |
| Triploidy (maternal) | ↔ | ↓ | ↓ | ? | |
| Smith-Lemli-Opitz syndrome | ↓ | ↓↓ | ↓ | ? | |

Second trimester markers: AFP, alpha-fetoprotein; uE3, unconjugated estriol; hCG, human chorionic gonadotropin; inh A, inhibin A. First trimester marker: PAPP-A, pregnancy-associated plasma protein A.

### Screening Recommendations
#### Summary of Recommendations and Conclusions
*The following recommendations are based on good and consistent scientific evidence (Level A):*

First-trimester screening using both nuchal translucency measurement and bio-chemical markers is an effective screening test for Down syndrome in the general population. At the same false-positive rates, this screening strategy results in a higher Down syndrome detection rate than does the second-trimester maternal serum triple screen and is comparable to the quadruple screen. Measurement of nuchal translucency alone is less effective for first-trimester screening than is the combined test (nuchal translucency measurement and biochemical markers).

Women found to have increased risk of aneuploidy with first-trimester screening should be offered genetic counseling and the option of chorionic villus sampling or second-trimester amniocentesis.

Specific training, standardization, use of appropriate ultrasound equipment, and ongoing quality assessment are important to achieve optimal nuchal translucency measurement for Down syndrome risk assessment, and this procedure should be limited to centers and individuals meeting these criteria. Neural tube defect screening should be offered in the second trimester to women who elect only first-trimester screening for aneuploidy.

**The following recommendations are based on limited or inconsistent scientific evidence (Level B):**

Screening and invasive diagnostic testing for aneuploidy should be available to all women who present for prenatal care before 20 weeks of gestation regardless of maternal age. Women should be counseled regarding the differences between screening and invasive diagnostic testing.

Integrated first- and second-trimester screening is more sensitive with lower false-positive rates than first-trimester screening alone.

Serum integrated screening is a useful option in pregnancies where nuchal translucency measurement is not available or cannot be obtained.

An abnormal finding on second-trimester ultrasound examination identifying a major congenital anomaly significantly increases the risk of aneuploidy and warrants further counseling and the offer of a diagnostic procedure.

Patients who have a fetal nuchal translucency measurement of 3.5 mm or higher in the first trimester, despite a negative aneuploidy screen, or normal fetal chromosomes, should be offered a targeted ultrasound examination, fetal echocardiogram, or both.

Down syndrome risk assessment in multiple gestation using first- or second-trimester serum analytes is less accurate than in singleton pregnancies.

First-trimester nuchal translucency screening for Down syndrome is feasible in twin or triplet gestation but has lower sensitivity than first-trimester screening in singleton pregnancies.

**The following recommendations are based primarily on consensus and expert opinion (Level C):**

After first-trimester screening, a subsequent second-trimester Down syndrome screening is not indicated unless it is being performed as a component of the integrated test, stepwise sequential, or contingent sequential test.

Subtle second-trimester ultrasonographic markers should be interpreted in the context of a patient's age, history, and serum screening results.

*Source:* ACOG Practice Bulletin Number 77. Screening for fetal chromosomal abnormalities. *Obstet Gynecol.* 2007;109(1):217–227.

# GENETICS

## Down Syndrome Risk Assessment Approaches

---

**First trimester**
Nuchal translucency, PAPP-A, hCG

**Second trimester**
Triple screen: MSAFP, hCG, uE$_3$
Quadruple screen: MSAFP, hCG, uE$_3$, inhibin-A
Genetic sonogram: ultrasound markers
Extended sonogram: serum + ultrasound markers

**Integrative (nondisclosure of first-trimester results)**
Integrated (NT, PAPP-A, quad screen)
Serum integrated (PAPP-A, quad screen)
Sequential (disclosure of first-trimester results)

**Independent: independent interpretation of first- and second-trimester tests**
Step-wise:
First-trimester test:
Positive: diagnostic test offered
Negative: second-trimester test offered; final risk estimate incorporates first- and second-trimester results
Contingent:
First-trimester test:
Positive: diagnostic test offered
Negative: no further testing
Intermediate: second-trimester test offered; final risk estimate incorporates first- and second-trimester results

---

hCG, human chorionic gonadotrophin; MSAFP, maternal serum alpha-fetoprotein; NT, nuchal translucency; PAPP-A, pregnancy-associated plasma protein A; uE$_3$, unconjugated estriol.
*Source:* Reprinted with permission from Reddy UM, Mennuti MT, eds. Introduction. Prenatal screening: incorporating the first trimester studies. *Semin Perinatol.* 2005; 29:189.

## Summary of Results from the SURUSS + FASTER Trials

| Test | Detection Rate (%) at 1% False-Positive Rate | | Detection Rate (%) at 5% False-Positive Rate | | False-Positive Rate[a] (%) to Achieve: | |
| | SURUSS | FASTER | SURUSS | FASTER | 85% Detection | 95% Detection |
|---|---|---|---|---|---|---|
| 2nd-Trimester triple marker | 56 | 45 | 77 | 70 | 14 | 32 |
| 2nd-Trimester quad marker | 64 | 60 | 83 | 80 | 7.3 | 22 |
| 1st-Trimester combined | 72 | 73 | 86 | 87 | 3.8 | 18 |
| Serum integrated test | 73 | 73 | 87 | 88 | 3.6 | 15 |
| Full integrated test | 86 | 88 | 94 | 96 | 0.6 | 4 |

FASTER, first- and second-trimester evaluation of risk; SURUSS, serum, urine, and ultrasound screening study.
[a]Based on FASTER trial only.
Reproduced with permission from Canick, JA. New choices in prenatal screening for Down syndrome. *OBG Management.* 2005;17:38. Copyright © 2005 Dowden Health Media.

## Combined First-Trimester Screening: Prospective Study Outcomes

| Study[a] | First-Trimester Detection Rate at 5% of False-Positive Rate | | |
| | Patients (n) | Down Syndrome Cases (n) | Detection Rate (%)[b] |
|---|---|---|---|
| BUN | 8216 | 61 | 79 |
| FASTER | 33,557 | 84 | 83 |
| SURUSS | 47,053 | 101 | 83 |
| OSCAR | 15,030 | 82 | 90 |
| Total | 103,856 | 328 | 84 |

BUN, biochemistry and fetal nuchal translucency screening; FASTER, first- and second-trimester evaluation of risk; OSCAR, one-stop clinic for assessment of risk; SURUSS, serum, urine, and ultrasound screening study.
[a]These numbers, presented at the time of the workshop, may differ from those presented in later publication.
[b]95% confidence interval 79.7–87.0%.
*Source:* Reprinted with permission from Wapner RJ. First trimester screening: the BUN Study. *Semin Perinatol.* 2005;29:237.

# GENETICS

## Prenatal Screening Alternatives for Down Syndrome

| Tests | Gestational Age (wks) | Description of Screening | Average DR/FP Rates of 5% Unless Otherwise Specified |
|---|---|---|---|
| Blood tests | | | |
| Triple test | 15–20 | β-hCG, estrogen, and AFP | DR: 65% Driscoll[a] |
| Quad screen | 15–20 | β-hCG, estrogen, AFP, and inhibin | DR: 81% Malone[b] |
| Serum integrated (individual screens combined to calculate one risk assessment: nondisclosure until screening is complete) | 9–14 and 15–20 | PAPP-A in first trimester AND quad screen in second trimester; patient receives result in second trimester | DR: up to 87%; FP: around 3% Knight[c] |
| Sonogram | | | |
| Nuchal translucency | 11–13 | Measures translucent space behind neck of fetus, which may be increased with DS and other chromosomal abnormalities. The finding of a nasal bone further decreases risk of DS. | DR: 76%; decreases to 57% at 14 weeks gestation Cuckle[d] |
| Level II sonogram | 18–20 | Markers include increased nuchal fold, a shortened humerus or femur, echogenic bowel, echocardiac foci, and renal pyelectases. Generally, these markers raise suspicion for DS when associated with structural abnormalities or when found in combination. | DR: Except for increased nuchal fold, individual markers alone do not usually offer a good indication for invasive testing; FP: high for each marker Ville[e] |
| First trimester | 11–14 | NT + serum markers PAPP-A and free β-hCG | DR: 85–90% Cuckle[d] |
| Fully integrated (nondisclosure until screening is complete) | 9–14 and 15–20 | NT + PAPP-A in the first trimester plus quad screen: in the second trimester: single risk reported in the second trimester | DR: 90–94% Cuckle[d] |

| | | | |
|---|---|---|---|
| Stepwise sequential | 9–14 and 15–20 | Offer invasive testing for screen positive first-trimester screens; screen negative first-trimester screens offered quad screen in second trimester. Risk assessment based on both first- and second-trimester results. | DR: 87–95% Malone[b] |
| Contingent sequential | 9–14 and 15–20 | Screen-negative first-trimester screens complete screening; offer invasive testing for screen positive; "borderline" first-trimester screens receive quad screen. | DR: 89–91%; FP: 2.1–3.1% Benn[f] |

AFP, alpha-fetoprotein; DR, detection rate; DS, Down syndrome; FP, false positive; hCG, human chorionic gonadotropin; NT, nuchal translucency; PAPP-A, pregnancy-associated plasma protein A.

[a]Driscoll DA, for the Professional Practice and Guidelines Committee. American College of Medical Genetics Policy Statement. Second trimester maternal serum screening for fetal open neural tube defects and aneuploidy. *Genet Med.* 2004;6:540–541.

[b]Malone FD, Canick JA, Ball RH, et al. First-trimester or second-trimester screening, or both, for Down's syndrome. *N Engl J Med.* 2005;353:2001–2011.

[c]Knight GJ, Palomaki GE, Neveux LM, et al. Integrated serum screening for Down Syndrome in primary obstetric practice. *Prenat Diagn.* 2005; 25:1162–1167.

[d]Cuckle HS, Arbuzova S. Multimarker maternal serum screening for chromosomal abnormalities. In: Milunsky A, ed. *Genetic Disorders and the Fetus: Diagnosis, Prevention, and Treatment.* 5th ed. Baltimore, MD: The Johns-Hopkins University Press; 2004. p. 795–835.

[e]Ville YG, Nicolaides KH, Campbell S. Prenatal diagnosis of fetal malformations by ultrasound. In: Milunsky A, ed. *Genetic Disorders and the Fetus: Diagnosis, Prevention, and Treatment.* 5th ed. Baltimore, MD: The Johns-Hopkins University Press; 2004. p. 836–900.

[f]Benn P, Weight D, Cuckle H. Practical strategies in contingent sequential screening for Down syndrome. *Prenat Diag.* 2005;25:645–652.

*Source:* Reprinted with permission from Shur N, Marion R, Gross SJ. A surprising postnatal diagnosis. *Obstet Gynecol.* 2006;108(1):189–195.

# GENETICS

## Chromosomal Abnormalities at Amniocentesis

| Maternal Age | Singleton Gestation | | Twin Gestation | |
|---|---|---|---|---|
| | Trisomy 21 | All Abnormalities | Trisomy 21 | All Abnormalities |
| 25 | 1/885 | 1/1533 | 1/481 | 1/833 |
| 26 | 1/826 | 1/1202 | 1/447 | 1/650 |
| 27 | 1/769 | 1/943 | 1/415 | 1/509 |
| 28 | 1/719 | 1/740 | 1/387 | 1/398 |
| 29 | 1/680 | 1/580 | 1/364 | /310 |
| 30 | 1/641 | 1/455 | 1/342 | 1/243 |
| 31 | 1/610 | 1/357 | 1/324 | 1/190 |
| 32 | 1/481 | 1/280 | 1/256 | 1/149 |
| 33 | 1/389 | 1/219 | 1/206 | 1/116 |
| 34 | 1/303 | 1/172 | 1/160 | 1/91 |
| 35 | 1/237 | 1/135 | 1/125 | 1/71 |
| 36 | 1/185 | 1/106 | 1/98 | 1/56 |
| 37 | 1/145 | 1/83 | 1/77 | 1/44 |
| 38 | 1/113 | 1/65 | 1/60 | 1/35 |
| 39 | 1/89 | 1/51 | 1/47 | 1/27 |
| 40 | 1/69 | 1/40 | 1/37 | 1/21 |
| 41 | 1/55 | 1/31 | 1/29 | 1/17 |
| 42 | 1/43 | 1/25 | 1/23 | 1/13 |
| 43 | 1/33 | 1/19 | 1/18 | 1/10 |
| 44 | 1/26 | 1/15 | 1/14 | 1/8 |
| 45 | 1/21 | 1/12 | 1/11 | 1/6 |

*Source:* Meyers C, Adam R, Dungan J, Prenger V. Aneuploidy in twin gestations: When is maternal age advanced? *Obstet Gynecol.* 1997;89:248–251. Reproduced with permission from the American College of Obstetricians and Gynecologists.

## Aneuploid Risk of Major Anomalies

| Structural Defect | Population Incidence | Aneuploidy Risk | Most Common Aneuploidy |
|---|---|---|---|
| Cystic hygroma | 1/120 EU – 1/6000 B | 60–70% | 45X (80%), 21, 18, 13, XXY |
| Hydrops | 1/1500–4000 B | 30–80%* | 13, 21, 18, 45X |
| Hydrocephalus | 3–8/10,000 LB | 3–8% | 13, 18, triploidy |
| Hydranencephaly | 2/1000 IA | Minimal | |
| Holoprosencephaly | 1/16,000 LB | 40–60% | 3, 18, 18p– |
| Cardiac defects | 7–9/1000 LB | 5–30% | 21, 18, 13, 22, 8, 9 |
| Complete atrioventricular canal | | 40–70% | 21 |
| Diaphragmatic hernia | 1/3500–4000 LB | 20–25% | 13, 18, 21, 45X |
| Omphalocele | 1/5800 LB | 30–40% | 13, 18 |
| Gastroschisis | 1/10,000–15,000 LB | Minimal | |
| Duodenal atresia | 1/10,000 LB | 20–30% | 21 |
| Bowel obstruction | 1/2500–5000 LB | Minimal | |
| Bladder outlet obstruction | 1–2/1000 LB | 20–25% | 13, 18 |
| Prune belly syndrome | 1/35,000–50,000 LB | Low | 18, 13, 45X |
| Facial cleft | 1/700 LB | 1% | 13, 18, deletions |
| Limb reduction | 4–6/10,000 LB | 8% | 18 |
| Club foot | 1.2/1000 LB | 6% | 18, 13, 4p–, 18q– |
| Single umbilical artery | 1% | Minimal | |

B, birth; EU, early ultrasound: IA, infant autopsy; LB, livebirth.
*30% if diagnosed 24 wks; 80% if diagnosed <17 wks.
*Source:* Data from Shipp TD, Benacerraf BR. The significance of prenatally identified isolated club-foot: is amniocentesis indicated? *Am J Obstet Gynecol.* 1998;178:600-602; and Nyberg DA. Crane JP. Chromosomal abnormalities. In: Nyberg DA, Mahony BS. Pretorius DH. *Diagnostic Ultrasound of Fetal Anomalies: Text and Atlas.* Chicago: Year Book Medical, 1990:676–724.
*Source:* Prenatal diagnosis of fetal chromosomal abnormalities. Obstet Gynecol. 2001 May;97 (5 Pt 1):suppl 1–12. ACOG Practice Bulletin 27.

# GENETICS

## FEATURES OF COMMON SEX CHROMOSOME ABNORMALITIES

| Karyotype; Name | Expected Phenotype |
|---|---|
| 47,XXY; Klinefelter syndrome | 1 in 500 newborn males.<br>Most common cause of hypogonadism and infertility.<br>Normal at birth, normal genitalia.<br>Normal puberty, testicular size reduced, need for testosterone supplementation beginning in adolescence and through adulthood, infertility, risk for gynecomastia.<br>Heterosexual orientation.<br>Tall stature, slim, expressive language deficits.<br>Risk of learning disabilities, especially in reading; 50% may have dyslexia. |
| 47,XY/47,XXY; Klinefelter mosaic | Usually normal in appearance.<br>Fertility possible in many cases.<br>Developmental risks reduced consistent with 47,XXY. |
| 47,XXX; Triple X | "Super female."<br>1 in 1000 newborn females.<br>Normal in appearance, tall stature.<br>Normal puberty although poor ovarian function and early menopause.<br>Risk for learning disabilities and hyperactivity, risk for depression, variable menses.<br>No ↑ incidence of aggression. |
| 45,X; Turner syndrome | At birth, may have congenital lymphedema; risk for cardiac malformations; webbing of neck; kidney malformations.<br>Growth delay, short stature, risk for obesity.<br>Ovarian dysgenesis and absence of sexual development; hormone supplementation usually begun in adolescence.<br>At risk for otitis media cerebrovascular disease, hypertension, diabetes mellitus, thyroid disorders, obesity.<br>Risk for learning disabilities, especially those involving spatial relations and perception; depression and decreased social skills and self-esteem. |
| 45,X/46,XX; Turner mosaic | Often normal in appearance, may have slightly short stature.<br>Fertility possible in many cases; at risk for spontaneous losses and early menopause.<br>Developmental risks reduced compared with 45,X. |
| 46,XX/47,XXX; Triple X mosaic | Usually normal in appearance, and fertility is likely.<br>Developmental risks reduced compared with 47,XXX. |

| Karyotype; Name | Expected Phenotype |
|---|---|
| 45,X/4XY | Mixed gonadal dysgenesis. |
| | Gonads: one streak gonad (as in 45,X) and one poorly developed testis. |
| | Varying degrees of male-type genitalia due to varying testicular hormone production. |
| | Short stature as in 45,X. |
| | Wide spectrum of phenotype: normal male genitalia to mixed gonadal dysgenesis and ambiguous external genitalia to normal female external genitalia. |
| 47,XYY | 1 in 840 newborn males. |
| | Majority phenotypically normal. |
| | Accelerated growth in mid-childhood; km-normal intelligence quotient, possible (hearing disability, speech delay common; poor musculature; behavior problems: hyperactivity and tantrums (aggression *not* a problem). |
| | Heterosexual. |
| | Puberty delayed by 6 mos. |
| Fragile X syndrome | X-linked autosomal-dominant inheritance; most common inherited cause of mental retardation. |
| | Caused by expanded CGG repeat sequence in the FMR1 gene; direct DNA analysis. |
| | Carrier frequency in women, 1 in 2–50. |
| | Almost all males and approximately $1/2$ of females with the full mutation have significant mental retardation (1 in 2000 males; 1 in 4000 females). |
| | Screen those with developmental disability of unknown etiology: Autism. |
| | Family history of unexplained mental retardation or fragile X syndrome. |
| | Premature ovarian failure ($1/4$ are fragile X carriers). |
| Triploidy 6 9,XXY or 69,XYY | Rare and usually observed in aborted embryos/fetuses. |
| | If liveborn, demise is rapid (newborns with ambiguous genitalia). |

*Source:* Adapted from Linden MG, Bender BG, Robinson A. Intrauterine diagnosis of sex chromosome aneuploidy. *Obstet Gynecol.* 1996;87(3):468.

# GENETICS

## α AND β THALASSEMIA

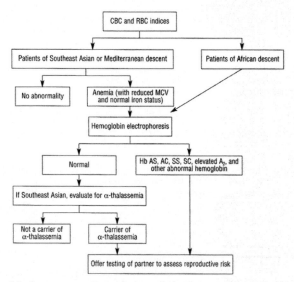

Specialized antepartum evaluation for hematologic assessment of patients in African, Southeast Asian, or Mediterranean descent. Patients of Southeast Asian or Mediterranean descent should undergo electrophoresis if their blood test results reveal anemia. CBC, complete blood count; Hb, hemoglobin; MCV, mean corpuscular volume; RBC, red blood cell.
*Source:* Adapted from ACOG Practice Bulletin Number 78. Hemoglobinopathies in pregnancy. *Obstet Gynecol.* 2007;109(1):229–237.

## Hematologic Features of Main Hemoglobinopathies

| Disorder | Heterozygous State | Homozygous State | DNA Analysis |
|---|---|---|---|
| α⁺ Thalassemia (−α) | 0–2% Hb Bart's at birth | 5–10% Hb Bart's in the neonatal period, low MCV | S. blot: α-gene probe, abnormal band with Bam H1 |
| α⁰ Thalassemia (−) | 5–10% Hb Bart's in the neonatal period, low MCV, normal Hb A₂ | Hb Bart's hydrops fetalis | S. blot or PCR: absence of: α-gene band in homozygote |
| β⁰ Thalassemia | Low MCH & MCV, Hb A₂ 3.5-7.0% | Thalassemia major: Hb F 98%  Hb A₂ 2% | PCR, ASO—dot blot, S. blot  β-Gene probe |
| β⁺ Thalassemia (severe) | Low MCH & MCV, Hb A₂ 3.5-7.0% | Thalassemia major: Hb F 70–95% | PCR, ASO—dot blot, S. blot  β-Gene probe |
| β⁺ Thalassemia (mild) | Low MCH & MCV, Hb A₂ 3.5-7.0% | Thalassemia intermedia: Hb F 20-40% | PCR, ASO—dot blot, S. blot  β-Gene probe |
| Hb S | Hb A, Hb S, Hb A₂ | Hb S, Hb F (1–15%), Hb A₂ | PCR: Dde 1 digestion PCR, ASO—dot blot |
| Hb S/β-Thalassemia | — | If β⁰ thalassemia, severe sickle cell anemia; if β⁺ thalassemia, less severe | PCR,: Dde 1 digestion PCR, ASO—dot blot |
| Hb E/β-Thalassemia | — | Thalassemia major or intermedia: Hb F 60-70% Hb F 10-40% | PCR: Hb E by Mn1 1 digestion |

ASO, allele specific oligonucleotide; Hb, hemoglobin; MCH, mean corpuscular hemoglobin; MCV, mean corpuscular volume; PCR, polymerase chain reaction; S. blot, Southern blot.

*Source:* Modified from Milunsky A, MB.B.Ch., D.Sc., F.R.C.P., F.A.C.M.G., D.C.H., ed. *Genetic disorders and the fetus: diagnosis, prevention, and treatment.* 5th ed. p. 665. Copyright 2004 Aubrey Milunsky. Reprinted with permission of the Johns Hopkins University Press.

## Classification of Alpha-Thalassemias

| Number of Globin Genes | Genotype | Description | Clinical Features |
|---|---|---|---|
| 4 | αα/αα | Normal | Normal |
| 3 | α−/αα | Heterozygous α⁺-thalassemia | Asymptomatic |
| 2 | α−/α− | Homozygous α⁰-thalassemia | Mild anemia |
|  | αα/−− | Heterozygous α⁺-thalassemia |  |
| 1 | α−/−− | α⁺-Thalassemia/α⁰-thalassemia | Hb H disease hemolytic anemia |
| 0 | −−/−− | Homozygous α⁰-thalassemia | Hb Bart's disease hydrops fetalis |

*Source:* Reprinted with permission from ACOG Practice Bulletin Number 78: Hemoglobinopathies in pregnancy. *Obstet Gynecol.* 2007;109(1):229–37.

# GENETICS

## TERATOLOGY
### Agents Not Documented as Teratogens
*Paternal exposure to any agent has not been shown to be teratogenic.

| Drugs and chemicals | Occupational chemical agents |
|---|---|
| Acetaminophen | Oral contraceptives |
| Acyclovir | Pesticides |
| Antiemetics (e.g., phenothiazines, trimethobenzamide) | Trimethoprim-sulfamethoxazole |
| | Vaginal spermicides |
| Antihistamines (e.g., doxylamine) | Zidovudine |
| Aspartame | *Infections* |
| Aspirin | Herpes simplex type 2 virus |
| Caffeine | Parvovirus B19 |
| Hair spray | Electromagnetic fields from video display terminals |
| Marijuana | Heat |
| Metronidazole | |
| Minor tranquilizers (e.g., meprobamate, chlordiazepoxide, fluoxetine) | |

## Sources of Current Teratogen Information

REPRORISK system.

This is a commercially-available CD-ROM that contains electronic versions of REPRO-TEXT, REPROTOX, Shepard's Catalog, and TERIS. The system is available from Micromedex, Inc. (http://www.micromedex.com)

REPROTEXT: Reproductive Hazard Reference by Betty Dabney.

Available on CD-ROM as part of the REPRORISK system.

This database includes reviews of the reproductive, carcinogenic, and genetic effects of acute and chronic exposures to over 600 commonly-encountered industrial chemicals. The reviews include a numerical scale that ranks the general toxicity and a "grade-card" scale that suggests the level of reproductive hazard associated with each chemical.

REPROTOX: Reproductive Hazard Information by Anthony R. Scialli.

Available online, in a disk-based version for MS-DOS personal computers, and CD-ROM format from the Reproductive Toxicology Center, Columbia Hospital for Women Medical Center, Washington, DC. The database is also available on CD-ROM as part of the REPRORISK system. (http://www.reprotox.org)

Shepard's Catalog of Teratogenic Agents by Thomas H. Shepard.

Available online from the Department of Pediatrics, Box 356320, University of Washington, Seattle WA 98195. The database is also available online and in a disk-based version for MS-DOS personal computers in conjunction with the TERIS database and on CD-ROM as part of the REPRORISK system (http://depts.washington.edu/terisweb/teris/index.html). This is a frequently-updated version of Shepard's Catalog.

TERIS: Teratogen Information System by J.M. Friedman and Janine E. Polifka.

Available online and in a disk-based version for MS-DOS personal computers from Janine E. Polifka, TERIS Box 357920, University of Washington, WA 98195-7920 and as part of the REPRORISK system. (http://depts.washington.edu/terisweb/teris/index.html).

## Teratology

| Agent | Effects | Comments |
| --- | --- | --- |
| Alcohol | Growth restriction before and after birth, mental retardation, microcephaly, midfacial hypoplasia producing atypical facial appearance, renal and cardiac defects, various other major and minor malformations. | Nutritional deficiency, smoking, and multiple drug use confound data. Risk due to ingestion of one to two drinks per day is not well defined but may cause a small reduction in average birth weight. Fetuses of women who ingest six drinks per day are at a 40% risk of developing some features of the fetal alcohol syndrome. |
| Androgens and testosterone derivatives (e.g., danazol) | Virilization of female, advanced genital development in males. | Effects are dose-dependent and related to the stage of embryonic development at the time of exposure. Given before 9 weeks of gestation, labioscrotal fusion can be produced; clitoromegaly can occur with exposure at any gestational age. Risk related to incidental brief androgenic exposure is minimal. |
| Angiotensin-converting enzyme (ACE) inhibitors (e.g., enalapril, captopril) | Fetal renal tubular dysplasia, oligohydramnios, neonatal renal failure, lack of cranial ossification, intrauterine growth restriction. | Incidence of fetal morbidity is 30%. The risk increases with second- and third trimester use, leading to in utero-fetal hypotension, decreased renal blood flow, and renal failure. |
| Coumarin derivatives (e.g., warfarin) | Nasal hypoplasia and stippled bone epiphyses are most common; other effects include broad short hands with shortened phalanges, ophthalmologic abnormalities, intrauterine growth restriction, developmental delay, anomalies of neck and central nervous system. | Risk for a seriously affected child is considered to be 15–25% when anticoagulants that inhibit vitamin K are used in the first trimester, especially during 6–9 wks of gestation. Later drug exposure may be associated with spontaneous abortion, stillbirths, central nervous system abnormalities, abruptio placentae, and fetal or neonatal hemorrhage. |
| Carbamazepine | Neural tube defects, minor craniofacial defects, fingernail hypoplasia, microcephaly, developmental delay, intrauterine growth restriction. | Risk of neural tube defects, most lumbosacral, is 1–2% when used alone during first trimester and increased when used with other antiepileptic agents. |

*(continued)*

## Teratology (continued)

| Agent | Effects | Comments |
|-------|---------|----------|
| Folic acid antagonists (methotrexate and aminopterin) | Increased risk for spontaneous abortions, various anomalies. | These drugs are contraindicated for the treatment of psoriasis in pregnancy and must be used with extreme caution in the treatment of malignancy. Cytotoxic drugs are potentially teratogenic. Effects of aminopterin are well documented. Folic acid antagonists used during the first trimester produce a malformation rate of up to 30% in fetuses that survive. |
| Cocaine | Bowel atresias; congenital malformations of the heart, limbs, face, and genitourinary tract; microcephaly, intrauterine growth restriction; cerebral infarctions. | Risk may be affected by other factors and concurrent abuse of multiple substances. Maternal and pregnancy complications include sudden death and placental abruption. |
| Diethylstilbestrol | Clear cell adenocarcinoma of the vagina or cervix, vaginal adenosis, abnormalities of cervix and uterus, abnormalities of the testes, possible infertility in males and females. | Vaginal adenosis is detected in more than 50% of women whose mothers took these drugs before 9 wks of gestation. Risk for vaginal adenocarcinoma is low. Males exposed in utero may have a 25% incidence of epididymal cysts, hypotrophic testes, abnormal spermatozoa, and induration of the testes. |
| Lead | Increased abortion rate, stillbirths. | Fetal central nervous system development maybe adversely affected. Determining preconception lead levels for those at risk may be useful. |
| Lithium | Congenital heart disease, in particular, Ebstein anomaly. | Risk of heart malformations due to first-trimester exposure is low. The effect is not as significant as reported in earlier studies. Exposure in the last month of gestation may produce toxic effects on the thyroid, kidneys, and neuromuscular systems. |
| Organic mercury | Cerebral atrophy, microcephaly, mental retardation, spasticity, seizures, blindness. | Cerebral palsy can occur even when exposure is in the third trimester. Exposed individuals involve consumers of fish and grain contaminated with methyl mercury. |

| Agent | Effects | Comments |
|-------|---------|----------|
| Phenytoin | Intrauterine growth restriction, mental retardation, microcephaly, dysmorphic craniofacial features, cardiac defects, hypoplastic nails, and distal phalanges. | The full syndrome is seen in less than 10% of children exposed in utero, but up to 30% have some manifestations. Mild to moderate mental retardation is found in some children who have severe physical stigmata. The effect may depend on whether the fetus inherits a mutant gene that decreases production of epoxide hydrolase, an enzyme necessary to decrease the teratogen phenytoin epoxide. |
| Streptomycin and kanamycin | Hearing loss, eight-nerve damage. | No ototoxicity has been reported from use of gentamicin or vancomycin. |
| Tetracycline | Hypoplasia of tooth enamel, incorporation of tetracycline into bone and teeth, permanent yellow-brown discoloration of deciduous teeth. | Drug has no known effect unless exposure occurs in second or third trimester. |
| Thalidomide | Bilateral limp deficiencies, anotia and microtia, cardiac and gastrointestinal anomalies. | Of children whose mothers use thalidomide between 35 and 50 days gestation, 20% show the effect. |
| Trimethadione and paramethadione | Cleft lip or cleft palate; cardiac defects; growth deficiency; microcephaly; mental retardation; characteristic facial appearance; ophthalmologic, limb, and genitourinary tract abnormalities. | Risk of defects or spontaneous abortion is 60–80% with first-trimester exposure. A syndrome including V-shaped eyebrows, low-set ears, high arched palate, and irregular dentition has been identified. These drugs are no longer used during pregnancy due to the availability of more effective, less toxic agents. |
| Valproic acid | Neural tube defects, especially spina bifida; minor facial defects. | Exposure must occur prior to normal closure of neural tube during first trimester to produce open defect (incidence of approximately 1%). |
| Vitamin A and its derivatives (e.g., isotretinoin, etretinate and retinoids) | Increased abortion rate, microtia, central nervous system defects, thymic agenesis, cardiovascular effects, craniofacial dysmorphism, microphthalmia, cleft lip and palate, mental retardation. | Isotretinoin exposure before pregnancy is not a risk because the drug is not stored in tissue. Etretinate has a long half-life and effects occur long after drug is discontinued. Topical application does not have a known risk. |

*(continued)*

## Teratology (continued)

| Agent | Effects | Comments |
|-------|---------|----------|
| Cytomegalovirus | Hydrocephaly, microcephaly, chorioretinitis, cerebral calcifications, symmetric intrauterine growth restriction, microphthalmos, brain damage, mental retardation, hearing loss. | Most common congenital infection. Congenital infection rate is 40% after primary infection and 14% after recurrent infection. Of infected infants, physical effects as listed are present in 20% after primary infection and 8% after secondary infection. No effective therapy exists. |
| Rubella | Microcephaly, mental retardation, cataracts, deafness, congenital heart disease; all organs may be affected. | Malformation rate is 50% if the mother is infected during first trimester. Rate of severe permanent organ damage decreases to 6% by midpregnancy. Immunization of children and nonpregnant adults is necessary for prevention. Immunization is not recommended during pregnancy, but the live attenuated vaccine virus has not been shown to cause the malformations of congenital rubella syndrome. |
| Syphilis | If severe infection, fetal demise with hydrops; if mild, detectable abnormalities of skin, teeth, and bones. | Penicillin treatment is effective for *Treponema pallidum* eradication to prevent progression of damage. Severity of fetal damage depends on duration of fetal infection; damage is worse if infection is greater than 20 weeks. Prevalence is increasing need to rule out other sexually transmitted diseases. |
| Toxoplasmosis | Possible effects on all systems but particularly central nervous system; microcephaly, hydrocephaly, central nervous system: microcephaly, hydrocephaly, cerebral calcifications. Chorioretinitis is most common. Severity of manifestations depends on duration of disease. | Low prevalence during pregnancy (0.1–0.5%); initial maternal infection must occur during pregnancy to place fetus at risk. *Toxoplasma gondii* is transmitted to humans by raw meat or exposure to infected cat feces. In the first trimester, the incidence of fetal infection is as low as 9% and increases to approximately 59% in the third trimester. The severity of congenital infection is greater in the first trimester than at the end of gestation. Treat with pyrimethamine, sulfadiazine, or spiramycin. |

| Agent | Effects | Comments |
|-------|---------|----------|
| Varicella | Possible effects on all organs, including skin scarring, chorioretinitis, cataracts, microcephaly, hypoplasia of the hands and feet, and muscle atrophy. | Risk of congenital varicella is low, approximately 2–3% and occurs between 7 and 21 wks of gestation. Varicella-zoster immune globulin is available regionally for newborns exposed in utero during 4–7 days of gestation. No effect from herpes zoster. |
| Radiation | Microcephaly, mental retardation. | Medical diagnostic radiation delivering less than 0.05 Gy to the fetus has no teratogenic risk. Estimated fetal exposure of common radiologic procedures is 0.01 Gy or less (e.g., intravenous pyelography, 0.0041 Gy). Note: 1 Gray (Gy) = 100 rad. |

*Source:* American College of Obstetricians and Gynecologists. *Teratology.* ACOG Educational Bulletin, Number 236, April 1997. Copyright 1997 American College of Obstetricians and Gynecologists.

# GENETICS

## NEURAL TUBE DEFECTS

### Neural Tube Defect Pathophysiology

| Neural Tube Defect | Malformation |
| --- | --- |
| Cranial | |
| Anencephaly | Failure of fusion of cephalic portion of neural folds; absence of all or part of brain, neurocranium, and skin |
| Exencephaly | Failure of scalp and skull formation; exteriorization of abnormally formed brain |
| Encephalocele | Failure of skull formation; extrusion of brain tissue into membranous sac |
| Iniencephaly | Defect of cervical and upper thoracic vertebrae; abnormally formed brain tissue and extreme retroflexion of upper spine |
| Spinal | |
| Spina bifida | Failure of fusion of caudal portion of neural tube, usually of 3–5 contiguous vertebrae; spinal cord or meninges or both exposed to amniotic fluid |
| Meningocele | Failure of fusion of caudal portion of neural tube; meninges exposed |
| Meningomyelocele | Failure of fusion of caudal portion of neural tube; meninges and neural tissue exposed |
| Myeloschisis | Failure of fusion of caudal portion of neural tube; flattened mass of neural tissue exposed |
| Holorachischisis | Failure of fusion of vertebral arches; entire spinal cord exposed |
| Craniorachischisis | Co-existing anencephaly and rachischisis |

*Source:* Reprinted with permission from ACOG practice bulletin. Clinical management guidelines for obstetrician gynecologist. Number 44. *Obstet Gynecol.* 2003;102(1):203–213.

## Summary of Recommendations
*The following recommendations are based on good and consistent scientific evidence (Level A):*
- Periconceptional folic acid supplementation is recommended because it has been shown to reduce the occurrence and recurrence of neural tube defects (NTDs).
- For low-risk women, folic acid supplementation of 400 mcg per day currently is recommended because nutritional sources alone are insufficient. Higher levels of supplementation should not be achieved by taking excess multivitamins because of the risk of vitamin A toxicity.
- For women at high risk of NTDs or who have had a previous pregnancy with an NTD, folic acid supplementation of 4 mg per day is recommended.
- Maternal serum alpha-fetoprotein evaluation is an effective screening test for NTDs and should be offered to all pregnant women.

*The following recommendations are based on limited or inconsistent scientific evidence (Level B):*
- Women with elevated serum AFP levels should have a specialized ultrasound examination to further assess the risk of NTDs.
- The fetus with an NTD should be delivered at a facility that has personnel capable of handling all aspects of neonatal complications.

*The following recommendations are based primarily on consensus and expert opinion (Level C):*
- The ideal dose for folic acid supplementation has not been appropriately evaluated in prospective clinical studies. A 400-mcg supplement currently is recommended for women capable of becoming pregnant.
- The route of delivery for the fetus with an NTD should be individualized because data are lacking that any one route provides a superior outcome.

(*Source:* ACOG Practice Bulletin Number 44.) Neural tube defects. July 2003.

# ULTRASOUND

## FETAL ANATOMIC LANDMARKS

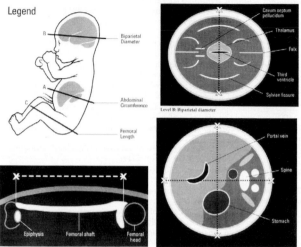

Legend

Level B: Biparietal diameter

Cavum septum pellucidum
Thalamus
Falx
Third ventricle
Sylvian fissure

Biparietal Diameter
Abdominal Circumference
Femoral Length

Level C: Femoral length

Epiphysis
Femoral shaft
Femoral head

Level A: Abdominal circumference

Portal vein
Spine
Stomach

Reproduced with permission from Advanced Technology Laboratories (ATL), Bothell, Washington. *Clinical source:* Jeanne Crowley, RDMS, and Sabrina Craigo, MD, Center for Prenatal Diagnosis, New England Medical Center, Boston, Massachusetts.

## INTRACRANIAL ANATOMY

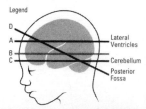

Legend

D
A — Lateral Ventricles
B
C — Cerebellum
— Posterior Fossa

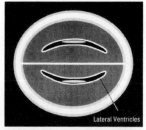

Level A: Lateral Ventricles

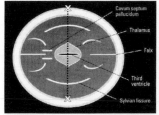

Level B: Biparietal diameter

Cavum septum pellucidum

Thalamus

Falx

Third ventricle

Sylvian fissure

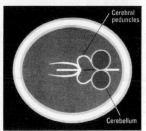

Level C: Cerebellum

Cerebral peduncles

Cerebellum

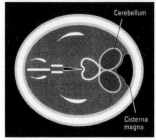

Level D: Posterior Fossa

Cerebellum

Cisterna magna

Reproduced with permission from Advanced Technology Laboratories (ATL), Bothell, Washington. *Clinical source:* Jeanne Crowley, RDMS, and Sabrina Craigo, MD, Center for Prenatal Diagnosis, New England Medical Center, Boston, Massachusetts.

# ULTRASOUND

## ENDOVAGINAL ULTRASONOGRAPHY

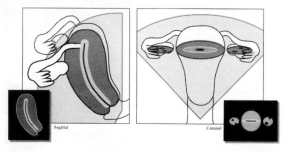

Reproduced with permission from Advanced Technology Laboratories (ATL), Bothell, Washington. *Clinical source:* Kris M. Holoska, RDMS, Antenatal Testing Unit, Pennsylvania Hospital, Philadelphia, Pennsylvania.

## ANATOMY

### Uterus
- Check the cervix with the probe pulled back slightly.
- Scan and measure the size of the uterus in the sagittal and coronal views.
- Check for posterior masses and fluid in the cul-de-sac.

### Ovaries
- Usually adjacent to the femoral vessels.
- Check for free fluid around the tubes and ovaries.
- Scan completely through the ovary in two planes.
- Normal ovarian volume is 6–14 cm$^3$.

### Endometrium
- Begins to thicken during the follicular phase of the cycle.
- Around ovulation can usually identify a "triple line."
- During the secretory phase of the cycle the endometrium is thick (8–12 mm) and echogenic.
- Should not measure >6–8 mm in postmenopausal patients.
- Abnormalities may indicate hyperplasia or neoplasia.

# FETAL ECHOCARDIOGRAPHY

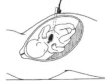

### 1. General

First determine situs:
- Identify fetal position
- Locate fetal stomach and other abdominal organs
- Verify relationship of fetal stomach to fetal heart
- Apex of heart should be to the left

### 2. Four-Chamber

Obtain a four-chamber view. Locate and verify:
- An intact interventricular septum
- Right and left atria approximately the same size
- Right and left ventricles approximately equal sizes
- Free movement of mitral and tricuspid valves
- Foramen ovale flap in left atrium

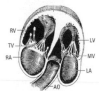

### 3. Long Axis Left Ventricle

Obtain a long axis view of the left ventricle. Locate and verify:
- Intact interventricular septum
- Continuity of the ascending aorta with
  - Mitral valve posterior
  - Interventricular septum anterior

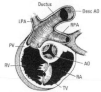

### 4. Short Axis of Great Vessels

Obtain the short axis view of the great vessels. Locate:
- Pulmonary artery which should exit the anterior (right) ventricle and bifurcate

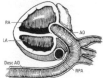

### 5. Aortic Arch

Locate the aortic arch and verify that:
- The aorta exits from the posterior (left) ventricle (not shown)
- Three head and neck vessels should branch from the aorta

### 6. Pulmonary Artery-Ductus Arteriosus

Locate the descending aorta and confirm:
- Continuity of the ductus arteriosus with the descending aorta

*Clinical source:* Joshua A. Copel, MD, Director, Division of Maternal-Fetal Medicine, Department of Obstetrics and Gynecology, Yale University School of Medicine, New Haven, CT. Reproduced courtesy of Advanced Technology Laboratories (ATL), Bothell, Washington.

# CONTRACEPTION

## CONTRACEPTIVE CHOICES

### Summary Table of Contraceptive Efficacy

| Method[a] | % of Women Experiencing an Unintended Pregnancy within the First Yr of Use | | % of Women Continuing Use at 1 Yr |
|---|---|---|---|
| | Typical Use 1[b] | Perfect Use 2[c] | [d] |
| No method[d] | 85 | 85 | |
| Spermicides[e] | 29 | 18 | 42 |
| Withdrawal | 27 | 4 | 43 |
| Periodic abstinence | 25 | | 51 |
| Calendar | | 9 | |
| Ovulation method | | 3 | |
| Sympto-thermal[f] | | 2 | |
| Post-ovulation | | 1 | |
| Cap 7 | | | |
| Parous women | 32 | 26 | 46 |
| Nulliparous women | 16 | 9 | 57 |
| Sponge | | | |
| Parous women | 32 | 20 | 46 |
| Nulliparous women | 16 | 9 | 57 |
| Diaphragm[g] | 16 | 6 | 57 |
| Condom[h] | | | |
| Female (Reality) | 21 | 5 | 49 |
| Male | 15 | 2 | 53 |
| Combined pill and minipill | 8 | 0.3 | 68 |
| Evra Patch | 8 | 0.3 | 68 |
| NuvaRing | 8 | 0.3 | 68 |
| Depo-Provera | 3 | 0.3 | 56 |
| Intrauterine device | | | |
| ParaGard (copper T) | 0.8 | 0.6 | 78 |
| Mirena (LNG-IUS) | 0.1 | 0.1 | 81 |
| Implanon (3 yr) 40 mm by 2 mm (matchstick) | 0.1 | 0.1 | 87 |
| Norplant and Norplant-2 | 0.05 | 0.05 | 84 |
| Female sterilization | 0.5 | 0.5 | 100 |
| Male sterilization | 0.15 | 0.10 | 100 |

**Emergency Contraceptive Pills:** Treatment initiated within 72 hours after unprotected intercourse reduces the risk of pregnancy by at least 75%.[i]

**Lactational Amenorrhea Method:** LAM is a highly effective, *temporary* method of contraception.

*Source:* Trussell J. Contraceptive efficacy: In Hatcner RA, Trussell J, Stewart F, Nelson A, Cates W, Guest F, Kowal D. *Contraceptive Technology: Eighteenth Revised Edition.* New York NY: Ardent Media, 2004. Reproduced with the permission of the publisher.

[a]Among *typical* couples who initiate use α method (not necessarily for the first time), the percentage who experience an accidental pregnancy during the first year if they do not stop use for any other reason. Estimates of the probability of pregnancy during the first year of typical use for spermicides, withdrawal, periodic abstinence, the diaphragm, the male condom, the pill, and Depo-Provera are taken from the 1995 National Survey of Family Growth corrected for underreporting of abortion; see the text for the derivation of estimates for the other methods.

[b]Among couples who initiate use of a method (not necessarily for the first time) and who use it *perfectly* (both consistently and correctly), the percentage who experience an accidental pregnancy during the first year if they do not stop use for any other reason. See the text for the derivation of the estimate for each method.

[c]Among couples attempting to avoid pregnancy, the percentage who continue to use a method for 1 year.

[d]The percentages becoming pregnant in columns 2 and 3 are based on data from populations where contraception is not used and from women who cease using contraception in order to become pregnant. Among such populations, about 89% become pregnant within 1 year. This estimate was lowered slightly (to 85%) to represent the percentage who would become pregnant within 1 year among women now relying on reversible methods of contraception if they abandoned contraception altogether.

[e]Foams, creams, gels, vaginal suppositories, and vaginal film.

[f]Cervical mucus (ovulation) method supplemented by calendar in the pre-ovulatory and basal body temperature in the post-ovulatory phases.

[g]With spermicidal cream or jelly.

[h]Without spermicides.

[i]The treatment schedule is one dose within 120 hrs after unprotected intercourse, and a second dose 12 hrs after the first dose. However, recent research indicates that both doses of Plan B can be taken at the same time. Plan B (1 dose is 1 white pill) is the only dedicated product specifically marketed for emergency contraception. The Food and Drug Administration has in addition declared the following 18 brands of oral contraceptives to be safe and effective for emergency contraception: Ogestrel or Ovral (1 dose is 2 white pills), Alesse, Lessina, or Levlite, (1 dose is 5 pink pills), Levlen or Nondette (1 dose is 4 light-orange pills), Cryselle, Levora, Low-Ogestrel, or Lo/Ovral (1 dose is 4 white pills), Tri-Levlen or Triphasil (1 dose is 4 yellow pills), Portia, Trivora, or Seasonale (1 dose is 4 pink pills), Aviane (one dose is 5 orange pills), and Empresse (one dose is 4 orange pills).

# CONTRACEPTION

## Contraceptive Selection for Women with Risk Factors for Cardiovascular Disease

| Risk Factor | Combination Hormonal Methods (COCs, patch, Vaginal Ring) | Progestin-Only Methods (POPs, DMPA) | Other (Copper IUC, LNG-IUS) |
|---|---|---|---|
| Smoking | Yes, if age <35 | Yes, any age | Yes, any age |
| Hypertension | Yes, if controlled, age <35, nonsmoker | Yes, if controlled | Yes, controlled/ uncontrolled |
| Obesity | Yes; patch may be less effective in obese women | Yes | Yes |
| Diabetes with vascular disease | Contraindicated | Yes (POPs)/No (DMPA) | Yes |
| Diabetes without vascular disease | Yes, if age <35 | Yes | Yes |
| SLE | No | Yes | Yes |
| Dyslipidemias | Contraindicated in severe hypercholesterolemia or hypertriglyceridemia | Yes | Yes |
| Known inherited thrombophilia | No | Yes | Yes |
| Acquired thrombophilia | No | Yes | Yes |
| Age ≥35 | Yes[a] | Yes | Yes |
| Migraine without aura | Yes[a] | Yes | Yes |
| Migraine with aura | Contraindicated | Yes | Yes |
| Strong family history of MI, stroke, VTE | Consider hypercoagulability testing: if positive, no; if negative, yes | Yes | Yes |
| Multiple CVD risk factors | No | Yes | Yes |

Yes, appropriate selection; No, alternative selections preferable.

[a] In the absence of other risk factors for CVD.

COCs, combination oral contraceptives; CVD, cardiovascular disease; DMPA, depot medroxyprogesterone acetate; IUC, intrauterine contraception; IUS, intrauterine system; LNG, levonorgestrel; MI, myocardial infarction; POPs, progestin-only oral contraceptives; SLE, systemic lupus erythematosus; VTE, venous thrombosis and embolism.

*Source:* Reprinted with permission from Burkman RT, Wysocki SJ. Contraception for women with risk factors for venous and arterial thrombosis. *Dialogues in Contraception.* 2005;9(4):4–5.

## Migraine Types

| Migraine with Aura | Migraine |
|---|---|
| Visual disturbance in both eyes (i.e., homonymous hemianopsia) | Nausea ± vomiting |
| | Photophobia |
| Flashing or moving scotoma | Phonophobia |
| Unilateral numbness | Watery eyes |
| "Pins & needles" in extremities | Taste or smell sensations |
| Unilateral weakness | |
| Aphasia or other speech difficulties | |

*Source:* Adapted from Hatcher R, Cwiak C. When a chronically ill patient needs contraceptives. *Cont OB/GYN.* 2003;Oct:70–82.

## Reductions in Cancer Risks with Use of Specific Contraceptive Methods Compared with Nonusers

| | Use Duration | Risk Reduction |
|---|---|---|
| *Endometrial Cancer* | | |
| Combination hormonal methods | 1 yr | 40% |
| | 12 yrs | 72% |
| | 20 yrs after discontinuation | 50% |
| DMPA | Ever-use | 79% |
| | Protection persists ≥8 years after discontinuation | |
| IUDs | Limited data | 40–60% |
| *Ovarian Cancer* | | |
| Combination hormonal methods | 3–6 mos | 40% |
| | >5 yrs | 50% |
| | Protection persists ≥30 yrs after discontinuation | |
| *Colorectal Cancer* | | |
| Combination hormonal methods | Ever-use | 16–18% |
| | 96 mos | 40% |

DMPA, depot medroxyprogesterone acetate; IUD, intrauterine device.
*Source:* Reprinted with permission from Kavnitz AM, Speroff L. Contraception in the perimenopasal woman. *Dialogues in Contraception.* 2005;9(1):1–3.

# CONTRACEPTION

## BARRIER CONTRACEPTIVES

### Diaphragm
- Safe method with rare side effects.
- Urinary tract infection twice as common.
- Reduces rate of sexually transmitted infections (STIs).
- Successful fitting is crucial to efficacy.
- Insert no longer than 6 hours prior to coitus.
- Remove 6–24 hours after coitus.
- Use with spermicide.
- Assess fit annually.

### Cervical Cap (Prentif)
- Safe method with rare side effects.
- Only 4 sizes and harder to place.
- Insert 20 minutes to 4 hours prior to coitus.
- Successful fitting is crucial to efficacy.
- Can leave in place for 24–36 hours.

### Spermicides
- Nonoxynol-9, Octoxynol-9, Mefegol.
- Proven STI protection.
- Apply 10–30 minutes prior to coitus.
- High failure rate.

### Condoms
- 6 billion used worldwide annually.
- Latex condoms 0.3–0.8 mm thick.
- Natural skin condoms do **not** protect against HIV and other STIs.
- Do not use with oil-based lubricants.
- Inconsistent use accounts for most failures.

## ORAL CONTRACEPTIVES

### Summary of Guidelines for the Use of Combination Estrogen-Progestin Oral Contraceptives in Women with Characteristics That Might Increase the Risk of Adverse Effects[a]

| Variable | AGOG Guidelines | WHO Guidelines |
|---|---|---|
| Smoker, >35 yrs of age | | |
| <15 cigarettes/day | Risk unacceptable | Risk usually outweighs benefit |
| ≥15 cigarettes/day | Risk unacceptable | Risk unacceptable |
| Hypertension | | |
| Blood pressure controlled | Risk acceptable; no definition of blood-pressure control | Risk usually outweighs benefit if systolic blood pressure is 140–159 mm Hg and diastolic blood pressure is 90–99 mm Hg |
| Blood pressure uncontrolled | Risk unacceptable; no definition of uncontrolled blood pressure | Risk unacceptable if systolic blood pressure is ≥160 mm Hg or diastolic blood pressure is ≥100 mm Hg |
| History of stroke, ischemic heart disease, or venous thromboembolism | Risk unacceptable | Risk unacceptable |
| Diabetes | Risk acceptable if no other cardiovascular risk factors and no end-organ damage | Benefit outweighs risk if no end-organ damage and diabetes is of ≤20 yrs duration |
| Hypercholesterolemia | Risk acceptable if LDL cholesterol <160 mg/dL and no other cardiovascular risk factors | Benefit-risk ratio is dependent on the presence or absence of other cardiovascular risk factors |
| Multiple cardiovascular risk factors | Not addressed | Risk usually outweighs benefit or risk unacceptable, depending on risk factors |
| Migraine headache | | |
| Age ≥35 yrs | Risk usually outweighs benefit | Risk usually outweighs benefit |
| Focal symptoms | Risk unacceptable | Risk unacceptable |
| Breast cancer | | |
| Current disease | Risk unacceptable | Risk unacceptable |
| Past disease, no active disease for 5 yrs | Risk unacceptable | Risk usually outweighs benefit |
| Family history of breast or ovarian cancer | Risk acceptable | Risk acceptable |

[a]The American College of Obstetricians and Gynecologists (ACOG) guidelines recommend the use of formulations containing less than 50 mcg of ethinyl estradiol with the "lowest progestin dose," without mention of the type of progestin. The World Health Organization (WHO) guidelines pertain explicitly to formulations containing 35 mcg or less of ethinyl estradiol and do not mention the dose or type of progestin. To convert values for low-density lipoprotein (LDL) cholesterol to millimoles per liter, multiply by 0.02586.

*Source:* Reprinted with permission from Petitti DB. Combination estrogen-progestin oral contraceptives. *N Engl J Med.* 2003;349(14):1443–1450. Copyright © 2003 Massachusetts Medical Society. All rights reserved.

# CONTRACEPTION

## Types of Progestin in Combination Estrogen–Progestin Oral Contraceptives Marketed in the United States or Mentioned in Studies of Types of Progestin and Cardiovascular Disease

| Type of Progestin | Generation | | Brand Names of Selected Products[a] |
|---|---|---|---|
| | According to Time of Market Introduction[b] | According to Published Studies of Vascular Disease | |
| Ever marketed in the United States | | | |
| Chlormadinone acetate[c,d] | First | Other | C-Quens |
| Desogestrel | Third | Third | Desogen, Ortho-Cept, Apri (monophasic) |
| | | | Cyclessa (triphasic) |
| Dimethisterone[c,d] | First | Not mentioned | Oracon |
| Drospirenone | Fourth | Not studied | Yasmin (monophasic) |
| Ethynodiol diacetate | First | First or second | Demulen 1/35, Zovia 1/35E (monophasic) |
| Levonorgestrel | Second | Second | Levlen, Levora, Nordette, Portia (monophasic) |
| | | | Alesse, Aviane, Lessina, Levlite (monophasic) |
| | | | Empresse, Tri-Levlen, Triphasil, Trivora (triphasic) |
| Medroxyprogesterone acetate[c] | First | Not mentioned | Provest |
| Norethindrone | First | First or second | Necon 1/35, Norinyl 1+35, Nortrel 1/35, Ortho-Novum 1/35 (monophasic) |
| | | | Brevicon, Modicon, Neocon 0.5/35, Nortrel 0.5/35 (monophasic) |
| | | | Ovcon-35 (monophasic) |
| | | | Necon 7/7/7, Ortho-Novum 7/7/7, Nortrel 7/7/7, Tri-Norinyl (triphasic) |
| Norethindrone acetate[c] | First | First or second | Loestrin 21 1.5/30, Loestrin Fe 1.5/30, Microgestin Fe 1.5/30 (monophasic) |
| | | | Loestrin 21 1/20, Loestrin Fe 1/20, Microgestin Fe 1/20 (monophasic) |
| | | | Estrostep 21, Estrostep Fe (triphasic) |

*(continued)*

| | Generation | | |
| Type of Progestin | According to Time of Market Introduction[b] | According to Published Studies of Vascular Disease | Brand Names of Selected Products[a] |
|---|---|---|---|
| Norethynodrel[c] | First | First | Enovid |
| Norgestimate[c] | Third | Second, third, or other | Mononessa, Ortho-Cyclen, Sprintec (monophasic) |
| | | | Ortho Tri-Cyclen, Ortho Tri-Cyclen Lo (triphasic) |
| Norgestrel | First | First or second | Cryselle, Lo/Ovral, Low-Ogestrel (monophasic) |
| **Never marketed in the United States** | | | |
| Gestodene | Third | Third | — |
| Lynestrenol | First | First or second | — |

[a]Among products currently marketed in the United States, the lists include only monophasic and triphasic formulations containing less than 50 mcg of ethinyl estradiol: each list of monophasic formulations containing a given type of progestin includes products containing the same amount of estrogen and progestin: separate lists of monophasic preparations containing a given type of progestin appear in order of decreasing dose of ethinyl estradiol or progestin. The listed products are provided as examples and were not selected on the basis of cost or market share.

[b]According to this classification, the first generation includes contraceptives approved for marketing in the United States before 1973, the second generation those approved for marketing in the United States between 1973 and 1989, the third generation those approved for marketing in the United States or Europe between 1990 and 2000, and the fourth generation those approved for marketing in the United States after 2000.

[c]This type of progestin is not contained in any combination estrogen progestin oral contraceptives currently marketed in the United States.

[d]In the United States, this type of progestin has been marketed only in combination oral contraceptives involving the sequential administration of estrogen and progestin.

*Source:* Reprinted with permission from Petitti DB. Combination estrogen-progestin oral contraceptives. *N Engl J Med.* 2003;349(14):1443–1450. Copyright © 2003 Massachusetts Medical Society. All rights reserved.

# CONTRACEPTION

## Oral Contraceptive Management

- Start on 1st Sunday of cycle (monophasics) or 1st day of period (triphasics).
- Protected from pregnancy after 5 days.
- If 1 pill is missed, take missed pill as soon as possible, take next pill at usual time.
- If 2 pills are missed during 1st 2 weeks, take 2 pills as soon as possible, then 2 pills the next day, then return to usual schedule but use additional barrier contraception for that month.
- If 2 pills are missed during 3rd week or 3 pills at any time during month then immediately start a new pack without having a pill-free interval and use back-up method for 7 days.
- Breakthrough bleeding (BTB) common in 1st 3 months.
    - If BTB still a problem after that then change to different oral contraceptive.
    - Higher estradiol and progestin doses have lower rates of BTB.

## Pharmacologic Profiles of Progesterone and Various Progestins

| Progesterone/ Progestins | Pharmacologic Activity | | | |
|---|---|---|---|---|
| | Progestogenic | Androgenic | Antiandro-genic | Antimineralo-corticoid |
| Progesterone | + | – | (+) | + |
| Drospirenone | + | – | + | + |
| Gestodene[a] | + | (+) | – | (+) |
| Norgestimate[b] | + | (+) | – | – |
| Levonorgestrel | + | (+) | – | – |
| Desogestrel[c] | + | (+) | – | – |
| Dienogest[a] | + | – | + | – |
| Cyproterone acetate[a] | + | – | + | – |

+, effect; (+), negligible effect at therapeutic doses; –, no effect.
[a]Not available in the United States.
[b]Main metabolite levonorgestrel.
[c]Active metabolite 3-ketodesogestrel.
*Source:* Adapted from Krattenmacher R. Drospirenone: pharmacology and pharmacokinetics of a unique progestogen. *Contraception.* 2000;62:29–38.

## Interaction of Antiinfective Agents and Combination Oral Contraceptives

| |
|---|
| Antiinfective agent that decreases steroid levels in women taking combination oral contraceptives |
| Rifampin |
| Antiinfective agents that do not decrease steroid levels in women taking combination oral contraceptives |
| Ampicillin |
| Doxycycline |
| Fluconazole |
| Metronidazole |
| Miconazole[a] |
| Quinolone antibiotics |
| Tetracycline |

[a]Vaginal administration does not lower steroid levels in women using the contraceptive vaginal ring.
*Source:* Reprinted with permission from ACOG Practice Bulletin Number 73, June 2006. Use of hormonal contraception in women with coexisting medical conditions. *Obstet Gynecol.* 2006;107(6):1453–1472.

# CONTRACEPTION

## Interaction of Anticonvulsants and Combination Oral Contraceptives

| Anticonvulsants that decrease steroid levels in women taking combination oral contraceptives |
|---|
| Barbiturates (including phenobarbital and primidone) |
| Carbamazepine and oxcarbazepine |
| Felbamate |
| Phenytoin |
| Topiramate |
| Vigabatrin |
| **Anticonvulsants that do not decrease steroid levels in women taking combination oral contraceptives** |
| Ethosuximide[a] |
| Gabapentin[b] |
| Lamotrigine[b] |
| Levetiracetam |
| Tiagabine[b] |
| Valproic acid |
| Zonisamide |

[a]No pharmacokinetic data are available.
[b]Pharmacokinetic study used anticonvulsant dose lower than that used in clinical practice.
*Source:* Reprinted with permission from ACOG Practice Bulletin Number 73, June 2006. Use of hormonal contraception in women with coexisting medical conditions. *Obstet Gynecol.* 2006;107(6):1453–1472.

## Pharmacokinetic Combination Oral Contraceptive-Antiretroviral Drug Interactions

| Antiretroviral Levels | Contraceptive Steroid Levels | Antiretroviral |
|---|---|---|
| *Protease inhibitors* | | |
| Neflinavir | ↓ | No data |
| Ritonavir | ↓ | No data |
| Lopinavir/ritonavir | ↓ | No data |
| Atazanavir | ↑ | No data |
| Amprenavir | ↑ | ↓ |
| Indinavir | ↑ | No data |
| Saquinavir | No data | No change |
| *Nonnucleoside reverse transcriptase inhibitors* | | |
| Nevirapine | ↓ | No change |
| Efavirenz | ↓ | No change |
| Delavirdine | ? ↑ | No data |

*Source:* Reprinted with permission from ACOG Practice Bulletin Number 73, June 2006. Use of hormonal contraception in women with coexisting medical conditions. *Obstet Gynecol.* 2006;107(6):1453–1472.

## COMMON HORMONAL CONTRACEPTIVES

### Oral Contraceptives—Combined

| Monophasic Extended Cycle | | |
|---|---|---|
| **Product (No. of tabs)** | **Estrogen (mcg)** | **Progestin (mg)** |
| Seasonale (91) (Duramed) | 30 EE | 0.15 LNG |
| 84 days of estrogen-progestin tab followed by 7 days of inert tab | | |
| Seaonique (91) (Duramed)/33 EE/0.15 LNG | | |
| 84 days of estrogen-progestin tab followed by 7 days 10 mcg EE | | |

| Monophasic Products (arranged from lowest to highest estrogen dose) | | |
|---|---|---|
| **Product (No. of tabs)** | **Estrogen (mcg)** | **Progestin (mg)** |
| Alesse (28) (Wyeth) | 20 EE | 0.1 LNG |
| Lutera (28) (Watson) | 20 EE | 0.1 LNG |
| Aviane (28) (Barr) | 20 EE | 0.1 LNG |
| Lessina (21/28)[a] (Barr) | 20 EE | 0.1 LNG |
| Levlite (28) (Berlex) | 20 EE | 0.1 LNG |
| Loestrin 1/20 (21) (Barr) | 20 EE | 1 NEA |
| Loestrin Fe 1/20 (28) (Barr) | 20 EE | 1 NEA |
| Loestrin 24 Fe (28) (Warner Chilcott) | 20 EE | 1 NEA |
| Junel 1/20 (Barr) | 20 EE | 1 NEA |
| Junel Fe 1/20 (Barr) | 20 EE | 1 NEA |
| Microgestin 1/20 (21) (Watson) | 20 EE | 1 NEA |
| Microgestin Fe 1/20 (28) (Watson) | 20 EE | 1 NEA |
| Levlen (21/28)[a] (Berlex) | 30 EE | 0.15 LNG |
| Levora (21/28)[a] (Watson) | 30 EE | 0.15 LNG |
| Nordette (21/28)[a] (King) | 30 EE | 0.15 LNG |
| Portia (28) (Barr) | 30 EE | 0.15 LNG |
| Desogen (28) (Organon) | 30 EE | 0.15 DSG |
| Ortho-Cept (28) (Ortho-McNeil) | 30 EE | 0.15 DSG |
| Apri (28) (Barr) | 30 EE | 0.15 DSG |
| Cryselle (28) (Barr) | 30 EE | 0.3 NOR |
| Lo/Ovral (28) (Wyeth) | 30 EE | 0.3 NOR |
| Low-Ogestrel (28) (Watson) | 30 EE | 0.3 NOR |
| Loestrin 1.5/30 (21) (Barr) | 30 EE | 1.5 NEA |
| Loestrin Fe 1.5/30 (21/28)[a] (Barr) | 30 EE | 1.5 NEA |
| Junel 1.5/30 (21) (Barr) | 30 EE | 1.5 NEA |
| Junel Fe 1.5/30 (28) (Barr) | 30 EE | 1.5 NEA |
| Microgestin Fe 1.5/30 (28) (Watson) | 30 EE | 1.5 NEA |
| Yasmin (28) (Berlex) | 30 EE | 3 DRO |
| Yaz (28) (Bayer) | 20 EE | 3 DRO |
| MonoNessa (28) (Watson) | 35 EE | 0.25 NGM |
| Ortho-Cyclen (28) (Ortho-McNeil) | 35 EE | 0.25 NGM |
| Previfem (28) (Teva) | 35 EE | 0.25 NGM |
| Sprintec (28) (Barr) | 35 EE | 0.25 NGM |

*(continued)*

# CONTRACEPTION

## Oral Contraceptives—Combined *(continued)*

| Monophasic Products (arranged from lowest to highest estrogen dose) | | |
|---|---|---|
| **Product (No. of tabs)** | **Estrogen (mcg)** | **Progestin (mg)** |
| Femcon (*chewable*) (28) (Warner Chilcott) | 35 EE | 0.4 NE |
| Ovcon 35 (21/28)[ab] (Warner Chilcott) | 35 EE | 0.4 NE |
| Brevicon (28) (Watson) | 35 EE | 0.5 NE |
| Modicon (28) (Ortho-McNeil) | 35 EE | 0.5 NE |
| Necon 0.5/35 (21/28)[a] (Watson) | 35 EE | 0.5 NE |
| Nortrel 0.5/35 (28) (Barr) | 35 EE | 0.5 NE |
| Necon 1/35 (21/28)[a] (Watson) | 35 EE | 1 NE |
| Norinyl 1+35 (28) (Watson) | 35 EE | 1 NE |
| Nortrel 1/35 (21/28)[a] (Barr) | 35 EE | 1 NE |
| Ortho-Novum 1/35 (28) (Ortho-McNeil) | 35 EE | 1 NE |
| Demulen 1/35 (21/28)[a] (Pfizer) | 35 EE | 1 ED |
| Zovia 1/35 (21/28)[a] (Watson) | 35 EE | 1 ED |
| Ovral (21/28)[a] (Wyeth) | 50 EE | 0.5 NOR |
| Ogestrel 0.5/50 (28) (Watson) | 50 EE | 0.5 NOR |
| Demulen 1/50 (21/28)[a] (Pfizer) | 50 EE | 1 ED |
| Zovia 1/50 (21/28)[a] (Watson) | 50 EE | 1 ED |
| Ovcon 50 (28) (Warner Chilcott) | 50 EE | 1 NE |
| Necon 1/50 (21/28)[a] (Watson) | 50 MES | 1 NE |
| Norinyl 1+50 (28) (Watson) | 50 MES | 1 NE |
| Ortho-Novum 1/50 (28) (Ortho-McNeil) | 50 MES | 1 NE |

| Biphasic Products with 2-Day Hormone-Free Interval | | |
|---|---|---|
| **Product (No. of tabs)** | **Estrogen (mcg)** | **Progestin (mg)** |
| Kariva (28) (Barr) | 20 EE/10 EE | 0.15 DSG (white tab only) |
|    1 white tab daily for 21 days, followed by 1 inert tab for 2 days then 1 blue tab for 5 days | | |
| Mircette (28) (Organon) | 20 EE/10 EE | 0.15 DSG (white tab only) |
|    1 white tab daily for 21 days, followed by 1 inert tab for 2 days then 1 yellow tab for 5 days | | |

| Biphasic Products | | |
|---|---|---|
| **Product (No. of tabs)** | **Phase 1 Days 1–10 (Tablet Color)** | **Phase 2 Days 11–21 (Tablet Color)** |
| Necon 10/11 (21/28) (Watson) | 35 mcg EE/0.5 mg NE (light yellow) | 35 mcg EE/1 mg NE (dark yellow) |
| Ortho-Novum 10/11 (28) (Ortho-McNeil) | 35 mcg EE/0.5 mg NE (white) | 35 mcg EE/1 mg NE (peach) |

234

| Triphasic Products: Constant Estrogen with a Phasic Progestin Dose (arranged from lowest to highest estrogen dose) | | | |
|---|---|---|---|
| Product (No. of tabs) | Phase 1 (No. of tabs, color, shape— if applicable) | Phase 2 (No. of tabs, color, shape—if applicable) | Phase 3 (No. of tabs, color, shape—if applicable) |
| Cyclessa (28) (Organon) | 25 mcg EE/0.1 mg DSG (7 light yellow) | 25 mcg EE/0.125 mg DSG (7 orange) | 25 mcg EE/0.15 mg DSG (7 red) |
| Velivet (28) (Barr) | 25 mcg EE/0.1 mg DSG (7 beige) | 25 mcg EE/0.125 mg DSG (7 orange) | 25 mcg EE/0.15 mg DSG (7 pink) |
| Ortho Tri-Cyclen Lo (28) (Ortho-McNeil) | 25 mcg EE/0.18 mg NGM (7 white) | 25 mcg EE/0.215 mg NGM (7 light blue) | 25 mcg EE/0.25 mg NGM (7 dark blue) |
| Ortho Tri-Cyclen (28)[c] (Ortho-McNeil) | 35 mcg EE/0.18 mg NGM (7 white) | 35 mcg EE/0.215 mg NGM (7 light blue) | 35 mcg EE/0.25 mg NGM (7 dark blue) |
| Tri-Previfem (28) (Teva) | 35 mcg EE/0.18 mg NGM (7 white) | 35 mcg EE/0.215 mg NGM (7 light blue) | 35 mcg EE/0.25 mg NGM (7 blue) |
| TriNessa (28) (Watson) | 35 mcg EE/0.18 mg NGM (7 white) | 35 mcg EE/0.215 mg NGM (7 light blue) | 35 mcg EE/0.25 mg NGM (7 blue) |
| Tri-Sprintec (28) (Barr) | 35 mcg EE/0.18 mg NGM (7 gray) | 35 mcg EE/0.215 mg NGM (7 light blue) | 35 mcg EE/0.25 mg NGM (7 blue) |
| Ortho-Novum 7/7/7 (28) (Ortho-McNeil) | 35 mcg EE/0.5 mg NE (7 white) | 35 mcg EE/0.75 mg NE (7 light peach) | 35 mcg EE/1 mg NE (7 peach) |
| Nortrel 7/7/7 (28) (Barr) | 35 mcg EE/0.5 mg NE (7 light yellow) | 35 mcg EE/0.75 mg NE (7 light blue) | 35 mcg EE/1 mg NE (7 peach) |
| Necon 7/7/7 (28) (Watson) | 35 mcg EE/0.5 mg NE (7 white) | 35 mcg EE/0.75 mg NE (7 light peach) | 35 mcg EE/1 mg NE (7 peach) |
| Aranelle (28) (Watson) | 35 mcg EE/0.5 mg NE (7 light yellow) | 35 mcg EE/1 mg NE (9 white) | 35 mcg EE/0.5 mg NE (5 light yellow) |
| Tri-Norinyl (28) (Watson) | 35 mcg EE/0.5 mg NE (7 blue) | 35 mcg EE/1 mg NE (9 yellow-green) | 35 mcg EE/0.5 mg NE (5 light blue) |

*(continued)*

| Triphasic Products: Phasic Estrogen Dose with a Phasic Progestin Dose (arranged from lowest to highest estrogen dose) | | | |
|---|---|---|---|
| Product (No. of tabs) | Phase 1 (No. of tabs, color, shape— if applicable) | Phase 2 (No. of tabs, color, shape— if applicable) | Phase 3 (No. of tabs, color, shape— if applicable) |
| Trivora (28) (Watson) | 30 mcg EE/0.05 mg LNG (6 blue) | 40 mcg EE/0.075 mg LNG (5 white) | 30 mcg EE/0.125 mg LNG (10 pink) |
| Triphasil (21/28)[a] (Wyeth) | 30 mcg EE/0.05 mg LNG (6 brown) | 40 mcg EE/0.075 mg LNG (5 white) | 30 mcg EE/0.125 mg LNG (10 light yellow) |
| Tri-Levlen (21/28) (Berlex) | 30 mcg EE/0.05 mg LNG (6 brown) | 40 mcg EE/0.075 mg LNG (5 white) | 30 mcg EE/0.125 mg LNG (10 light yellow) |
| Enpresse (28) (Barr) | 30 mcg EE/0.05 mg LNG (6 pink) | 40 mcg EE/0.075 mg LNG (5 white) | 30 mcg EE/0.125 mg LNG (10 orange) |
| Triphasic Products: Constant Progestin with a Phasic Estrogen Dose | | | |
| Estrostep 21 (21) (Warner Chilcott) | 20 mcg EE/1 mg NEA (5 white triangular) | 30 mcg EE/1 mg NEA (7 white square) | 35 mcg EE/1 mg NEA (10 white round) |
| Estrostep Fe (28) (Warner Chilcott) | 20 mcg EE/1 mg NEA (5 white triangular) | 30 mcg EE/1 mg NEA (7 white square) | 35 mcg EE/1 mg NEA (10 white round) |

[a]The 21-day version of this product does not include inert tablets.

*Source:* Reprinted with permission from Mancano M. Overview of contraceptive methods. OB/GYN Special Ed. 2005:51–58.

### Oral Contraceptives—Progestin Only
#### Progestin Pills Currently Available
- Ovrette (28) (Wyeth) 0.075 NOR (yellow)
- Ovrette (28) (Barr) 0.35 NE (light pink)
- Errin (28) (Barr) 0.35 NE (yellow)
- Nor-QD (28) (Watson) 0.35 NE (yellow)
- Jolivette (28) (Watson) 0.35 NE (light green)
- Nora-BE (28) (Watson) 0.35 NE (white)
- Ortho-Micronor (28) (Ortho-McNeil) 0.35 NE (green)

#### Mechanism of Action
- Prevents ovulation; thickens cervical mucus; causes endometrial changes that may prevent implantation (rare); reduces activity of cilia in the fallopian tube

# CONTRACEPTION

### Side Effects
- Similar to COCs—though estrogen-related side effects (e.g., nausea, breast tenderness, bloating) are diminished; menstrual irregularity (most common); irregular bleeding; prolonged bleeding episodes; amenorrhea

### Serious Adverse Reactions
- Similar to COCs with reduced risk of clotting problems; potential cardiovascular effects are controversial; ectopic pregnancy (rare)

### Contraindications/Precautions
- Undiagnosed genital bleeding; current CAD or cerebrovascular disease; known or suspected hormone-dependent neoplasia; history of benign or malignant liver neoplasm

### Key Counseling Points
- Does not protect against STIs or HIV infection.
- Taken daily, with no hormone-free interval.
- Take pills at the same time each day for maximum effectiveness.
- Appropriate action if:
  - *Pill is taken 3 hours late*
    - ⇨ Take pill as soon as possible. If taken the next day, take 2 pills, and complete the cycle pack.
    - ⇨ Use backup contraception for 48 hours.
  - ≥1 *pill is missed:* Stop taking pills. Discard cycle pack.
    - ⇨ Use EC if necessary (see pg. 244). Menses should begin within 2–3 weeks (unless pregnant).
    - ⇨ Start a new cycle pack on the day menses begins. Use backup contraception from the time the error is discovered until the third day of the new cycle pack.

### Additional Considerations
- **Initial Dose:** Can be started on any day of the week once pregnancy is ruled out.
- **Return of Fertility:** No delay
- **1-Year Failure Rate, Typical vs. Perfect Use**[a]**:** 8% vs 0.3%
- **Drug Interactions:** Similar to COCs
- Data indicate that the cervical mucus becomes impenetrable rapidly, so backup contraception is only needed until the third consecutive pill taken at the same time each day is ingested.[b]

COC, combined oral contraceptive; EC, emergency contraceptive; STI, sexually transmitted infection.
[a]In clinical studies, failure rates have been reported as high as 13%. (*Source:* McCann MF, Lotter LS. Progestin-only contraception: a comprehensive review. *Contraception.* 1994:50[suppl 1]:S34–S41.)
[b]McCann MF, Potter LS. Progestin-only contraception: a comprehensive review. *Contraception.* 1994;50(6 suppl 1): S1–S195.

# CONTRACEPTION

## ORAL CONTRACEPTIVE GUIDELINES

### Practice Guidelines for Oral Contraceptive Selection When Initiating Use, Based on Patient Characteristics and Side Effects

✓ represents panel's first choice (consensus opinion) of agent category for most women with the listed characteristic; other agents may also be appropriate in light of individual circumstances and/or clinician's judgment.

| Patient Characteristic | Preferred Dose of Ethinyl Estradiol (EE) | | |
|---|---|---|---|
| | 20 mcg EE | 25 mcg EE | 30–35 mcg EE |
| General Formulation Selections for Women Initiating Oral Contraceptive Use | | | |
| New start (all women except where noted in the next table) | ✓ | ✓ | ✓ |
| Adolescent | ✓a,b,c | ✓a,b | ✓a,b |
| Perimenopause | ✓a,c | ✓a | ✓a |
| Postpartum (lactating) | If no supplemental feedings and no menses, conception unlikely for 3 months; if oral contraceptive desired, progestin-only pill recommended beginning 6 weeks after childbirth. Replace with combination pill when any supplemental feeding introduced. | | |
| Postpartum (nonlactating) (start at 2–3 wks)d | ✓ | ✓ | ✓ |
| Formulation Selections for Minimizing or Managing Unwanted OC Side Effects | | | |
| Acne/hirsutism | ✓a,e | ✓a,e | ✓a,e |
| Breast tenderness | ✓ | ✓ | |
| Headache/common migrainef | ✓ | ✓ | ✓ |
| Intermenstrual bleeding | | | ✓ |
| Mood changef | ✓ | ✓ | |
| Nausea | ✓ | ✓ | |

aA formulation containing a progestin with km androgenic activity remains the agent of first choice, but evidence for a significant advantage for this clinical characteristic is lacking.
bA sizable minority of consensus faculty did not agree that formulations with low androgenic activity remain the agent of first choice in adolescents.
cA sizable minority of consensus faculty did not agree that formulations with 20 mcg EE are agents of first choice due to higher rates of intermenstrual bleeding, except the formulation containing 20 mcg EE with 0.15 mg desogestrel which has demonstrated an acceptable bleeding profile.
dCombination OC product labeling indicates start at 4 weeks; however, because ovulation can occur at 4 weeks postpartum, OC use at 2 to 3 weeks is recommended.
eThe OC formulations containing triphasic norgestimate with 35 mcg EE, norethindrone acetate with triphasic EE, and 20 mcg EE with 0.1 mg levonorgestrel are the only ones shown in published, randomized trials to improve acne significantly more than placebo; only the first two formulations are approved by the FDA to treat acne vulgaris. Thiboutot D et al. *Fertil Steril.* 2001;76:461–468; Lucky AW et at *J Am Acad Dematol.* 1997;37:746-754; Redmond G et al, *Obstet Gynecol.* 1997;89:613–622; Gilliam M et al. *Obstet Gynecol.* 2001;97(suppl):S9.
fIf headache or mood change occurs exclusively during the pill-free interval, use daily, continuous, combined monophasic OCs without pill-free interval.
*Source:* Reprinted with permission from *Dialogues in Contraception.* 2002:7;6–9.

## Practice Guidelines for Oral Contraceptive Selection When Initiating Use, Based on Patients' Medical Conditions and/or Risk Factors

| Patient Characteristic | Preferred Dose of Ethinyl Estradiol (EE) | | |
|---|---|---|---|
| | 20 mcg EE | 25 mcg EE | 30–35 mcg EE |
| Hypertension (uncontrolled) | | | |
| Inherited thrombophilias without personal history of thrombosis[a] | Conditions considered by consensus faculty to be contraindications in addition to those stated in product labeling; please see labeling for individual formulations. | | |
| Migraine (classic)[b] | | | |
| Smoker more than 35 yrs of age | | | |
| Acne/hirsutism | ✓[c,d] | ✓[c,d] | ✓[c,d] |
| Anticoagulant user (including those with prosthetic heart valves)[e] | ✓ | ✓ | ✓ |
| Anticonvulsant use[f] | | | |
| Benign breast disease | ✓ | ✓ | ✓ |
| Breast cancer (family history of) | ✓ | ✓ | ✓ |
| Cervical dysplasia | ✓ | ✓ | ✓ |
| Chronic hyperandrogenic anovulation/PCOS | | | ✓[d] |
| CHD (family history of) | ✓[d] | ✓[d] | ✓[d] |
| Depression | ✓ | ✓ | ✓ |
| Diabetes/gestational diabetes without vascular disease (except those with PCOS) | ✓[d] | ✓[d] | |
| Dysfunctional uterine bleeding | | | ✓[g] |
| Dyslipidemia (excluding hypertriglyceridemia) | | | ✓[h] |
| Dysmenorrhea[i,j] | ✓ | ✓ | ✓ |
| Endometriosis (pain)[i] | ✓[k] | ✓[k] | ✓[k] |
| Excessive uterine bleeding with blood dyscrasias[i] | | | ✓ |
| Functional ovarian cysts (history of symptomatic) | | | ✓[l] |
| Gestational trophoblast disease (history of) | ✓ | ✓ | ✓ |
| Hemoglobinopathies (including sickle cell disease and trait) | ✓ | ✓ | ✓ |
| Hepatitis (past history)[m] | ✓ | ✓ | ✓ |
| Hypertension | ✓ | ✓ | |
| Migraine (common)[i] | ✓ | ✓ | ✓ |
| Mittelschmerz | ✓ | ✓ | ✓ |

# CONTRACEPTION

| Patient Characteristic | Preferred Dose of Ethinyl Estradiol (EE) | | |
| --- | --- | --- | --- |
| | 20 mcg EE | 25 mcg EE | 30–35 mcg EE |
| Mitral valve prolapse (unless associated atrial fibrillation or thrombosis) | ✓ | ✓ | ✓ |
| Obesity (BMI >29)[n] | | ✓[d] | ✓[d] |
| Ovarian cancer (family history of) | | | ✓[o] |
| Premature ovarian failure[i] | ✓ | ✓ | ✓ |
| Premenstrual dysphoric disorder[j] | ✓ | ✓ | ✓ |
| Systemic lupus erythematosus without vascular or renal disease, and no anti-cardiolipin antibody or lupus anticoagulant antibody | ✓ | ✓ | ✓ |
| Thyroid disease[p] | ✓ | ✓ | ✓ |
| Uterine leiomyomata[a] | ✓ | ✓ | ✓ |

BMI, body mass index; CHD, coronary heart disease; OC, oral contraceptive; PCOS, polycystic ovary syndrome.
[a]Some panel members consider oral contraceptive use acceptable in some cases of mild thrombophilias; family history and clinician agreement are required.
[b]Focal neurologic symptoms or aura lasting more than one hour or with documented vascular involvement.
[c]The oral contraceptive formulations containing triphasic norgestimate with 35 mcg EE, norethindrone acetate with triphasic EE, and 20 mcg EE with 0.1 mg levonorgestrel are the only ones shown in published, randomized trials to improve acne significantly more than placebo; only the first two formulations are approved by the FDA to treat acne vulgaris. Thiboutot D, et al. Fertil Steril. 2001;76:461–468; Lucky AW, et al. J Am Acad Dermatol. 1997;89:615–622. Gilliam M, et al. Obstet Gynecol. 2007;97(suppl):89.
[d]A formulation containing a progestin with low androgenic activity remains the agent of first choice, but evidence for a significant advantage for this clinical characteristic is lacking.
[e]If anticoagulation is maintained at a therapeutic level, use of a combination OC will not increase thrombotic risk.
[f]For concomitant use of anticonvulsants except valproic acid in epilepsy or bipolar disorder, formulation containing 50 mcg estrogen may be preferable to reduce intermenstrual bleeding. There are no data indicating compromised OC efficacy with concomitant use of anticonvulsants.
[g]One randomized study found that triphasic norgestimate/35 mcg EE was significantly more effective than placebo in treating dysfunctional uterine bleeding. Davis, et al. Obstet Gynecol. 2000;94:913–920.
[h]OC-induced alterations in cholesterol and lipoprotein values are related to the androgenicity of the progestin component and the estrogen-progestin ratio. OCs containing norgestimate and desogestrel raise HDL and lower LDL levels. Speroff, et al. Obstet Gynecol. 1993;81:1034–1047.
[i]If symptoms occur during the pill-free interval, use daily, continuous, combined monophasic OCs to avoid cyclicity.
[j]If dysmenorrhea persists, add a prostaglandin synthetase inhibitor or diagnostic tests to rule out endometriosis.
[k]Although little data exist, a formulation containing a progestin with medium or high androgenic activity is preferred for treating endometriosis with pain.
[l]If cysts recur, a monophasic 50-mcg-EE OC may be preferable.
[m]Monitor with liver function tests.
[n]Obesity is an independent risk factor for VTE. There is no epidemiologic evidence indicating that there is a difference in risk of venous thrombosis with OCs containing 20 to 25 mcg EE and OCs containing 30 to 35 mcg EE.
[o]All OCs ≥30 mcg EE have been shown to reduce risk of ovarian cancer. Ness, et al. Am J Epidemiol. 2000;152:233–241. One study suggests that combination OCs with high-progestin potency are associated with a greater reduction in ovarian cancer risk than those with low-progestin potency. Schildkraut, et al. J Natl Cancer Inst. 2002;94:32–38.
[p]OCs are not contraindicated in thyroid disease. Recheck TSH 6 to 12 weeks after starting or discontinuing OCs.
Source: Reprinted with permission from Dialogues in Contraception. 2002:7;6–9.

## Transdermal Contraceptive
- Ortho Evra (Ortho-McNeil)

### Description
- 3-layer patch delivers 0.15 mg/d of norelgestromin and 20 mcg/day of EE

### Mechanism of Action
- Similar to COCs

### Application Issues
- Applied 1×/week for 3 weeks followed by a patch-free week.
- May be applied to 4 areas: lower abdomen, buttocks, upper outer arm and upper torso, excluding breasts.
- New patch is applied to a different area of skin, on the same day of the week as previous patch.
- Initial Use: Can be started on any day of the week once pregnancy is ruled out.
- If >5 days since start of menstrual bleeding, or postpartum, or postabortion, backup contraceptive method is recommended for 7 days.

### Side Effects: Serious Adverse Effects
- Similar to COCs
- Skin irritation

### Key Counseling Points
- Does not protect against lower genital tract STIs or HIV infection.
- Spotting or BTB may occur during the first 3 cycles of use.
- Contact healthcare provider if pregnancy is suspected, or if any of the following occur: sudden severe headache; visual disturbances, numbness in an arm or leg, severe abdominal pain, prolonged episodes of bleeding, or amenorrhea.
- **Appropriate action if patch is detached:**
  - *<24 hours*
    ⇨ Patch should be reapplied to the same body location or, if not adhering well, a new patch should be applied immediately. No backup contraception is needed.
  - *24 hours*
    ⇨ Apply a new patch.
    ⇨ Use backup contraception method for 7 days.

### Additional Considerations
- **Return of Fertility:** No delay
- **1-Year Failure Rate, Perfect Use**[a]**:** 0.3%
- **Contraindications/Precautions:**
  - Similar to COCs
- **Drug Interactions:** Similar to COCs
- **Noncontraceptive Health Benefits:** Studies have not been conducted that confirm long-term benefits because the patch has been available for <2 years

BTB, breakthrough bleeding; COC, combined oral contraceptive; STI, sexually transmitted infection.
[a]Typical-use failure rate is not available, since the transdermal patch was not available at the time of the 1995 National Survey of Family Growth.

# CONTRACEPTION

## Injectable Contraceptive
### Product
- Depo-Provera (Pfizer)
- Depo-subQ Provera 104 (Pfizer)

### Description
- 150 mg/1 mL suspension of DMPA (injected intramuscularly only)
- 104 mg/0.65 mL medroxyprogesterone acetate (Injected subcutaneously only)

### Mechanism of Action
- Prevents ovulation by inhibiting luteinizing hormone surge; thickens cervical mucus to block sperm entry into the upper reproductive tract; slows tubal motility; causes endometrial changes that may prevent implantation (rare).

### Administration Issues
- Only use as a long-term birth control method (for example, longer than 2 years) if other birth control methods are inadequate for the patient.
- First injection can be administered on any day, as long as pregnancy is ruled out.
- If >5 days since start of menses, postpartum, or postabortion, backup contraceptive method is recommended for 7 days.
- Pregnancy should be ruled out if the woman returns for repeat injection more than 13 weeks after the last injection.
- Shake vial vigorously before use to ensure uniform suspension.

### Duration of Efficacy
- 3 months

### Side Effects/Serious Adverse Effects
- Irregular bleeding, weight gain, breast tenderness, headaches.
- Prolonged use may result in significant loss of bone density with greater loss the longer the drug is administered. This bone density loss may not be completely reversible after discontinuation.

### Contraindications
- Undiagnosed abnormal genital bleeding; known or suspected pregnancy; acute liver disease; benign or malignant liver tumors; known or suspected malignancy of the breast.

### Key Counseling Points
- Does not protect against lower genital tract STIs or HIV infection.
- Most women experience irregular unpredictable bleeding during the first year.
- Return every 3 months for repeat injection.
- Contact your healthcare provider if pregnancy is suspected, or if any of the following occur: sudden severe headache, visual disturbances, numbness in an arm or leg, severe abdominal pain, prolonged episodes of bleeding, or amenorrhea.

### Additional Considerations
- **Return of Fertility:** Delayed; as many as 30% of women may not conceive within 12 months; delay may be >2 years
- **1-Year Failure Rate, Typical vs Perfect Use:** 0.3% vs 0.3%
- **Drug Interactions:** Aminoglutethimide may significantly depress MPA levels and reduce efficacy; contraceptive efficacy is not reduced with antiepileptic (phenobarbital and carbamazepine) use

DMPA, depot medroxyprogesterone acetate; MPA, medroxyprogesterone acetate; STI, sexually transmitted infection. *Sources:* Kaunitz A. Injectable long-acting contraceptives. *Clin Obstet Gynecol.* 2001;44:82–84; Speroff L. Bone mineral density and hormonal contraception. *Dialogues in Contraception.* 2002;7:2–3.

## Vaginal Contraceptive Ring

### Device
• NuvaRing (Organon)

### Description
• Flexible, ethylene vinylacetate ring approximately 54 mm in diameter; releases 0.12 mg etonogestrel and 15 mcg EE daily

### Mechanism of Action
• Similar to COCs

### Use Issues
• **Initial Use:** Can be inserted on any day of the week once pregnancy is ruled out.
• If >5 days since start of menstrual bleeding, or postpartum, or postabortion, backup contraceptive method is recommended for 7 days.
• Self-inserted ring is left in place for 3 weeks, then removed for 1 week.
• Menses is expected during the ring-free week.

### Side Effects/Serious Adverse Effects
• Similar to COCs

### Key Counseling Points
• Does not protect against lower genital tract STIs or HIV infection.
• Spotting or BTB may occur during the first 3 cycles of use.
• Contact healthcare provider if pregnancy is suspected, or if any of the following occur: sudden severe headache, visual disturbances, numbness in an arm or leg, severe abdominal pain, prolonged episodes of bleeding, or amenorrhea.
• **Appropriate action if ring is removed:**
  ▪ *>3 hours*
     ⇨ Backup contraceptive method must be used until the ring has been used continuously for 7 days.

### Additional Considerations
• **Return of Fertility:** No delay
• **1-Year Failure Rate, Perfect Use**[a]**:** 0.3%
• **Contraindications/Precautions:** Similar to COCs
• **Drug Interactions:** Similar to COCs
• **Noncontraceptive Health Benefits:** Because the patch has been available for <2 years, studies have not been conducted that confirm long-term benefits.

BTB, breakthrough bleeding; COC, combined oral contraceptive; STI, sexually transmitted infection.
[a]Typical-use failure rate is not available, since the vaginal ring was not available at the time of the 1995 National Survey of Family Growth.

# CONTRACEPTION

## EMERGENCY POST-COITAL ORAL CONTRACEPTION
### Fast Facts

- Safety confirmed in several large multicenter trials.
- Appropriate candidate is reproductive-age women within 72 hours of unprotected coitus.
  - Often associated with failure of barrier contraception
- Treatment reduces pregnancy rate by 75% (range 55%–94%) based on published studies.
  - Effective pregnancy rate ~2%
- Other option: midcycle IUD placement
  - Failure rate 0.1%
- 98% of patients will menstruate by 21 days after treatment (mean 7–9 days).

| Brand | Company | Pills per Dose[a] | Ethinyl Estradiol per Dose (mcg) | Levonorgestrel per Dose (mg) |
|---|---|---|---|---|
| Plan B[b] | Barr | 1 white pill | 0 | 0.75 |
| Ovral | Wyeth-Ayerst | 2 white pills | 100 | 0.50 |
| Ogestrel | Watson | 2 white pills | 100 | 0.50 |
| Cryselle | Barr | 4 white pills | 120 | 0.60 |
| Levora | Watson | 4 white pills | 120 | 0.60 |
| Lo/Ovral | Wyeth-Ayerst | 4 white pills | 120 | 0.60 |
| Low-Ogestrel | Watson | 4 white pills | 120 | 0.60 |
| Levien | Berlex | 4 light orange pills | 120 | 0.60 |
| Nordette | Wyeth-Ayerst | 4 light orange pills | 120 | 0.60 |
| Portia | Barr | 4 pink pills | 120 | 0.60 |
| Seasonale | Barr | 4 pink pills | 120 | 0.60 |
| Trivora | Watson | 4 pink pills | 120 | 0.50 |
| Tri-Levlen | Berlex | 4 yellow pills | 120 | 0.50 |
| Triphasil | Wyeth-Ayerst | 4 yellow pills | 120 | 0.30 |
| Enpresse | Barr | 4 orange pills | 120 | 0.50 |
| Alesse | Wyeth-Ayerst | 5 pink pills | 100 | 0.50 |
| Lessina | Barr | 5 pink pills | 100 | 0.50 |
| Levlite | Berlex | 5 pink pills | 100 | 0.50 |
| Lutera | Watson | 5 white pills | 100 | 0.50 |
| Aviane | Barr | 5 orange pills | 100 | 0.50 |
| Ovrette | Wyeth-Ayerst | 20 yellow pills | 0 | 0.75 |

[a]The treatment schedule is one dose as soon as possible after unprotected intercourse, and another dose 12 hrs later. However, recent research has found that both doses of Plan B or Ovrette can be taken at the same time.
[b]Plan B is the only dedicated product specifically marketed for emergency contraception in the United States. Preven, combined emergency contraception pill, is no longer available on the U.S. market.
*Source:* Reprinted with permission from ACOG Practice Bulletin Number 69, December 2005. Emergency contraception. *Obstet Gynecol.* 2005;106(6):1443–1452.

## INTRAUTERINE DEVICE

### Fast Facts

- Most widely used reversible contraceptive in the world.
- <1% of U.S. couples use this excellent method of contraception.
- 2 IUD choices now available in the United States: copper IUD, levonorgestrel IUS (20 micrograms levonorgestrel released per day).

### Contraindications

- PID currently or within the past 3 months; history of recurrent PID; postabortion or postpartum endometritis or septic abortion within the past 3 months; known or suspected, untreated endocervical gonorrhea, chlamydia, or mucopurulent cervicitis; undiagnosed abnormal vaginal bleeding; pregnancy or suspicion of pregnancy; severely distorted uterine cavity; suspected or known uterine perforation occurring with placement of a uterine sound during the current insertion procedure; history of symptomatic actinomycosis confirmed by culture, but not asymptomatic colonization; known cervical cancer that has yet to be treated; known endometrial cancer; known pelvic tuberculosis; acute liver disease or liver tumor (benign or malignant); known or suspected breast cancer.

### Five-Year Cumulative Pregnancy Rates and Side Effects Leading to Discontinuation of IUD

| Side Effect | Levonorgestrel IUD | Copper IUD |
|---|---|---|
| Pregnancy | 0.5% | 5.9% |
| Bleeding problems | 13.7% | 20.9% |
| Amenorrhea | 6.0% | 0% |
| Hormonal side effects | 12.1% | 2.0% |
| Pelvic inflammatory disease | 0.8% | 2.2% |

*Source:* Leonhardt KK. 2001 Guide to Contraceptive Management. *Ob/Gyn Special Edition.* 2001;4:17–22. Reproduced with permission of McMahon Publishing Group.

### Available IUDs

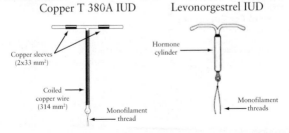

Copper T 380A IUD

Copper sleeves (2x33 mm²)

Coiled copper wire (314 mm²)

Monofilament thread

Duration of use: 10 years

Levonorgestrel IUD

Hormone cylinder

Monofilament threads

Duration of use: 5 years

# CONTRACEPTION

## Levonorgestrel IUD (Mirena)

### Description
- T-shaped device, containing 52 mg LNG covered by silicone that releases 20 mcg/day of LNG

### Mechanism of Action
- Levonorgestrel causes cervical mucus to become thicker, so sperm cannot reach ovum. Endometrial alteration may prevent implantation of fertilized ovum.

### Insertion Issues
- Must be inserted into the uterus by a healthcare professional.
- Insertion can occur anytime in a woman's cycle as long as pregnancy is ruled out. It can be inserted immediately postabortion and up to 48 hours postdelivery.
- May cause cramping and pain after insertion.

### Duration of Efficacy
- 5 years

### Side Effects/Serious Adverse Effects
- Bleeding irregularities common during the first 3–6 months of use; 20% experience amenorrhea after 1 year of use; PID, infertility; perforation of uterus.
- During the first few wks after insertion, PID may occur because of contamination of the endometrial cavity during insertion. After this time, PID occurs because of exposure to STIs.

### Key Counseling Points
- Does not protect against STIs or HIV infection.
- No increased risk of PID in monogamous couples.
- Healthcare provider should be contacted if woman experiences very heavy vaginal bleeding, bleeding lasting longer than 14 days, or non–menstrual-related lower abdominal or pelvic pain—especially if continuous and associated with fever; concern regarding pregnancy; suspected or detected full or partial expulsion; failure to feel the string.

### Additional Considerations
- Alternative to hysterectomy in women with hypermenorrhea.
- May be used as treatment for endometrial hyperplasia, adenomyosis, leiomyomas.
- **1-Year Failure Rate, Typical vs. Perfect Use:** 0.1% vs. 0.1%
- Given duration of efficacy, considered to be a good alternative to sterilization.

## Copper T IUD (ParaGard)

### Description
- A T-shaped device made of radiopaque polyethylene with added barium for x-ray visibility.

### Mechanism of Action
- Copper works as a functional spermicide, inhibiting sperm motility and acrosomal enzyme activation.

### Duration of Efficacy
- 10 years

### Side Effects/Serious Adverse Effects
- PID, infertility, perforation of uterus, possible increase of menstrual cramping and bleeding.
- During the first few weeks after insertion, PID may occur because of contamination of the endometrial cavity during insertion. After this time period, PID occurs because of exposure to STIs.

### Additional Considerations
- Given duration of efficacy, considered to be a good alternative to sterilization.
- **1-Year Failure Rate, Typical vs. Perfect Use:** 0.8% vs. 0.6%
- Should not be used in patients with copper allergies or Wilson's disease.

[a]Recent data indicate that device is highly effective for 12 years. (*Source:* United Nations Development Programme/United Nations Population Fund, World Health Organization/World Bank, Special Programme of Research, Development and Research Training in Human Reproduction. Long-term reversible contraception: twelve years of experience with the Tcu380A and Tu220C. *Contraception.* 1997;56:341–352.)

# CONTRACEPTION

## World Health Organization Eligibility Criteria for *Initiating* Use of Intrauterine Contraception

| Condition | Copper IUC | LNG-IUS |
|---|---|---|
| Obesity (BMI >30 kg/m²) | 1 | 1 |
| Multiple risk factors for CVD | 1 | 2 |
| **Hypertension** | | |
| Controlled | 1 | 1 |
| Uncontrolled | 1 | 1 (systolic 140–159 or diastolic 90–99) |
| | | 2 (systolic ≥160 or diastolic ≥100) |
| Ischemic heart disease (past/current) | 1 | 2 |
| Stroke history | 1 | 2 |
| **Diabetes** | | |
| No vascular disease/non-insulin | 1 | 2 |
| With vascular disease | 1 | 2 |
| Known thrombogenic mutations (e.g., factor V Leiden) | 1 | 2 |
| History of DVI/PE | 1 | 2 |
| Current DVI/PE | 1 | 3 |
| **Breast cancer** | | |
| Current | 1 | 4 |
| No cancer for 5 yrs | 1 | 3 |
| **Smoking** | | |
| Age <35 yrs | 1 | 1 |
| Age >35 yrs | 1 | 1 |
| Nonmigraine headaches | 1 | 1 |
| Migraines aged ≥35 yrs, no aura | 1 | 2 |
| Migraine with aura, any age | 1 | 2 |
| **Drug interactions** | | |
| Rifampicin | 1 | 1 |
| Griseofulvin | 1 | 1 |
| Antiretroviral (ARV) | | |
| Clinically well on ARV | 2 | 2 |
| Not clinically well on ARV | 3 | 3 |
| Other antibiotics | 1 | 1 |
| Certain anticonvulsants: barbiturates, carbamazepine, oxcarbazepin, phenytoin, primidone, topiramate | 1 | 1 |

BMI, body mass index; Copper IUC, copper T380A intrauterine contraceptive; CVD, cardiovascular disease; DVI, deep vein thrombosis; LNG-IUS, levonorgestrel-releasing intrauterine system; PE, pulmonary embolism.

Rating Scale:
1 = Can use the method. No restriction on use.
2 = Can use the method. Advantages generally outweigh theoretical or proven risks. If method is chosen, more than usual follow-up may be needed.
3 = Should not use the method unless clinician makes clinical judgment that the patient can safely use it. Theoretical or proven risks usually outweigh the advantages of method. Method of last choice, for which regular monitoring may be needed.
4 = Should not use the method. Condition represents an unacceptable health risk if method is used.

*Source:* Reprinted with permission from *Dialogues in Contraception.* 2006;10(2):3.

## TUBAL LIGATION

### Fast Facts
- Most frequent indication for laparoscopy in United States.
- Preoperative counseling is essential (including failure rate).
- Reversal of sterilization dependent on procedure performed.
  - Clips/bands have highest reversal success rates (>70%).
  - Incurs increased risk of ectopic pregnancy.

### Laparoscopic Tubal Ligation
- Performed as an interval procedure.
- Must clearly identify fimbria/tube.
  - Falope rings applied to the round ligament do not prevent pregnancies
- Perform prior to ovulation to prevent conception around the time of surgery.
- Most popular techniques.
  - Fulguration (with or without division), thermocautery, Falope rings, clips

### Postpartum Tubal Ligation
- Either at time of cesarean section or after vaginal delivery.
- Patient selection important.
  - No history of pelvic adhesions
  - No history of significant PID
  - Body habitus
- If patient is ambivalent, then defer to interval procedure.
- Empty bladder prior to performing procedure.
- Informed consent should always be documented.
- Be sure to follow up on path report to ensure the tubes were indeed excised.
- Uchida/Irving have lowest failure rates.

# CONTRACEPTION

## Types of Tubal Ligation

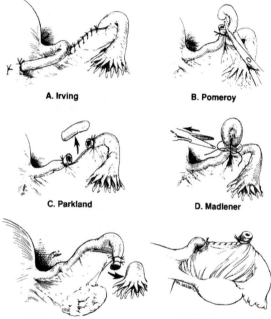

**A. Irving**

**B. Pomeroy**

**C. Parkland**

**D. Madlener**

**E. Kroener fimbriectomy**

**F. Uchida**

*Source:* Cunningham FG, MacDonald PC, Gant NF et al. Family planning. In: *Williams Obstetrics.* 20th ed. Stamford, Conn.: Appleton & Lange, 1997, and Depp R. Cesarean delivery and other surgical procedures. In: Gabbe SG, Niebyl JR, Simpson JL, ed. *Obstetrics: Normal and Problem Pregnancies.* 2nd ed. New York: Churchill Livingstone, 1991. Reproduced with the permission of the publishers.

## Hysteroscopic Sterilization (Essure Procedure)
- New hysteroscopic non-hormonal method to provide permanent sterilization.
- 99.8% effective—most effective method of permanent sterilization available.
- Usually done under local anesthesia and takes 5–30 minutes.
- Small 4 mm by 1 mm polyester/nickel/titanium/steel implants placed in proximal fallopian tube.
- Scarring forms around implant over 3 months and prevents sperm to enter fallopian tube.
- Need to do a hysterosalpingogram 3 months after insertion to verify tubal occlusion.
- Minimal menstrual changes and no hormonal changes.

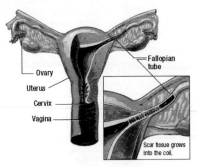

*Source:* Figure reproduced with permission from the Mayo Foundation for Medical Education and Research. All rights reserved.

### Failure Rates

| Method | Failures/1000 Procedures (95% CI) | |
|---|---|---|
| | < 30 Yrs Old | >30 Yrs Old |
| Bipolar coagulation | 31.9 (15.2–48.7) | 7.6 (1.9–13.2) |
| Unipolar coagulation | 5.9 (0.0–17.5) | 0.0 |
| Silicone rubber-band application | 11.1 (0.0–23.4) | 6.9 (0.2–13.7) |
| Spring-clip application | 7.8 (0.0–17.8) | 5.8 (0.0–14.9) |
| Interval partial salpingectomy | 14.6 (0.0–34.7) | 3.7 (0.0–11.1) |
| Postpartum partial salpingectomy | 1.2 (0.0–35) | 1.8 (0.0–5.2) |

*Source:* Modified from Peterson HB, Zhisen X, Hughes JM et al. The risk of ectopic pregnancy after tubal sterilization. *N Engl J Med.* 1997;336:762–767.

# GYNECOLOGY

## ABNORMAL UTERINE BLEEDING

### Definition
- *Dysfunctional uterine bleeding* is simply abnormal uterine bleeding (AUB) unrelated to systemic medical illness, endocrinopathy, or structural uterine anomaly → *diagnosis of exclusion.*

### Types of Abnormal Uterine Bleeding

| Term | Menses Pattern |
| --- | --- |
| Oligomenorrhea | >38-day cycle length |
| Polymenorrhea | <24-day cycle length |
| Menorrhagia | ↑Flow[a] or duration at regular intervals |
| Metrorrhagia | Regular flow at irregular intervals |
| Menometrorrhagia | ↑Flow or duration at irregular intervals |

[a]Blood loss >80 mL.

### Endometrial Sloughing
- Intense spiral arteriole vasoconstriction (prostaglandin [PG] $E_2$ and $PGF_{2\alpha}$) precedes the onset of menses (Markee, 1940).
- Two theories for the trigger of menstruation:
  1. Apoptosis, tissue regression, and release of PGs and proteases
  2. Spiral arteriole constriction and necrosis
- More than 90% of menstrual blood loss occurs during the first 3 days (Haynes et al., 1977).
- Different hemostatic mechanisms in the endometrium compared to the rest of the body:
  - Initial suppression of platelet adhesion.
  - With ↑ blood extravasation, damaged vessels are sealed by intravascular plugs of platelets and fibrin.
  - 20 hours after the onset of menses, hemostasis is achieved by further intense spiral arteriole vasoconstriction.
  - 36 hours after the start of menses, tissue regeneration is initiated.

## Systemic Etiologies for Abnormal Uterine Bleeding

Coagulation disorders
    von Willebrand's disease
    Thrombocytopenia
    Acute leukemia
    Advanced liver disease

Endocrinopathies
    Thyroid disease, hyperprolactinemia
    Polycystic ovary syndrome or elevated circulating androgens
    Cushing's syndrome

Anovulation or oligoovulation
    Idiopathic
    Stress, exercise, obesity, rapid weight changes
    Polycystic ovary syndrome or endocrinopathies as above

Drugs
    Contraception: oral/transdermal/vaginal contraceptive, intrauterine device, medroxyprogesterone acetate (Depo-Provera)
    Anticoagulants
    Antipsychotics
    Chemotherapy
    Drugs related to dopamine metabolism: tricyclic antidepressants, phenothiazines, antipsychotic drugs

Trauma
    Sexual intercourse
    Sexual abuse
    Foreign bodies
    Pelvic trauma

Other
    Urinary system disorders: urethritis, cystitis, bladder cancer
    Inflammatory bowel disease, hemorrhoids

## Genital Tract Disorders Leading to Abnormal Uterine Bleeding

|  | Uterus | Cervix | Vagina | Vulva |
|---|---|---|---|---|
| Infection | Endometritis | Cervicitis | Bacterial vaginosis, STDs, atrophic vaginitis | STD |
| Benign | Polyps, endometrial hyperplasia, adenomyosis, leiomyomas | Polyps, ectropion, endometriosis | Gartner's duct cysts, polyps, adenomyosis | Skin tags, condylomata, angiokeratoma |
| Cancer | Adenocarcinoma, sarcoma | Invasive or metastatic cancer | Vaginal cancer | Vulvar cancer |

STD, sexually transmitted disease.

# GYNECOLOGY

## Causes of Abnormal Uterine Bleeding by Age Group

- Neonates
  - Estrogen withdrawal
- Premenarchal
  - Foreign body
  - Adenomyosis
  - Trauma, abuse
  - Vulvovaginitis
  - Cancer (i.e., sarcoma botryoides)
  - Precocious puberty
- Early postmenarche
  - Anovulation: hypothalamic immaturity (>90% of cases)
  - Stress: exercise induced
  - Pregnancy
  - Infection
  - Coagulation disorder
- Reproductive age
  - Anovulation
  - Pregnancy
  - Endocrine disorder
  - Polyps/fibroids/adenomyosis
  - Medication related (oral contraceptives)
  - Infection
  - Sarcoma, ovarian
  - Coagulation disorder
- Perimenopausal
  - Anovulation leading to unopposed estrogen and hyperplasia
  - Polyp/fibroid/adenomyosis
  - Cancer
- Postmenopausal
  - Atrophy
  - Cancer/polyp
  - Estrogen therapy
  - Selective estrogen receptor modulators

*Source:* APGO Educational Series on Women;s Health. *Abnormal Uterine Bleeding.* 2002.

## Initial Evaluation

### History
- Timing: frequency, temporal pattern, last menstrual period
- Nature of bleeding: duration, postcoital, quantity, temporal pattern
- Associated symptoms: pain, fever, vaginal discharge, changes in bowel/bladder function
- Pertinent medical history, history of bleeding disorders (family history as well), and medication history
- Changes in weight, excessive exercise, chronic illness, stress

### Physical Examination
- General: signs of systemic illness, ecchymosis, thyromegaly, evidence of hyperandrogenism (hirsutism, acne, male pattern balding), acanthosis nigricans
- Pelvic: determine site of bleeding; assess contour, size, and tenderness of the uterus; any suspicious lesions or tumors

### Laboratory Testing
- Urine pregnancy test to rule out pregnancy-related bleeding
  - Serum β-human chorionic gonadotropin (β-hCG) if there has been a recent pregnancy (rule out trophoblastic disease)
- Pap smear
- Complete blood count (CBC) and platelets
- Thyroid-stimulating hormone to exclude hypothyroidism
- If history of menorrhagia since onset of menses, mucocutaneous bleeding, or family history of coagulopathy (Kouides et al., 2000), check prothrombin time/partial thromboplastin time, factor VIII, and von Willebrand's factor antigen (especially in adolescents)
- Liver function tests in those with chronic liver or renal disease
- Determine ovulatory status
  - Menstrual cycle charting: >10 days of variance from one cycle to the next suggests anovulatory cycles.
  - Normal menstrual cycle length: 24–35 days.
  - Luteinizing hormone (LH) urine predictor kit: False positives include premature ovarian failure, menopause, and polycystic ovary syndrome (on occasion).

### Endometrial Biopsy
- Perform in all women >35 years of age
- History of unopposed estrogen exposure
- Risk factors for endometrial hyperplasia:
  - Obesity, chronic anovulation, history of breast cancer, selective estrogen receptor modulator (tamoxifen) use
  - Family history of endometrial, ovarian, breast, or colon cancer (Farquhar et al., 1999)

# GYNECOLOGY

## Summary of Initial Evaluation

| |
|---|
| History and physical |
| Pregnancy tests: exclude pregnancy or trophoblastic disease |
| Pap smear |
| CBC/PLTs |
| TSH |
| LFTs (those with chronic liver or renal disease) |
| PT/PTT, factor VIII, von Willebrand's factor antigen (if suspicious history) |
| Ovulatory status |
|    Menstrual charting |
|    Luteal phase length (24–35 days) |
|    LH urine predictor kits |
| Endometrial biopsy |
| Transvaginal ultrasound (possible sonohysterogram or hysteroscopy) |

CBC, complete blood count; LFT, liver function tests; PLT, platelet; PT/PTT, prothrombin time and partial thromboplastin time; TSH, thyroid-stimulating hormone.

## Secondary Evaluation

- **Transvaginal ultrasound** (TVS) evaluates for structural lesions in the setting of abnormal pelvic examination or normal endometrial biopsy.
  - Can demonstrate a thickened endometrial lining; cannot reliably distinguish between submucous fibroids, polyps, adenomyosis, and neoplastic change.
  - Utility of TVS in excluding endometrial abnormalities is more reliable in postmenopausal women.
  - In premenopausal women, TVS should be performed on cycle days 4–6; if returns with an endometrial stripe >5 mm → obtain sonohysterogram.
  - In 200 premenopausal women with AUB, 16 of 80 women (20%!) with an endometrial stripe <5 mm had an endometrial polyp or submucosal fibroid seen on sonohysterogram (Breitkopf et al., 2004).
- **Sonohysterography** allows for careful evaluation of cavity by infusing sterile saline into the endometrial cavity and monitoring by TVS.
  - Can better detect smaller lesions such as polyps or small submucosal fibroids
  - Advantage: higher sensitivity in detecting polyps than TVS alone (94% vs. 75%, respectively) (Kamel et al., 2000)
  - Disadvantage: no tissue for histologic diagnosis
- **Hysteroscopy:** direct visualization of the endometrial cavity
  - Considered the gold standard for the diagnosis of abnormal uterine bleeding
  - Can biopsy or excise lesions identified

## Treatment

### Acute Menorrhagia

- High-dose intravenous, intramuscular, or oral estrogen
- 30-cc Foley balloon catheter (tamponade) until medical or surgical therapy can be performed
- Resuscitate with blood transfusion as needed
- Surgical: if persistent heavy vaginal bleeding, may consider dilatation and curettage

### Chronic Menorrhagia

### Medical Options

|  | ↓ Blood Flow (%) | Comments |
|---|---|---|
| Oral contraceptives | 50 | Continuous or cyclic[a] |
| Levonorgestrel intrauterine device | 80–90 | May induce amenorrhea |
| Nonsteroidal antiinflammatory drugs | 20–50 | Effective in ovulatory women |
| Cyclic progestin | — | Particularly in anovulatory bleeding |
| Antifibrinolytics (tranexamic acid, 1 g qid cycle days minus 1–4) | 50 | Side effects: nausea, leg cramps, potential deep venous thrombosis risk |
| Gonadotropin-releasing hormone agonists and antagonists | — | Hypoestrogenemia side effects: hot flashes, osteopenia; limit use to 6 mos |

[a]May need an oral contraceptive with a more estrogenic progestin, such as ethynodiol diacetate; if the endometrium is thick on oral contraceptives, then a higher dose of progestin (1 mg norethindrone) may be necessary.

### Failed Medical Therapy or Known Surgical Indication

- Hysteroscopy/dilatation and curettage.
- Endometrial ablation.
- Approximately 20% of patients require further surgery, with 10% needing hysterectomy.
- Hysterectomy: definitive surgery.

# GYNECOLOGY

## Evaluation of Pre-Menopausal Abnormal Bleeding

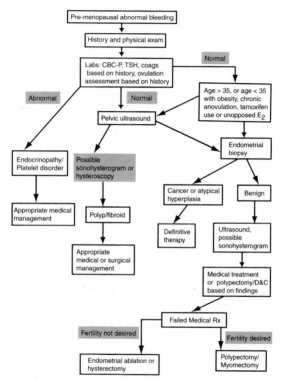

CBC-P, complete blood count/platelets; coags, coagulation disorders; D&C, dilatation and curettage; E₂, estradiol; Rx, treatment; TSH, thyroid-stimulating hormone.

**Evaluation of Post-Menopausal Abnormal Bleeding**

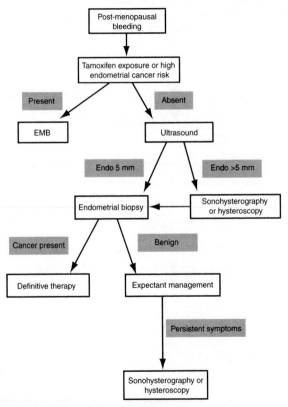

EMB, endometrial biopsy; Endo, endometrium.

# GYNECOLOGY

## ENDOMETRIAL ABLATION

### Device Comparisons Based upon Initial FDA Randomized Trials

| Device | Cervical Dilatation (mm) | Cavity Limits (cm) | Approximate Treatment Time (min) | Pretreatment Used |
|---|---|---|---|---|
| ThermaChoice (thermal balloon) | 5 | 4–10 | 8 | 3-min suction curettage |
| Hydro ThermAblator (circulated hot fluid) | 8 | 10.5 or less | 10 | GnRH agonist |
| Her Option (cryotherapy) | 5 | 10 or less | 10–18 | GnRH agonist |
| NovaSure (RF electrosurgery) | 8 | 6–10[a] | 1.5 | None |
| MEA (microwave energy) | 8.5 | 6–14 | 3.5 | GnRH agonist |

FDA, U.S. Food and Drug Administration; GnRH, gonadotropin-releasing hormone; MEA, Microsulis Endometrial Ablation; RF, radiofrequency.
[a]Cavity length: 4–6.5 cm from internal os.

### Patient Satisfaction and Amenorrhea Rates Associated with Nonresectoscopic Endometrial Ablation Compared with Resectoscopic Ablation at 12 Months[a]

| Device | Satisfaction Rate | Amenorrhea Rate[b] | Diary Success (Score: 75 or Less) |
|---|---|---|---|
| ThermaChoice (thermal balloon) | 96/99[c] | 13.2/27.2 | 80.2/84.3 |
| Hydro ThermAblator (heated free fluid) | —[d] | 35.3/47.1 | 68.4/76.4 |
| Her Option (cryotherapy) | 86/88[e] | 22.2/46.5 | 67.4/73.3 |
| NovaSure (radiofrequency electricity) | 92/93[c] | 36/32.2 | 77.7/74.4 |
| Microwave Endometrial Ablation System (microwave energy) | 92/93[c] | 55.3/45.8 | 87/83.2 |

[a]Based on the U.S. Food and Drug Administration pivotal trials.
[b]Based on intent to treat.
[c]Patients reported being satisfied or very satisfied.
[d]Quality-of-life scores compared with baseline only.
[e]Patients reported being very or extremely satisfied.
Source: Adapted from Sharp HT. Assessment of new technology in the treatment of idiopathic menorrhagia and uterine leiomyomata. Obstet Gynecol. 2006;108:990–1003.

## Contraindications to Global Endometrial Ablation

| |
|---|
| Pregnancy or desire to be pregnant in the future |
| Known or suspected endometrial carcinoma |
| Premalignant change of the endometrium[a] |
| Active pelvic inflammatory disease or hydrosalpinx[a] |
| Prior classic cesarean delivery or transmural myomectomy |
| Uterine anomaly, e.g., septate uterus, bicornuate uterus, or unicornuate uterus |
| Intrauterine device in place |
| Active urinary tract infection at the time of treatment[a] |

[a]Relative contraindications.

## Recommended Preoperative Checklist for Global Endometrial Ablation

| |
|---|
| Document-failure, refusal, or intolerance to medical management. |
| Confirm that patient does not desire future pregnancy. |
| Establish a plan for contraception. |
| Exclude endometrial hyperplasia or malignancy with a tissue sample. |
| Perform adequate endometrial imaging to exclude a lesion that would preclude the use of global endometrial ablation. |
| Exclude pregnancy. |

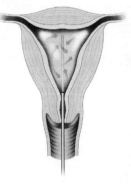

ThermaChoice uterine balloon therapy. Heated fluid circulates within the Therma-Choice uterine balloon. Illustration: John Yanson.

# GYNECOLOGY

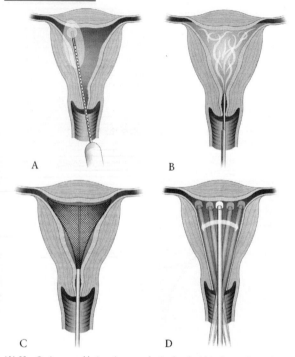

A

B

C

D

(A) Her Option cryoablation. A cryoprobe is placed within the uterine cavity near the cornu, resulting in ice ball formation. (B) Hydro Thermablation. A hysteroscope and the hydrothermablation sheath are inserted into the uterine cavity to allow heated fluid to circulate within the uterine cavity. (C) NovaSure radiofrequency ablation. The electrode fans out to fit within the uterine cavity. (D) Microwave Endometrial Ablation. The Microsulis Endometrial Ablation wand is inserted into the uterine fundus and moved back and forth while it is being withdrawn. Illustrations: John Yanson.

# ECTOPIC PREGNANCY

## Fast Facts
- Ectopic pregnancies represent 9% of all maternal deaths.
- Prior pelvic inflammatory disease, especially related to *C. trachomatis*, is the major risk factor.

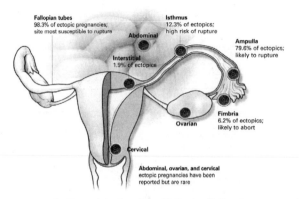

*Source:* Reprinted with permission from Buster JE, Barnhart K. Ectopic pregnancy: a 5-step plan for medical management. *OBG Management.* 2004;74–86. Artist: Scott Bodell.

## Diagnosis
- Serum β-hCG positive 8–9 days after ovulation, produced from cytotrophoblasts.
- β-hCG rises >53% in 48 hours with normal intrauterine pregnancy.
- Rule of 10s for normal pregnancies:
  - β-hCG = 100 mIU/mL at time of missed menses
  - β-hCG = 100,000 mIU/mL at 10 weeks (peak)
  - β-hCG = 10,000 mIU/mL at term
- β-hCG elimination half-life = approximately 1 day.
- 90% of ectopics have β-hCG <6500 mIU/mL.

# GYNECOLOGY

## Treatment Outcomes for Ectopic Pregnancy

| Method | Number of Studies | Number of Patients | Number with Successful Resolution |
|---|---|---|---|
| Conservative laparoscopic surgery | 32 | 1626 | 1516 (93%) |
| Variable-dose methotrexate | 12 | 338 | 314 (93%) |
| Single-dose methotrexate | 7 | 393 | 340 (87%) |
| Direct-injection methotrexate | 21 | 660 | 502 (76%) |
| Expectant management | 14 | 628 | 425 (68%) |

| Method | Tubal Patency Rate | Subsequent Fertility Rate Intrauterine Pregnancy | Ectopic |
|---|---|---|---|
| Conservative laparoscopic surgery | 170/223 (76%) | 366/647 (57%) | 87/647 (13%) |
| Variable-dose methotrexate | 136/182 (75%) | 55/95 (58%) | 7/95 (7%) |
| Single-dose methotrexate | 61/75 (81%) | 39/64 (61%) | 5/64 (8%) |
| Direct-injection methotrexate | 130/162 (80%) | 87/152 (57%) | 9/152 (6%) |
| Expectant management | 60/79 (76%) | 12/14 (86%) | 1/14 (7%) |

*Source:* Data from Pisarska MD, Carson SA, Buster JE. Ectopic pregnancy. Lancet 1998;351:1115–1120.

**Ectopic Pregnancy—Management Algorithm**

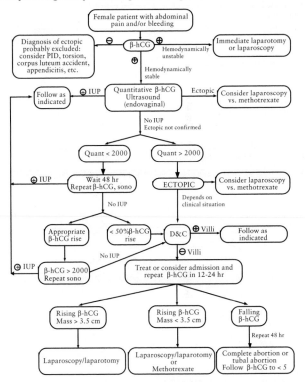

*Source:* Adapted from Carson SA, Buster JE. Ectopic pregnancy. N Engl J Med 1993; 329(16):1174–1181, and Stovall TG, Ling FW. Ectopic pregnancy. Diagnostic and therapeutic algorithms minimizing surgical intervention. J Reprod Med 1993;38(10):807–812.

# GYNECOLOGY

## Methotrexate Therapy for Ectopic Pregnancy

- Reported success rates of 67–100% in selected patients
- Indications/contraindications to methotrexate (MTX)

| Indications |
| --- |
| Unruptured |
| Ectopic mass <3.5 cm (exceptions noted) |
| No FCA (exceptions noted) |
| β-Human chorionic gonadotropin <6500 mIU/mL (exceptions noted) |
| **Contraindications** |
| Abnormal labs (creatinine [>1.3 mg/dL], liver function tests [>50 IU/L]) |
| Alcoholism, alcoholic liver disease, chronic liver disease |
| Preexisting blood dyscrasias |
| Active pulmonary disease |
| Peptic ulcer disease |
| Hepatic, renal, or hematologic dysfunction |

- Single-dose protocol (stop prenatal vitamins and folate):

| Day 1: MTX, 50 mg/m$^2$ | β-hCG, ALT, Cr, CBC, type and screen | Rh$_o$(D) immune globulin (RhoGAM; 300 mcg IM) if Rh negative. |
| --- | --- | --- |
| Day 4 | β-hCG | Usually > than initial β-hCG. |
| Day 7 | β-hCG, ALT, Cr, CBC | If not ↓ by 15% from day 4, give 2nd MTX dose (50 mg/m$^2$) or consider laparoscopy. |
| Weekly | β-hCG | Continue until <5 mIU/mL.[a] |

ALT, alanine aminotransferase; β-hCG, β-human chorionic gonadotropin; CBC, complete blood count; Cr, creatinine; MTX, methotrexate.
[a]If <15% decline in any follow-up week, protocol is repeated.

- Multidose protocol (stop prenatal vitamins and folate):

| Day 0: MTX, 1 mg/kg IM or IV | β-hCG, ALT, Cr, CBC, type and screen | RhoGAM (300 mcg IM) if Rh negative. |
| --- | --- | --- |
| Day 1: LEU, 0.1 mg/kg IM or IV | β-hCG | If not ↓ by 15% from day 0, give 2nd MTX dose on day 2. |
| Day 2: MTX | — | |
| Day 3: LEU | β-hCG | If not ↓ by 15% from day 1, give 3rd MTX dose on day 4. |
| Day 4: MTX | — | |
| Day 5: LEU | β-hCG | If not ↓ by 15% from day 3, give 4th MTX dose on day 6. |
| Day 6: MTX | — | |
| Day 7: LEU | β-hCG, ALT, Cr, CBC | If not ↓ by 15% from day 5, laparoscopy. |
| Weekly | β-hCG | Continue until <5 mIU/mL.[a] |

ALT, alanine aminotransferase; β-hCG, β-human chorionic gonadotropin; CBC, complete blood count; Cr, creatinine; LEU, leucovorin; MTX, methotrexate; RhoGAM, Rh$_o$(D) immune globulin.
[a]Discontinue treatment when there is a decline in two consecutive βhCG titers or after four doses, whichever comes first.

- Average time to resolution (β-hCG <15 mIU/mL) for those successfully treated with MTX = approximately 35 days, although it can take up to 109 days (Lipscomb et al., 1998).
- Longest interval between initial treatment and rupture = 42 days (Lipscomb et al., 2000).
- Pretreatment β-hCG level is the only significant prognosticator of failure (Lipscomb et al., 1999).
- Previous EP appears to be an independent risk factor for MTX failure (failure rate of 18.6% in those with a prior EP compared to a 6.8% failure rate for first-time EP) (Lipscomb et al., 2004).

| β-Human Chorionic Gonadotropin Level (mIU/mL) | Failure Rate (%) |
|---|---|
| <1000 | 1.7 |
| 1000–9999 | 7–13 |
| 10,000–14,999 | 18 |
| >15,000 | 32 |

*Source:* Adapted from Lipscomb GH, McCord ML, Stovall TG, et al. Predictors of success of methotrexate treatment in women with tubal ectopic pregnancies. *N Engl J Med*. 1999;341:1974. Copyright © 1999 Massachusetts Medical Society. All rights reserved.

- If the initial β-hCG <1000 mIU/mL, 88% resolve without MTX (this is equivalent to MTX efficiency) (Trio et al., 1995).

## BODY SURFACE AREA NOMOGRAM

| Height | Surface area | Weight |
|---|---|---|
| cm 200 — 79 in<br>78<br>195 — 77<br>76<br>190 — 75<br>74<br>185 — 73<br>72<br>180 — 71<br>70<br>175 — 69<br>68<br>170 — 67<br>66<br>165 — 65<br>64<br>160 — 63<br>62<br>155 — 61<br>60<br>150 — 59<br>58<br>145 — 57<br>56<br>140 — 55<br>54<br>135 — 53<br>52<br>130 — 51<br>50<br>125 — 49<br>48<br>120 — 47<br>46<br>115 — 45<br>44<br>110 — 43<br>42<br>105 — 41<br>40<br>cm 100 — 39 in | 2.80 m²<br>2.70<br>2.60<br>2.50<br>2.40<br>2.30<br>2.20<br>2.10<br>2.00<br>1.95<br>1.90<br>1.85<br>1.80<br>1.75<br>1.70<br>1.65<br>1.60<br>1.55<br>1.50<br>1.45<br>1.40<br>1.35<br>1.30<br>1.25<br>1.20<br>1.15<br>1.10<br>1.05<br>1.00<br>0.95<br>0.90<br>0.85 m² | kg 150 — 330 lb<br>145 — 320<br>140 — 310<br>135 — 300<br>130 — 290<br>125 — 280<br>270<br>120 — 260<br>115 — 250<br>110 — 240<br>105 — 230<br>100 — 220<br>95 — 210<br>90 — 200<br>85 — 190<br>180<br>80 — 170<br>75 — 160<br>70 — 150<br>65 — 140<br>60 — 130<br>55 — 120<br>50 — 110<br>105<br>45 — 100<br>95<br>40 — 90<br>85<br>35 — 80<br>75<br>70<br>kg 30 — 66 lb |

*Source:* DiSaia PJ, Creasman WT. Epithelial ovarian cancer. In: *Clinical Gynecologic Oncology.* 4th ed. St. Louis: Mosby Year Book, 1993. Reproduced with the permission of the publisher.

## FALSE-POSITIVE BETA-HCG

- Frequency of false-positive β-hCG: between 1 in 10,000 and 1 in 100,000 tests.
- False-positive β-hCG usually <150 mIU/mL.
- Most false positives are due to interference by non-hCG substances (i.e., anti–animal immunoglobulin antibodies).
- Characteristically, the serum is positive, but the urine is negative because the heterophilic antibodies are usually immunoglobulins G with a molecular weight of ~160,000 diopter and are not easily filtered through the renal glomeruli. In addition, serial dilutions of serum are not parallel to the hCG standard.

### Causes of False-Positive Serum hCG

| |
|---|
| Interference by non-hCG substances |
|     Anti–animal heterophilic immunoglobulin antibodies |
|     hLH or hLH β-subunit |
|     Rheumatoid factor |
|     Nonspecific serum factors |
| Injection of exogenous hCG |
| Pituitary hCG-like substance |
| Assay contaminants |

hCG, human chorionic gonadotropin; hLH, human luteinizing hormone.

# GYNECOLOGY

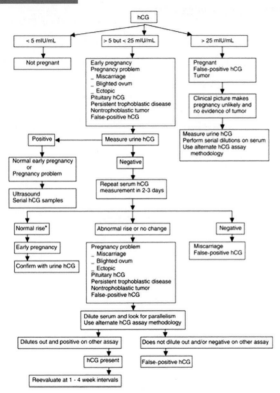

*Slowest or minimal rise of human chorionic gonadotropin (hCG) for a normal pregnancy: 1 day = 24%; 2 days = 53% (*Source:* Adapted from Braunstein, GD. False-positive serum human chorionic gonadotropin results: causes, characteristics, and recognition. *Am J Obstet Gynecol.* 2002;187[1]:217.)

## EVALUATION OF THE SEXUAL ASSAULT PATIENT

### Fast Facts

- Sexual assault is the most underreported crime in the United States.
- 50% of assaults occur in the victim's home.
- Ob/Gyn physicians are often required to provide ER evaluation of rape victims.
- Use of special consent forms and rape victim evaluation kit can be helpful.

### Rape Tray Contents

1. Sealed package of microscope slides with frosted tips
2. Eye dropper bottle with 0.9% normal saline
3. Six to twelve packages of sterile cotton swabs
4. Eight to twelve sterile tubes
5. Urine container
6. Sterile, unused, and packaged comb
7. Sterile scissors
8. Two to four Papanicolaou smear mailers
9. Package of gummed labels
10. Nail scraper
11. An outline for conducting the examination

### Evaluation

### History

1. Age
2. Marital status
3. Parity
4. Menstrual history
5. Contraceptive usage
6. Time of last coitus prior to assault
7. Condom use at last coitus prior to assault and/or douching afterward
8. Drug or alcohol use
9. Past or present venereal disease
10. Mental illness or deficiency
11. Gynecologic surgery
12. Drug allergies
13. Description of the assailant and any knowledge of his identity
14. Circumstances surrounding the assault, particularly:
    - Did the assailant's penis penetrate the vulva?
    - Did the assailant experience orgasm?
    - Did the assailant wear a condom?
    - Did extragenital acts occur?
    - Did the assailant display or use a weapon?
15. Location of the assault
16. Time and date of the assault
17. Any reasons the assailant may have targeted the patient
18. Patient's actions since the assault, particularly

| | | |
|---|---|---|
| • Douching | • Urination | • Brushing teeth |
| • Bathing or showering | • Defecation | • Changing clothes |

# GYNECOLOGY

## Examination
- Have patient disrobe while standing on white sheet.
- Place clothing in sealed plastic bag.

### Pelvic Examination
- Note
  - Condition of pubic hair (? matted, bloody, etc.).
  - Trauma to vulva.
  - Condition of hymen, anus, rectum.
  - Condition of vagina.
  - Condition of cervix.

## Laboratory Testing
- Saline prep for sperm (note motility)
- Papanicolaou smear or Gram's stain for sperm (request on sheet)
- Gonorrhea and *Chlamydia* smear/culture (including rectal if appropriate)
- Serologic testing for human immunodeficiency virus (HIV), syphilis, hepatitis B, cytomegalovirus, herpes simplex virus
- Serum pregnancy test
- Blood alcohol level, urine drug toxicology screen

## Options for Sexually Transmitted Disease Prophylaxis
- 250 mg ceftriaxone IM plus 100 mg of doxycycline orally bid × 7 days
- 2 g spectinomycin IM plus 100 mg of doxycycline orally bid × 7 days
- 500 mg of erythromycin tid or 1 g of azithromycin (for pregnant patients)

## HIV Postexposure Assessment of Adolescent and Adult Survivors within 72 Hours of Sexual Assault
- Assess risk for HIV infection in the assailant.
- Evaluate characteristics of the assault event that might increase risk for HIV transmission.
- Consult with a specialist in HIV treatment, if postexposure prophylaxis (PEP) is being considered.
- If the survivor appears to be at risk for HIV transmission from the assault, discuss antitetroviral prophylaxis, including toxicity and lack of proven benefit.
- If the survivor chooses to start antiretroviral PEP, provide enough medication to last until the next return visit; to evaluate the survivor 3–7 days after initial assessment and assess tolerance of medications.
- If PEP is started, perform CBC and serum chemistry at baseline (initiation of PEP should not be delayed, pending results).
- Perform HIV antibody test at original assessment; repeat at 6 weeks, 3 months, and 6 months.

## Protection against Pregnancy (Yuzpe Method)

• 2 doses taken 12 hours apart with an antiemetic (also see pg. 260)

## Follow-Up

• Only 20–30% of patients will return for follow-up.
• Consider arranging for patient to be seen by same MD in follow-up.

## Follow-Up Testing

> 2 weeks: Gonorrhea/*Chlamydia*
> 4 weeks: Hepatitis B
> 6 weeks: Pregnancy, *Trichomonas*, human papillomavirus, vaginosis
> 3 months: Gonorrhea/*Chlamydia*, HIV
> 6 months: Hepatitis B, HIV, rapid plasma reagin

*Sources:* Halbert, DR. Treating rape victims: are you prepared? *OBG Management.* 1995;7(11):39–50. Copyright 1995 Dowden Publishing Company, Montvale, NJ. Reproduced with permission. Antiretroviral postexposure prophylaxis after sexual, injection-drug use, or other nonoccupational exposure to HIV in the united states *MMWR* January 21, 2005;54(RR02):1–20.

# GYNECOLOGY

## PELVIC PAIN

### Fast Facts

- Frustrating disease for patient and physician
- Many possible etiologies
- Excessive use of narcotics can lead to drug dependency

### Etiology

### Gynecologic

Extrauterine
Adhesions
Chronic ectopic pregnancy
Chronic pelvic infection
Endometriosis
Residual ovary syndrome
Uterine
Adenomyosis
Chronic endometritis
Leiomyomata
Intrauterine contraceptive device
Pelvic congestion
Pelvic support defects
Polyps

### Urologic

Chronic urinary tract infection
Detrusor overactivity
Interstitial cystitis
Stone
Suburethral diverticulitis
Urethral syndrome

### Gastrointestinal

Cholelithiasis
Chronic appendicitis
Constipation
Diverticular disease
Enterocolitis
Gastric/duodenal ulcer
Inflammatory bowel disease (Crohn's disease, ulcerative colitis)
Irritable bowel syndrome
Neoplasia

**Musculoskeletal**
  Coccydynia
  Disk problems
  Degenerative joint disease
  Fibromyositis
  Hernias
  Herpes zoster (shingles)
  Low back pain
  Levator ani syndrome (spasm of pelvic floor)
  Myofascial pain (trigger points, spasms)
  Nerve entrapment syndromes
  Osteoporosis (fractures)
  Pain posture
  Scoliosis/lordosis/kyphosis
  Strains/sprains

**Other**
  Abuse (physical or sexual, prior or current)
  Heavy metal poisoning (lead, mercury)
  Hyperparathyroidism
  Porphyria
  Psychiatric disorders (depression, bipolar disorders, inadequate personality
    disorder)
  Psychosocial stress (marital discord, work stress)
  Sickle cell disease
  Sleep disturbances
  Somatoform disorders
  Substance use (especially cocaine)
  Sympathetic dystrophy
  Tabes dorsalis (third-degree syphilis)

*Source:* American College of Obstetricians and Gynecologists. *Chronic Pelvic Pain.* ACOG Technical Bulletin, Number 223, May 1996. Copyright 1996 American College of Obstetricians and Gynecologists. Reproduced with permission.

# GYNECOLOGY

## Gynecologic Conditions That May Cause or Exacerbate Chronic Pelvic Pain, by Level of Evidence

---

### Level A[a]

- Gynecologic malignancies (especially late stage)
- Ovarian retention syndrome (residual ovary syndrome)
- Ovarian remnant syndrome
- Pelvic congestion syndrome
- Pelvic inflammatory disease[b]
- Tuberculous salpingitis

### Level B[c]

- Adhesions[b]
- Benign cystic mesothelioma
- Leiomyomata[b]
- Postoperative peritoneal cysts

### Level C[d]

- Adenomyosis
- Atypical dysmenorrhea or ovulatory pain
- Adnexal cysts (nonendometriotic)
- Cervical stenosis
- Chronic ectopic pregnancy
- Chronic endometritis
- Endometrial or cervical polyps
- Endosalpingiosis
- Intrauterine contraceptive device
- Ovarian ovulatory pain
- Residual accessory ovary
- Symptomatic pelvic relaxation (genital prolapse)

---

[a]Level A: good and consistent scientific evidence of causal relation ship to chronic pelvic pain.
[b]Diagnosis frequently reported in published series of women with chronic pelvic pain.
[c]Level B: limited or inconsistent scientific evidence of causal relationship to chronic pelvic pain.
[d]Level C: causal relationship to chronic pelvic pain based on expert opinions.
*Source:* Reprinted with permission from ACOG Practice Bulletin Number 51. Chronic pelvic pain. *Obstet Gynecol.* 2004;103(3):589–605.

## Nongynecologic Conditions That May Cause or Exacerbate Chronic Pelvic Pain, by Level of Evidence

| Level of Evidence | Urologic | Gastrointestinal | Musculoskeletal | Other |
|---|---|---|---|---|
| Level A[a] | Bladder malignancy | Carcinoma of the colon | Abdominal wall myofascial pain (trigger points) | Abdominal cutaneous nerve entrapment in surgical scar |
| | Interstitial cystitis[b] | Constipation | Chronic coccygeal or back pain[b] | Depression[b] |
| | Radiation cystitis | Inflammatory bowel disease | Faulty or poor posture | Somatization disorder |
| | Urethral syndrome | Irritable bowel syndrome[c] | Fibromyalgia | |
| | | | Neuralgia of iliohypogastric, ilioinguinal, and/or genitofemoral nerves | |
| | | | Pelvic floor myalgia (levator ani or piriformis syndrome) | |
| | | | Peripartum pelvic pain syndrome | |
| Level B[c] | Uninhibited bladder contractions (detrusor dyssynergia) | — | Herniated nucleus pulposus | Celiac disease |
| | Urethral diverticulum | | Low back pain[b] | Neurologic dysfunction |
| | | | Neoplasia of spinal cord or sacral nerve | Porphyria |
| | | | | Shingles |
| | | | | Sleep disturbances |
| Level C[d] | Chronic urinary tract infection | Colitis | Compression of lumbar vertebrae | Abdominal epilepsy |
| | Recurrent, acute cystitis | Chronic intermittent bowel obstruction | Degenerative joint disease | Abdominal migraine |
| | Recurrent, acute urethritis | Diverticular disease | Hernias: ventral, inguinal, femoral, spigelian | Bipolar personality disorders |
| | Stone/urolithiasis | | Muscular strains and sprains | Familial Mediterranean fever |
| | | | Rectus tendon strain | |
| | Urethral caruncle | | Spondylosis | |

[a]Level A: good and consistent scientific evidence of causal relationship to chronic pelvic pain
[b]Diagnosis frequently reported in published series of women with chronic pelvic pain
[c]Level B: limited or inconsistent scientific evidence of causal relationship to chronic pelvic pain
[d]Level C: causal relationship to chronic pelvic pain based on expert opinions
*Source:* Reprinted with permission from ACOG Practice Bulletin Number 51. Chronic pelvic pain. *Obstet Gynecol.* 2004;103(3):589–605.

# GYNECOLOGY

## Strategies for Treating Primary Dysmenorrhea

| Strategy | Route/Dose | Advantages | Disadvantages |
|---|---|---|---|
| **Ovulation suppression** | | | |
| Hormonal contraceptives | Oral, transdermal, intravaginal | Provides contraception, regular bleeding, lighter flow | 21 days of medication for 2–4 days of relief, prescription required |
| **Prostaglandin suppression** | | | |
| Ibuprofen | Oral (800 mg to 1200 mg initial, 800 mg every 6 hrs) | Widely available, proven effective | Risk of gastrointestinal upset, prescription required |
| Mefenamic acid (Ponstel) | Oral (250 mg to 500 mg initial, 250 mg, every 6 hrs) | Proven effective in reducing uterine activity and subjective pain | Risk of gastrointestinal upset, prescription required |
| Naproxen sodium (Anaprox, Naprosyn) | Oral (250 mg to 500 mg initial, 250 mg twice daily) | Widely available, proven effective in reducing uterine activity and subjective pain, twice daily dosing | Risk of gastrointestinal upset, prescription required |
| **Continuous low-level topical heat** | | | |
| ThermaCare | Topical (low abdomen or back) | Non-prescription, no systemic side effects, proven effective in reducing uterine activity and subjective pain (comparable to prescription therapy), individual heat patches effective for 8–10 hrs | Effectiveness reduced if heat patch is deprived of oxygen |

*Source:* Reprinted with permission from Smith RP. Finding the best approach to dysmenorrhea. *Cont OB/GYN.* 2006;Nov:54–60. *Cont OB/GYN* is a copyrighted publication of Advanstar Communications Inc. All rights reserved.

**Evaluation and Treatment Algorithm**

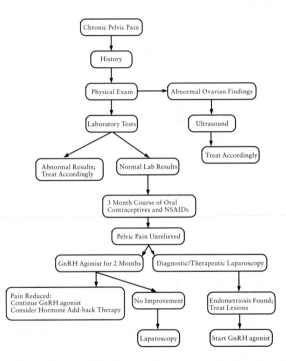

*Source:* Carter JE, Trotter JP, GnRH analogs in the treatment of endometriosis: clinical and economic considerations. *The Female Patient.* 1995;20:13–18. Adapted with permission.

# GYNECOLOGY

## ENDOMETRIOSIS

### Fast Facts

- Found in 5–15% of reproductive age women undergoing laparoscopy.
- $1/3$ of these have infertility concerns.
- Symptoms: none (!), cyclic pre- and peri-menstrual pain, dyspareunia (vaginal hyperalgesia), chronic pelvic pain, dyschezia, infertility.

### Etiology

- Sampson: retrograde flow (monkey studies)
- Halban: lymphatic-vascular spreading (lung, brain, pericardium)
- Meyer: coelomic (found in males and infants)
- Dmowski: decrease in cellular immunity

### Pathology

- Ectopic endometrial glands
- Ectopic endometrial stroma
- Adjacent hemorrhage
- Common locations: uterosacral ligament, ovary, cul-de-sac

### Treatment

#### Medical
##### Primary therapy
Gonadotropin-releasing hormone (GnRH) agonists

- Buserelin
- Triptorelin
- Decapeptyl
- Goserelin (Zoladex)
- Leuprolide (Lupron)
- Nafarelin (Synarel)

Consider treatment of hypoestrogenic side effects

- Daily medroxyprogesterone acetate 2.5 mg plus conjugated estrogens 0.625 mg
- Daily norethindrone 5.0 mg

##### Alternatives (side effects, costs, duration of treatment >6 months)
Continuous oral contraceptives for 6–12 months
Medroxyprogesterone acetate 30 mg PO q day (must provide additional contraception)
Depot medroxyprogesterone acetate subcutaneous-104 × 3 months
Danazol 200–800 mg PO q day × 6 months
Aromatase inhibitors (Femara 2.5 mg PO q day with continuous oral contraceptives)

## American Society for Reproductive Medicine Scoring System for Endometriosis

AMERICAN SOCIETY FOR REPRODUCTIVE MEDICINE
REVISED CLASSIFICATION OF ENDOMETRIOSIS

Patient's Name ........................................ Date ....................

Stage I (Minimal) - 1-5
Stage II (Mild) - 6-15
Stage III (Moderate) - 16-40
Stage IV (Severe) - >40
Total ..................

Laparoscopy............. Laparotomy............. Photography.............
Recommended Treatment....................................................

Prognosis....................................................

| PERITONEUM | ENDOMETRIOSIS | | <1cm | 1-3cm | >3cm |
|---|---|---|---|---|---|
| | Superficial | | 1 | 2 | 4 |
| | Deep | | 2 | 4 | 6 |
| OVARY | R | Superficial | 1 | 2 | 4 |
| | | Deep | 4 | 16 | 20 |
| | L | Superficial | 1 | 2 | 4 |
| | | Deep | 4 | 16 | 20 |

| | POSTERIOR CULDESAC OBLITERATION | | Partial | | Complete |
|---|---|---|---|---|---|
| | | | 4 | | 40 |

| | ADHESIONS | | <1/3 Enclosure | 1/3-2/3 Enclosure | >2/3 Enclosure |
|---|---|---|---|---|---|
| OVARY | R | Filmy | 1 | 2 | 4 |
| | | Dense | 4 | 8 | 16 |
| | L | Filmy | 1 | 2 | 4 |
| | | Dense | 4 | 8 | 16 |
| TUBE | R | Filmy | 1 | 2 | 4 |
| | | Dense | 4* | 8* | 16 |
| | L | Filmy | 1 | 2 | 4 |
| | | Dense | 4* | 8* | 16 |

*If the fimbriated end of the fallopian tube is completely enclosed, change the point assignment to 16.

Denote appearance of superficial implant types as red [(R), red, red-pink, flamelike, vesicular blobs, clear vesicles], white [(W), opacifications, peritoneal defects, yellow-brown], or black [(B) black, hemosiderin deposits, blue]. Denote percent of total described as R.....% W.....% and B.....%. Total should equal 100%.

Additional Endometriosis: ........................................

Associated Pathology: ........................................

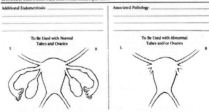

To Be Used with Normal Tubes and Ovaries

To Be Used with Abnormal Tubes and/or Ovaries

*Source:* Revised American Society for Reproductive Medicine classification of endometriosis: 1996. *Fertil Steril.* 1997;(67):817–821. Reproduced with the permission of the publisher, the American Society for Reproductive Medicine.

**EXAMPLES & GUIDELINES**

| STAGE I (MINIMAL) | STAGE II (MILD) | STAGE III (MODERATE) |
|---|---|---|

PERITONEUM
Superficial Endo – 1-3cm · 2
R. OVARY
Superficial Endo – < 1cm · 1
Filmy Adhesions – < 1/3 · 1
TOTAL POINTS 4

PERITONEUM
Deep Endo – >3cm · 6
R. OVARY
Superficial Endo – < 1cm · 1
Filmy Adhesions – < 1/3 · 1
L. OVARY
Superficial Endo – < 1cm · 1
TOTAL POINTS 9

PERITONEUM
Deep Endo – >3cm · 6
CULDESAC
Partial Obliteration · 4
L. OVARY
Deep Endo – 1-3cm · 16
TOTAL POINTS 26

| STAGE III (MODERATE) | STAGE IV (SEVERE) | STAGE IV (SEVERE) |
|---|---|---|

PERITONEUM
Superficial Endo – >3cm · 4
R. OVARY
Filmy Adhesions – < 1/3 · 1
R. OVARY
Filmy Adhesions – < 1/3 · 1
L. TUBE
Dense Adhesions – < 1/3 · 16*
L. OVARY
Deep Endo – < 1 cm · 4
Dense Adhesions – < 1/3 · 4
TOTAL POINTS 30

PERITONEUM
Superficial Endo – >3cm · 4
L. OVARY
Deep Endo – 1-3cm · 32**
Dense Adhesions – < 1/3 · 8**
L. TUBE
Dense Adhesions – < 1/3 · 8**
TOTAL POINTS 52

PERITONEUM
Deep Endo – >3cm · 6
CULDESAC
Complete Obliteration · 40
R. OVARY
Deep Endo – 1-3cm · 16
Dense Adhesions – < 1/3 · 4
L. TUBE
Dense Adhesions – >2/3 · 16
L. OVARY
Deep Endo – 1-3cm · 16
Dense Adhesions – >2/3 · 16
TOTAL POINTS 114

*Point assignment changed to 16
**Point assignment doubled

Determination of the stage or degree of endometrial involvement is based on a weighted point system. Distribution of points has been arbitrarily determined and may require further revision or refinement as knowledge of the disease increases.

To ensure complete evaluation, inspection of the pelvis in a clockwise or counterclockwise fashion is encouraged. Number, size and location of endometrial implants, plaques, endometriomas and/or adhesions are noted. For example, five separate 0.5cm superficial implants on the peritoneum (2.5 cm total) would be assigned 2 points. (The surface of the uterus should be considered peritoneum.) The severity of the endometriosis or adhesions should be assigned the highest score only for peritoneum, ovary, tube or culdesac. For example, a 4cm superficial and a 2cm deep implant of the peritoneum should be given a score of 6 (not 8). A 4cm

deep endometrioma of the ovary associated with more than 3cm of superficial disease should be scored 20 (not 24).

In those patients with only one adnexa, points applied to disease of the remaining tube and ovary should be multiplied by two. **Points assigned may be circled and totaled. Aggregation of points indicates stage of disease (minimal, mild, moderate, or severe).

The presence of endometriosis of the bowel, urinary tract, fallopian tube, vagina, cervix, skin etc., should be documented under "additional endometriosis." Other pathology such as tubal occlusion, leiomyomata, uterine anomaly, etc., should be documented under "associated pathology." All pathology should be depicted as specifically as possible on the sketch of pelvic organs, and means of observation (laparoscopy or laparotomy) should be noted.

*Source:* Revised American Society for Reproductive Medicine classification of endometriosis: 1996. *Fertil Steril.* 1997;(67):817–821. Reproduced with the permission of the publisher, the American Society for Reproductive Medicine.

## GONADOTROPIN-RELEASING HORMONE ANALOGS

### Fast Facts

- Native GnRH is a decapeptide.
- Substitutions at position 6 produce various agonists.
- Native LH releasing hormone isolated 1971 by Schally and Guillemin.
- Secreted in pulsatile fashion by hypothalamus.
- Serum half-life 2–8 minutes.
- Initiates synthesis and release of LH and follicle-stimulating hormone.

### Analogs

- Most agonists substitution of D amino acid at position 6.
- Most antagonists substitutions and modification at position 2.
- Use of agonists results in transient upregulation of GnRH receptors followed by reversible downregulation and desensitization.

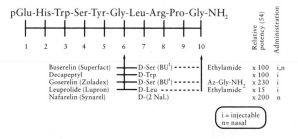

### Indications

- Endometriosis
- Leiomyomata (preoperative shrinkage)
- In vitro fertilization and other assisted reproductive technologies
- Precocious puberty
- Prostate carcinoma
- Breast carcinoma (many trials)

### Adverse Effects

- Hypoestrogenic state (hot flashes, decreased libido, vaginal dryness, decreased bone mass)
- Androgenic (acne, myalgias, edema, weight gain)

# GYNECOLOGY

## Add-Back Therapy for GnRH-a (Lupron) Patients

| Author (reference) | No. of Patients | Add-Back Therapy | Symptoms | Vasomotor Symptoms | Bone Mineral Density |
|---|---|---|---|---|---|
| Surrey et al. | 19 | a) NEt (10 mg/day) | ↓ | ↓ | No change |
| | | b) NEt (2.5 mg/day) + cyclic etidronate disodium (400 mg/day) | ↓ | ↓ | No change (DXA spine) |
| Hornstein et al. | 201 | a) NEt Ac (5 mg/day) | ↓ | ↓ | No change |
| | | b) NEt Ac (5 mg/day) + CEE (0.625 mg/day) | ↓ | ↓ | No change |
| | | c) NEt Ac (5 mg/day) + CEE (1.25 mg/day) | ↓ | ↓ | No change (DXA spine) (All less than GnRH-a alone) |

CEE, conjugated equine estrogens; DXA, dual energy x-ray absorptiometry; GnRH-a, gonadotropin-releasing hormone agonist; NEt, norethindrone; NEt Ac, norethindrone acetate.

## Add-Back Regimens

| GnRH-Agonist Use | Add-Back | Bone Density Scan | Recommended Agent |
|---|---|---|---|
| 6 mos | Optional | High-risk patients only | a) Norethindrone acetate 2.5 mg daily b) Conjugated equine estrogens 0.3–0.625 mg (or equivalent) + medroxy-progesterone acetate 5 mg daily |
| 6–12 mos | Required | Every 6–12 mos | Norethindrone acetate 5 mg daily |
| Retreatment | Required | Prior to retreatment | Norethindrone acetate 5 mg daily |

Source: Data from Surrey et al. Prolonged gonadotropin-releasing hormone agonist treatment of symptomatic endometriosis: the role of cyclic sodium etidronate and low-dose norethindrone "add-back" therapy. Fertil Steril 1995;63:747–755; and Hornstein et al. Leuprolide acetate depot and hormonal add-back in endometriosis: a 12-month study. Lupron Add-Back Study Group. Obstet Gynecol 1998;91:16–24.

## LAPAROSCOPY

### Fast Facts
- 1805 Bozzanie examines urethra with light reflector.
- 1910 Jocobaeus in Sweden creates pneumoperitoneum in humans and uses endoscope.
- 1968 Cohen and Fear write first American article in 30 years.
- 1970s Semm in Germany describes techniques for adhesion lysis, adnexectomy, and myomectomy.
- 1972 American Association of Gynecologic Laparoscopists founded.
- 1973 Shapiro and Adler describe laparoscopic removal of ectopic pregnancy.

### Indications

#### Diagnosis
- Evaluation of benign pelvic mass
- Pelvic pain
- Acute (torsion, pelvic inflammatory disease, ectopic, appendicitis, etc.)
- Infertility
- Evaluation of uterine perforation
- Evaluation of pelvis prior to vaginal hysterectomy

#### Therapy
- Sterilization
- Fulguration of endometriosis
- Ectopic pregnancy
- Gamete intrafallopian transfer
- Ovarian cystectomy
- Oophorectomy
- Lysis of adhesions
- Appendectomy
- ? Hysterectomy, myomectomy, incontinence surgery

### Pre-op Evaluation
- Patients must be well informed about all risks of planned procedure
- Routine history and physical
- Laboratory studies as indicated ($\beta$-hCG, CBC, etc.)
- Bowel prep where appropriate (GoLytely or Fleet's enema)
- Antibiotics at discretion of surgeon

### Critical Analysis
- Fair evidence to suggest superiority of laparoscopy in treatment of
  - Ectopic pregnancy
  - Endometriosis
  - Polycystic ovary syndrome resistant to clomiphene

*Superiority of laparoscopy over laparotomy in more advanced procedures requires further evaluation and is more surgeon-specific.*

# GYNECOLOGY

## HYSTEROSCOPY

### Fast Facts
- 1895 Bumm reports on uterine endoscope.
- 1914 Heineberg introduces improved uteroscope.
- 1925 Rubin describes using $CO_2$ as distention media.
- 1968 Menken uses high viscosity media.

### Indications

#### Abnormal Uterine Bleeding
- Diagnosis and therapy
  - Ablation of endometrium
  - Excision of endometrial polyps
  - Excision of submucous fibroids

#### Intrauterine Foreign Bodies
- Diagnosis and therapy
  - Location of displaced intrauterine device with visually directed removal of intrauterine device
  - Location of foreign bodies with visually directed removal of foreign bodies

#### Infertility or Recurrent Pregnancy Wastage
- Diagnosis and therapy
  - Resection of müllerian fusion defects
  - Division of endometrial adhesions

### Intrauterine Evaluation

| Anatomic Abnormality | Hysteroscopy | D&C | HSG | Ultrasound | MRI |
|---|---|---|---|---|---|
| Fibroids | | | | | |
| Intramural | + | – | + | +++ | +++ |
| Submucous | +++ | + | ++ | ++ | +++ |
| Intrauterine synechiae | +++ | | ++ | – | – |
| Bicornuate/septate uterus | +++ | + | +++ | + | +++ |
| Endometrial polyps | ++ | + | + | + | ++ |
| Endometrial hyperplasia | +++ | +++ | – | + | – |
| Endometrial cancer | ++ | +++ | + | + | – |
| Assessing tubal patency | +/– | | +++ | – | – |

–, not helpful; +, occasionally helpful; ++, often helpful; +++, very helpful.
D&C, dilatation and curettage; HSG, hysterosalpingogram.
*Sources:* Corfman RS. Indications for hysteroscopy. *Obstet Gynecol Clin NA.* 1988;15(1):41–49. Lavy G. Hysteroscopy as a diagnostic aid. *Obstet Gynecol Clin NA.* 1988;15(1):61–72.

## Comparison of Hysteroscopic Distention Media

| Medium | Benefits | Caveats | Complications |
|---|---|---|---|
| **Gas** | | | |
| $CO_2$ | Widely available<br>Safe<br>Rapidly absorbed | Limited diagnostic visibility due to bubbles and blood<br><br>Keep flow rate <100 mL/min and intra-uterine pressure <150 mm Hg | Gas embolism |
| **Hypotonic, electrolyte-free, nonconductive solutions** | | | |
| Glycine 1.5% (200 mosm)<br>Sorbitol/manitol (178 mosm)<br>Manitol 5% (280 mosm) | Electrolyte-free | Must be used for monopolar cautery | Hypotonic fluid overload leading to hyponatremia, hypoosmolarity, and cerebral edema |
| **Isotonic, electrolyte-containing solutions** | | | |
| Normal saline (308 mosm)<br>Lactated Ringers (273 mosm) | Aqueous<br>Safe<br>Fewer complications | Cannot be used for monopolar cautery | Isotonic fluid overload |
| **High-viscosity solutions** | | | |
| Hyskon (32% dextran) | Nonconductive and immiscible with blood<br>No electrolytes | Functions as a plasma expander | Anaphylaxis<br>Hypotonic fluid overload |

$CO_2$, carbon dioxide.

# GYNECOLOGY

## POST OPERATIVE MANAGEMENT

### Post-Operative Orders

1. Admit
2. Because... Diagnosis
3. Condition
4. Diet
5. Exercise... Activity
6. Fluids (IV)
7. Graphics (vitals, weights, urine output, etc.)
8. Hypersensitivities... Allergies
9. Input/Output
10. Junk (Foley, nasogastric tube, stereotactic catheter drainage, spirometry, drains)
11. Call house officer for...
12. Labs
13. Meds
14. Narcotics (see patient controlled analgesia [PCA] orders)
15. Oxygen
16. Position (semi-Fowler's, knee chest, etc.)
17. Respiratory therapy
18. X-rays

### Patient-Controlled Analgesia

| Drug | Bolus Dose (mg) | Lockout Interval (min) | Continuous Infusion (mg/h) |
|------|-----------------|------------------------|----------------------------|
| Agonists | | | |
| Fentanyl | 0.015–0.05 | 3–10 | 0.02–0.1 |
| Hydromorphone | 0.1–0.5 | 5–15 | 0.2–0.5 |
| Meperidine | 5–15 | 5–15 | 5–40 |
| Methadone | 0.5–3 | 10–20 | |
| Morphine | 0.5–3 | 5–20 | 1–10 |
| Sufentanil | 0.003–0.015 | 3–10 | 0.004–0.03 |
| Agonists-Antagonists | | | |
| Buprenorphine | 0.03–0.2 | 10–20 | |
| Pentazocine | 5–30 | 5–15 | 6–40 |

## Post-operative Pain Management

| Drug | Route | Maximum Daily Dose (mg) | Analgesic Effect Onset (hrs) | Peak (hrs) | Duration (hrs) |
|---|---|---|---|---|---|
| **Nonopioids** | | | | | |
| **Sylicylates** | | | | | |
| Aspirin | PO | 3600 | 0.5–1 | 0.5–2 | 2–4 |
| Diflunisal | PO | 2000 | 1–2 | 2–3 | 8–12 |
| **Propionic acids** | | | | | |
| Fenoprofen | PO | 3200 | 1 | 1–2 | 4–6 |
| Ibuprofen | PO | 3200 | 0.5 | 1–2 | 4–6 |
| Naproxen | PO | 1500 | 1 | 2–4 | 4–7 |
| **Indoles** | | | | | |
| Indomethacin | PO | 200 | 0.5 | 1–2 | 4–6 |
| Sulindac | PO | 400 | | 2–4 | |
| Ketorolac | IM | 120 | 0.5–1 | 1 | 4–6 |
| **Oxicams** | | | | | |
| Piroxicam | PO | 20 | 1 | 3–5 | 48–72 |
| **p-Aminophenols** | | | | | |
| Acetaminophen | PO | 1200 | 0.5 | 0.5–1 | 2–4 |
| Phenacetin | PO | 2400 | | 1 | |

| Drug | Route | Maximum Daily Dose (mg) | Analgesic Effect Onset (hrs) | Peak (hrs) | Duration (hrs) |
|---|---|---|---|---|---|
| **Opioids** | | | | | |
| Morphine | IV | 2.5 | Rapid | 0.125 | |
| Codeine | IM | 15–60 | 0.25–0.5 | 1–5 | 4–6 |
| | PO | 15–60 | 0.25–1 | 0.5–2 | 3–4 |
| Hydromorphone | IM | 1–4 | 0.3–0.5 | 1 | 2–3 |
| Oxycodone | PO | 5 | 0.5 | 1–2 | 3–6 |
| Methadone | PO | 2.5–10 | 0.5–1 | 1.5–2 | 4–8 |
| Propoxyphene | PO | 32–65 | 0.25–1 | 1–2 | 3–6 |
| Meperidine | IM | 0.3–0.6 | 0.12–0.5 | 1 | 2–4 |
| Buprenorphine | IM | 0.3–0.6 | 0.12 | 1 | 6–8 |
| Butorphanol | IM | 2–4 | 0.1–0.2 | 0.5–1 | 3–4 |
| Nalbuphine | IM | 10–20 | 0.25 | 1 | 3–6 |
| | IV | 1–5 | | | |
| Pentazocine | IM | 30–60 | 0.12–0.5 | 1–3 | 3–6 |
| | PO | 50 | | | 4–7 |

*Source:* Management of acute postoperative pain. In Barash PG, Cullen BF, Stoeling RK, eds. *Handbook of Clinical Anesthesia. 2nd edition.* Philadelphia: J.B. Lippincott, 1993. Reproduced with permission.

# GYNECOLOGY

## UROGYNECOLOGY

### Common Findings for the Different Types of Urinary Incontinence

| Finding | Stress Incontinence | Detrusor Instability | Intrinsic Sphincter Deficiency | Overflow Incontinence | Functional Incontinence |
|---|---|---|---|---|---|
| Loss with Valsalva | + | − | + | + | − |
| Difficulty starting stream | − | − | − | + | − |
| Urge incontinence | − | + | − | + | + |
| Constant wetness | − | − | + | + | − |
| Hypermobile Valsalva | + | +/− | +/− | +/− | +/− |
| Elevated postvoid residual | − | − | − | + | − |
| Neurologic disease | − | +/− | +/− | +/− | +/− |
| Severe genital prolapse | +/− | +/− | +/− | +/− | +/− |

## Differential Diagnosis of Urinary Incontinence in Women

**Genitourinary etiology**
- Filling and storage disorders
  - Urodynamic stress incontinence
  - Detrusor overactivity (idiopathic)
  - Detrusor overactivity (neurogenic)
  - Mixed types
- Fistula
  - Vesical
  - Ureteral
  - Urethral
- Congenital
  - Ectopic ureter
  - Epispadias

**Nongenitourinary etiology**
- Functional
  - Neurologic
  - Cognitive
  - Psychologic
  - Physical impairment
- Environmental
- Pharmacologic
- Metabolic

*Source:* Reprinted with permission from ACOG Practice Bulletin Number 63. Urinary incontinence in women. *Obstet Gynecol.* 2005;105(6):1533–1545.

## Common Causes of Transient Urinary Incontinence

- Urinary tract infection or urethritis
- Atrophic urethritis or vaginitis
- Drug side effects
- Pregnancy
- Increased urine production
  - Metabolic (hyperglycemia, hypercalcemia)
  - Excess fluid intake
  - Volume overload
- Delirium
- Restricted mobility
- Stool impaction
- Psychologic

*Source:* Reprinted with permission from ACOG Practice Bulletin Number 63. Urinary incontinence in women. *Obstet Gynecol.* 2005;105(6):1533–1545.

## DIAPPERS Mnemonic for Transient Causes of Urinary Incontinence

| | |
|---|---|
| D | Delirium or acute confusion |
| I | Infection (symptomatic urinary tract infection) |
| A | Atrophic vaginitis or urethritis |
| P | Pharmaceutical agents |
| P | Psychological disorder (depression, behavioral disturbance) |
| E | Excess urine output (due to excess fluid intake, diuretics, congestive heart failure, etc.) |
| R | Restricted mobility |
| S | Stool impaction |

*Source:* Reprinted with permission from Clinical management of urinary incontinence. APGO Educational Series on Women's Health Issues. 2004:8–21.

## Common Medications Used to Treat Urinary Incontinence

| Drug | Dosage |
|---|---|
| **Stress incontinence** | |
| Pseudoephedrine (Sudafed) | 15–30 mg, 3 times daily |
| Vaginal estrogen ring (Estring) | Insert into vagina once every 3 mos |
| Vaginal estrogen cream | 0.5–1 g, apply in vagina every night |
| **Overactive bladder** | |
| Oxybutynin ER (Ditropan XL) | 5–15 mg, every morning |
| Generic oxybutynin | 2.5–10 mg, 2–4 times daily |
| Tolterodine (Detrol) | 1–2 mg, a times daily |
| Imipramine (Tofranil) | 10–75 mg, every night |
| Dicyclomine (Bentyl) | 10–20 mg, 4 times daily |
| Hyoscyamine (Cystospaz) | 0.375 mg, 2 times daily |

*Source:* Reprinted with permission from Clinical management of urinary incontinence. APGO Educational Series on Women's Health Issues. 2004:8–21.

# GYNECOLOGY

## Therapy to Facilitate Urine Storage/Bladder Filling

*Bladder related (inhibiting bladder contractility, decreasing sensory input, or increasing bladder capacity)*

**Behavioral therapy**

Education

Fluid restriction

Bladder training

Timed bladder emptying or scheduled voiding

Pelvic floor physiotherapy with or without biofeedback

**Pharmacologic therapy**

Anticholinergic agents

Drugs with mixed actions

Calcium antagonists

Prostaglandin inhibitors

Beta-adrenergic agonists

Alpha-adrenergic antagonists

Tricyclic antidepressants: 5-hydroxy-tryptamine and norepinephrine reuptake inhibitors

Dimethyl sulfoxide

Capsaicin, resiniferatoxin, and like agents

**Electrical stimulation and neuromodulation**

**Acupuncture and electroacupuncture**

**Interruption of innervation**

Less central (sacral rhizotomy, elective sacral rhizotomy)

Peripheral motor and sensory block

**Augmentation cystoplasty (bowel, auto, tissue engineering)**

*Outlet related (increasing outlet resistance)*

**Behavioral therapy**

**Electrical stimulation**

**Pharmacologic therapy**

Alpha-adrenergic agonists

Tricyclic antidepressants; 5-hydroxy-tryptamine and norepinephrine uptake inhibitors

Beta-adrenergic antagonists, agonists

Estrogens

**Vaginal and perineal occlusive or supportive devices; urethral plugs**

**Nonsurgical periurethral compression**

**Periurethral bulking agents (polytef, collagen, or pyrolytic carbon-coated beads)**

**Vesicourethral suspension with or without prolapse repair (female)**

**Sling procedures with or without prolapse repair (female)**

**Closure of the bladder outlet**

**Artificial urinary sphincter**

**Bladder outlet reconstruction**

**Myoplasty**

*Circumventing the problem*

**Antidiuretic hormone-like agents**

**Short-acting diuretics**

**Intermittent catheterization**

**External collecting devices**

**Absorbent products**

**Continuous catheterization**

**Urinary diversion**

*Source:* Reprinted with permission from Clinical management of urinary incontinence. APGO Educational Series on Women's Health Issues. 2004:8–21.

## Medications That Can Affect Lower Urinary Tract Function

| Type of Medication | Lower Urinary Tract Effects |
| --- | --- |
| Diuretics | Polyuria, frequency, urgency |
| Caffeine | Frequency, urgency |
| Alcohol | Sedation, impaired mobility, diuresis |
| Narcotic analgesics | Urinary retention, fecal impaction, sedation, delirium |
| Anticholinergic agents | Urinary retention, voiding difficulty |
| Antihistamines | Anticholinergic actions, sedation |
| Psychotropic agents | |
|    Antidepressants | Anticholinergic actions, sedation |
|    Antipsychotics | Anticholinergic actions, sedation |
|    Sedatives and hypnotics | Sedation, muscle relaxation, confusion |
| Alpha-adrenergic blockers | Stress incontinence |
| Alpha-adrenergic agonists | Urinary retention, voiding difficulty |
| Calcium-channel blockers | Urinary retention, voiding difficulty |

*Source:* Reprinted with permission from ACOG Practice Bulletin Number 63. Urinary incontinence in women. *Obstet Gynecol.* 2005;105(6):1533–1545.

# GYNECOLOGY

## Diagnosis and Treatment Algorithm for Urinary Incontinence

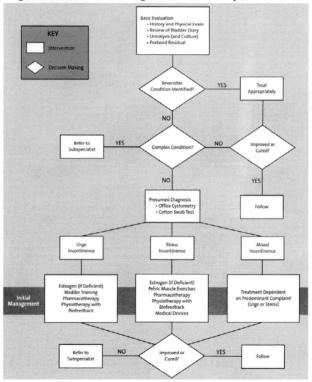

*Source:* Reprinted with permission from Clinical management of urinary incontinence. APGO Educational Series on Women's Health Issues. 2004:8–21.

## Evaluation/Treatment Algorithm for Urinary Incontinence

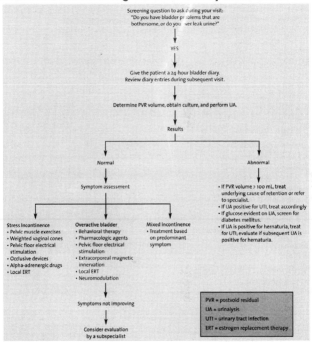

*Source:* Reprinted with permission from Clinical management of urinary incontinence. APGO Educational Series on Women's Health Issues. 2004:8–21.

# GYNECOLOGY

## VULVAR DYSTROPHIES

### Non-Neoplastic Epithelial Disorders
• New classification based on gross and histopathologic findings
I. Squamous cell hyperplasia (formerly hyperplastic dystrophy)
II. Lichen sclerosus
III. Other dermatoses

### Squamous Cell Hyperplasia
• Most represent lichen simplex chronicus
• Gross appearance variable
• Microscopic evaluation
  ▪ Hyperkeratosis
  ▪ Acanthosis
  ▪ Parakeratosis

### Lichen Sclerosus
• Classic lesion—crinkled (cigarette paper), parchment-like
• Biopsy
  ▪ Hyperkeratosis
  ▪ Epithelial thinning
• Often associated with foci of hyperplastic and thinning epithelium ("mixed dystrophy")
  ▪ Squamous cell hyperplasia found in 27–35%
  ▪ Intraepithelial neoplasia found in 5%

### Therapy
• Biopsy, biopsy, biopsy.

### Squamous Cell Hyperplasia
• Topical steroids (bid to tid)
• 0.025–0.01% triamcinolone acetonide
• 0.1% β-methasone valerate and crotamiton (Eurax) in 7:3 mix

### Lichen Sclerosus
• Topical testosterone no longer recommended
• Clobetasol (Temovate 0.05%) cream very effective
  ▪ Use bid × 1 month, then qhr × 2 months, then 2×/week for 3 months
  ▪ Complete regression can occur with this treatment
• Crotamiton (Eurax) 10% cream for pruritus

## VULVODYNIA
### Vulvodynia Treatment Algorithm

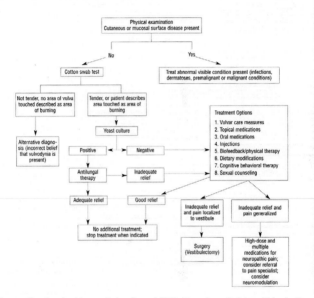

*Source:* Reprinted with permission from ACOG Committee Opinion. Vulvodynia. *Obstet Gynecol.* 2006;108(4):1049–1052.

## Treatment Options for Vulvodynia[a]

| Treatment | Dosage/Regimen | Side Effects |
| --- | --- | --- |
| *Topical* | | |
| Avoidance of topical irritants and allergens | Use mild soap or water for cleansing area, wear cotton underwear, and use fragrance-free sanitary products. | None |
| Estrogen (if estrogen-deficiency is indicated by parabasal cells on normal saline preparation) | Vaginal cream used daily for 3 wks, then 2–3 times/wk as needed. | Local: infrequent burning. Systemic: unclear |
| Topical lidocaine, 5% gel or cream | Topically to area of tenderness prior to intercourse, or nightly, applying lidocaine gel to a cotton ball that is then placed in the introitus and used overnight. Treatment duration is undetermined. | Occasional sensitivity/ irritation |
| Cromolyn cream, 4% | Apply three times/day to area of tenderness. | Sensitivity to the agent or vehicle |
| *Oral Agents (commonly started at first visit)* | | |
| Tricyclic antidepressants | Amitriptyline, starting at 25 mg/day at bedtime for 10 days, increasing by 25-mg increments as tolerated to typical dosage of 50–100 mg/day (maximum dosage, 250 mg/day). Desipramine or imipramine at similar dosage. Nortriptyline at similar dosage, but to maximum of 100 mg/day. | Oral dryness, constipation, fatigue, weight gain (less common). Occasional neurologic symptoms, cardiac arrhythmias, or urinary retention require discontinuation |
| Paroxetine | 10–20 mg/day, increasing as needed and tolerated to a maximum of 60 mg/day. | Occasional restlessness, weight gain, fatigue, anorgasmia |
| Venlafaxine | 37.5 mg/day for 10 days, increasing to 75 mg/day; may increase to maximum of 225 mg/day. | Anorgasmia, gastrointestinal problems, anxiety |
| Gabapentin | 300 mg/day, increasing every 4 days by 300 mg/day (divided into three doses) to a maximum of 900 mg three times/day. | Headache, nausea, vomiting, fatigue, dizziness |
| Calcium citrate (due to the citrate component) | Two tablets twice per day, increasing to 3–4 tablets twice/day. | Tablets are large and difficult for some to swallow. Not indicated for women with a history of calcium-based renal stones |

*(continued)*

## Treatment Options for Vulvodynia[a] *(continued)*

| Treatment | Dosage/Regimen | Side Effects |
|---|---|---|
| *Other Therapeutic Regimes* | | |
| Pelvic-floor physical therapy and/or biofeedback | Performed by physical therapist who has undergone appropriate training. | Discomfort, numerous visits, compliance with home exercises, possible high cost |
| Cognitive behavioral therapy | Sessions with a therapist; study included eight 2-hr group meetings over 12 wks, but may need ongoing treatment. | Time/commitment for full course of sessions |
| Low-oxalate diet | Ranges from highly restrictive diet to avoidance of a small number of high-risk foods. | Poor compliance |
| *Surgery (rarely used)* | | |
| Perineoplasty/ vestibulectomy (hypersensitive tissue is removed and replaced with vaginal mucosa advancement)· | Surgical procedure confined to the posterior introitus; for women who have not responded to other treatments. | Discomfort, recovery time; rare reports of bleeding, infection, hematoma, wound separation, vaginismus, vaginal stenosis |

[a]None of these options has been approved by the U.S. Food and Drug Administration specifically for the indication of vulvodynia.

*Source:* Reprinted with permission from Reed BD. Vulvodynia. *The Female Patient.* 2005;30:48–54.

# INFECTIOUS DISEASES

## GROUP B STREPTOCOCCUS

### Fast Facts

• A leading cause of life-threatening perinatal infections in United States.
• 15–30% of women are asymptomatic carriers.
• Infection rate has decreased from 1.8/1000 in 1990 to 0.34/1000 live births in 2004.
• Early onset infection (80% within 6 hours of delivery)—4% neonatal mortality of term infants and 23% mortality in preterm infants.

### Universal Screening Algorithm

Vaginal and rectal GBS screening cultures at 35–37 wks of gestation of ALL pregnant women (unless patient had GBS bacteriuria during the current pregnancy or a previous infant with invasive GBS disease)

| Intrapartum Prophylaxis Indicated | Intrapartum Prophylaxis Not Indicated |
|---|---|
| • Previous infant with invasive GBS disease<br><br>• GBS bacteriuria during current pregnancy<br><br>• Positive GBS screening culture during current pregnancy (unless a planned cesarean delivery, in the absence of labor or amniotic membrane rupture, is performed)<br><br>• Unknown GBS status (culture not done, incomplete, or results unknown) and any of the following:<br>  - Delivery at <37 weeks of gestation<br>  - Amniotic membrane rupture ≥18 hours<br>  - Intrapartum temperature ≥38°C [100.4° F] | • Previous pregnancy with a positive GBS screening culture, unless a culture was also positive during the current pregnancy<br><br>• Planned cesarean delivery performed in the absence of labor or membrane rupture, regardless of maternal GBS culture status<br><br>• Negative vaginal and rectal GBS screening culture in late gestation during the current pregnancy, regardless of intrapartum risk factors |

*Source:* Centers for Disease Control and Prevention (CDC). Prevention of perinatal group B streptococcal disease: revised guidelines from CDC. MMWR, 51(RR-11), August 16, 2002.

## Management Algorithm

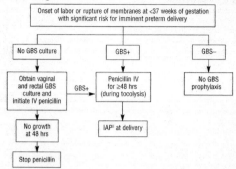

*If a hospital chooses to give antibiotics to prolong the latent period, a GBS culture should be obtained before initiating therapy and the results used to guide intrapartum management.

†Penicillin should be continued for a total of at least 48 hours in a GBS culture-positive woman if delivery has not yet occurred. For women who are GBS culture positive, antibiotic prophylaxis should be reinitiated when labor likely to proceed to delivery occurs or recurs.

‡If antibiotics are used to prolong the latent period, GBS cultures should be obtained prior to initiating therapy and the results used to guide intrapartum management.

§If delivery has not occurred within 4 weeks, a vaginal and rectal GBS screening culture should be repeated and the patient should be managed as described, based on the result of the repeat culture.

‖Intrapartum antibiotic prophylaxis.

Sample algorithm for group B streptococci (GBS) prophylaxis for women with threatened preterm delivery. This algorithm is not an exclusive course of management. Variations that incorporate individual circumstances or institutional preferences may be appropriate.

*Source:* Centers for Disease Control and Prevention (CDC). Prevention of perinatal group B streptococcal disease: revised guidelines from CDC. MMWR, 51(RR-11), August 16, 2002.

# INFECTIOUS DISEASES

## Comments on Prenatal Screening Algorithm

**New Recommendations in Centers for Disease Control and Prevention (CDC) Guidelines:**

- Universal prenatal culture-based screening for vaginal and rectal GBS colonization of all pregnant women at 35–37 wks of gestation.
- Updated prophylaxis regimens for women with penicillin allergy.
- Detailed instruction on prenatal specimen collection and expanded methods of GBS culture processing, including instructions on susceptibility testing.
- Recommendation against routine intrapartum antibiotic prophylaxis for GBS-colonized women undergoing planned cesarean deliveries who have not begun labor or had rupture of membranes.
- A suggested algorithm for management of patients with threatened preterm delivery.
- An updated algorithm for management of newborns exposed to intrapartum antibiotic prophylaxis.

**Recommendations That Remain the Same:**

- Penicillin is the first-line agent for intrapartum antibiotic prophylaxis, with ampicillin an acceptable alternative.
- Women whose culture results are unknown at the time of delivery should be managed according to the risk-based approach; the obstetric risk factors remain unchanged (i.e., delivery at <37 wk of gestation, duration of membrane rupture ≥18 h, or temperature ≥37° C [100.4° F]).
- Women with negative vaginal and rectal GBS screening cultures within 5 wks of delivery do not require intrapartum antimicrobial prophylaxis for GBS even if obstetric risk factors develop (i.e., delivery at <37 wk of gestation, duration of membrane rupture ≥18 h or temperature ≥38° C [100.4° F]).
- Women with GBS bacteriuria in any concentration during their current pregnancy or who previously gave birth to an infant with GBS disease should receive intrapartum antimicrobial prophylaxis.
- In the absence of GBS urinary tract infection, antimicrobial agents should not be used before the intrapartum period to treat asymptomatic GBS colonization.

Revised guidelines from CDC, Centers for Disease Control and Prevention. *MMWR Recomm Rep.* 2002;51 (RR-11):2.

*Source:* Reprinted with permission from the American College of Obstetricians and Gynecologists (ACOG). *Prolog: Obstetrics.* 5th ed. 2003, pg. 58.

## Recommend Regimens for Intrapartum Antimicrobial Prophylaxis for Perinatal Group B Streptococcal (GBS) Disease Prevention[a]

| | |
|---|---|
| Recommended | Penicillin G, 5 million units IV initial dose, then 2.5 million units IV every 4 hrs until delivery |
| Alternative | Ampicillin, 2 g IV initial dose, then 1 g IV every 4 hrs until delivery |
| **If penicillin allergic[b]** | |
| Patients not at high risk for anaphylaxis | Cefazolin, 2 g IV initial dose, then 1 g IV every 8 hrs until delivery |
| Patients at high risk for anaphylaxis[c] | |
|     GBS susceptible to clindamycin and erythromycin[d] | Clindamycin, 900 mg IV every 8 hrs until delivery OR Erythromycin, 500 mg IV every 6 hrs until delivery |
|     GBS resistant to clindamycin or erythromycin or susceptibility unknown | Vancomycin,[e] 1 g IV every 12 hrs until delivery |

[a]Broad-spectrum agents, including an agent active against GBS, may be necessary for treatment of chorio-amnionitis.

[b]History of penicillin allergy should be assessed to determine whether a high risk for anaphylaxis is present. Penicillin allergic patients at high risk for anaphylaxis are those who have experienced immediate hypersensitivity to penicillin including a history of penicillin-related anaphylaxis; other high-risk patients are those with asthma or other diseases that would make anaphylaxis more dangerous or difficult to treat, such as persons being treated with beta-adrenergic-blocking agents.

[c]If laboratory facilities are adequate, clindamycin and erythromycin susceptibility testing should be performed on prenatal GBS isolates from penicillin-allergic women at high risk for anaphylaxis.

[d]Resistance to erythromycin is often but not always associated clindamycin resistance. If a strain is resistant to erythromycin but appears susceptible to clindamycin, it may still have inducible resistance to clindamycin.

[e]Cefazolin is preferred over vancomycin for women with a history of penicillin allergy other than immediate hypersensitivity reactions, and pharmacologic data suggest it achieves effective intraamniotic concentrations. Vancomycin should be reserved for penicillin-allergic women at high risk for anaphylaxis.

*Source:* Centers for Disease Control and Prevention (CDC). Prevention of perinatal group B streptococcal disease: revised guidelines from CDC. MMWR, 51(RR-11), August 16, 2002.

# INFECTIOUS DISEASES

## INTRA-AMNIOTIC INFECTION

### Definition
A bacterial infection of the chorion, amnion and amniotic fluid often diagnosed during a prolonged labor.

### Diagnosis
Maternal temperature ≥100.7° F with no other obvious source and one of the following additional findings:
- Fetal tachycardia
- Maternal tachycardia
- Abdominal tenderness
- Foul-smelling amniotic fluid
- Leukocytosis
- Positive amniotic fluid culture

### Risk Factors
- Prolonged ruptured of membranes
- Multiple vaginal exams in labor and internal monitoring

### Antibiotics
Mezlocillin 4 g IV q4–6hrs or piperacillin 3–4 g IV q4hrs
Ticarcillin/clavulanic acid 3.1 g IV q6hrs
Ampicillin/sulbactam 3 g IV q4–6hrs
Ampicillin 2 g IV q6hrs **and** gentamicin 1.5 mg/kg load then 1.0 mg/kg q8hrs (if delivery by cesarean section **add** clindamycin 900 mg IV q6hrs)

### Comments
- Some continue antibiotics for 24–48 hours afebrile following delivery.
- Chorioamnionitis is **not** an indication for cesarean delivery.
- Fetal outcome is improved by maternal antibiotic therapy and ↓ temperature.
- Always consider other sources of maternal fever (pyelonephritis, pneumonia, appendicitis).
- Watch for postpartum hemorrhage and dystocia secondary to inadequate uterine action.
- Chorioamnionitis may represent a risk factor for cerebral palsy.

## FEBRILE MORBIDITY AND ENDOMYOMETRITIS

### Definition

Two temperature elevations to ≥38° C (100.4° F) (outside the 1st 24 hours after delivery)

or

A temperature of ≥38.7° C (101.5° F) at any time

### Etiology

Seven Ws of febrile morbidity

- Womb (endomyometritis)
- Wind (atelectesis, pneumonia)
- Water (urinary tract infection or pyelonephritis)
- Walk (deep vein thrombosis or pulmonary embolism)
- Wound (wound infection, episiotomy infection)
- Weaning (breast engorgement, mastitis, breast abscess)
- Wonder (drug fever—wonder drugs)

### Evaluation

Physical examination including pelvic exam to rule out hematoma or retained membranes

Complete blood count with differential, urinalysis, urine and blood cultures as indicated

Chest X-ray, ultrasound as indicated

### Treatment

Cefotetan 1–2 g IV q12hrs

Mezlocillin 4 g IV q4–6hr or piperacillin 3–4 g IV q4hrs

Ticarcillin/clavulanate 3.1 g IV q6hrs

Ampicillin/sulbactam 3 g IV q4–6hrs

Gentamicin 1.5 mg/kg load then 1.0 mg/kg q8hrs and clindamycin 900 mg IV q6hrs (plus ampicillin 2 g IV q6hrs as needed to cover enterococcus)

### Comments

- Continue IV antibiotics until 24–48 hours afebrile and improved physical exam.
- Oral antibiotics following IV antibiotics have not been shown to be of proven value.
- If unresponsive following 48–72 hours of IV antibiotics, reexamine the patient.
  - Consider pelvic abscess.
  - Consider septic pelvic thrombophlebitis.
  - Consider drug fever.

# INFECTIOUS DISEASES

## MASTITIS AND BREAST ABSCESS

### Fast Facts

- Affects 2–3% of nursing mothers
- Most frequently seen as a nonepidemic mammary cellulitis
- Usually *Staphylococcus aureus*
- Other pathogens: *b-hemolytic streptococci, H. influenzae, H. parainfluenzae, Escherichia coli, Klebsiella pneumoniae*
- Must distinguish between simple engorement and infectious process
- Outpatient antibiotic therapy usually successful but consider IV antibiotics if unresponsive or patient compliance/tolerance uncertain or patient appears septic

### Evaluation

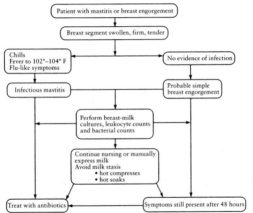

### Drug Regimens for Managing Mastitis

Cephalexin (Keflex) 500 mg orally every 6 hrs for 7 days
Amoxicillin/Clavulante potassium (Augmentin) 875 mg orally every 12 hrs for 7 days
Azithromycin (Zithromax) 500 mg initially, then 250 mg orally daily for 5–7 days
Dicloxacillin 250–500 mg orally every 8 hrs for 7 days
Clindamycin 300 mg orally every 8 hrs for 7 days

*Source:* Reprinted with permission from Hager, W. David. Managing mastitis. *Cont OB/GYN.* 2004;Jan;33–47. *Cont OB/GYN* is a copyrighted publication of Advanstar Communications Inc. All rights reserved.

- Breast abscess can form even on antibiotics; surgical drainage may be necessary or ultrasound guided needle aspiration could be considered.

## Prevention
- Avoid cracked or fissured nipples.
  - Use plain water to clean nipple area (NOT soap or alcohol).
  - Increase duration of nursing gradually to avoid soreness.
  - Use breast shield or topical cream to help healing of cracked nipples.
  - Place finger in corner of baby's mouth during feeding to break sucking force.
- Treat recurrent mastitis promptly but continue breastfeeding.

Adapted from from ACOG Educational Bulletin Number 258, July 2000. Breastfeeding: Maternal and Infant Aspects.

## Patient Information

### What to Do If You Develop Mastitis

If you have symptoms that suggest you have mastitis, you'll need to heed the following advice:

- Continue breastfeeding, starting on the affected side.
- If your baby doesn't feed well or will not feed on the affected breast, empty the breast using a piston-type, hospital breast pump.
- If possible, remain in bed for the first 48 hrs.
- Drink more fluids.
- Reduce your salt intake.
- Take acetaminophen or ibuprofen to reduce fever and discomfort so milk letdown will occur and the breast can be emptied.
- Apply moist heat to speed up milk letdown and ease soreness; cool packs may be used initially to decrease swelling.
- Apply gentle massage to move the milk forward and increase drainage from the infected area.
- Avoid breast shells and tight-fitting bras.
- Avoid tight clothing and underwire bras.
- Wash your hands before handling the infected breast.
- Lanolin creams may be used to treat nipples. Your physician may prescribe medication if you develop a fungal infection of the nipple.
- Make sure your baby is in a comfortable nursing position that does not pull excessively on your nipple; if necessary, talk to a lactation consultant to evaluate your nursing technique.
- If you have a fever, the doctor may prescribe antibiotics for 7–10 days. Schedule a follow-up appointment in 7 days so that the doctor can check for an abscess. If your symptoms don't respond within 48 hrs of antibiotic treatment, notify the physician.

*Source:* Reprinted with permission from Hager, W. David. Managing mastitis. *Cont OB/GYN.* 2004:Jan;33–47. *Cont OB/GYN* is a copyrighted publication of Advantar Communications Inc. All rights reserved.

## HEPATITIS

### Overview of Viral Hepatitis

| | A | B | C | D | E |
|---|---|---|---|---|---|
| Virus Family | Picornaviridae | Hepadnaviridae | Flaviviridae | N/A | Appears to be member of Caliciviridae |
| Transmission | Fecal-oral, permucosal | Percutaneous, permucosal | Percutaneous, permucosal | Percutaneous, permucosal | Fecal-oral (especially contaminated water) |
| Chronicity | None | 6–10% of adults | 75–85% | Average 6% | Unknown 25–50% of children (1–5 years of age) 70–90% of infants |
| Onset | Usually abrupt | Usually insidious | Insidious | Usually abrupt | Usually abrupt |
| Incubation | Average 28 days; range 15–45 days; −0.3% | Average 60–90 days; range 45–180 days | Average 6–7 wks; range 2–26 wks | 21–90 days | average 40 days; range 15–60 days |
| Mortality | | 0.5–1.0% | 0.2%–0.4% | 2–20% with coinfection, up to 30% with superinfection | About 1–2%; 15–20% in pregnant women |

*Source:* Reprinted with permission from Sexually Transmitted Infections Hepatitis B and C: The Ob/Gyn's Role. *APGO Educational Series on Women's Health Issues,* 2002:1–17.

## Hepatitis B Monitoring Panel

Positive test results on the acute viral hepatitis panel for HBsAg and anti-HBc IgM establish the diagnosis of acute hepatitis B infection. Serial testing with an HBV monitoring panel is then recommended. This panel consists of four hepatitis B markers:

1. HBsAg—persistence of this surface antigen provides prognostic information on a patient's likelihood of developing chronic HBV infection.
2. HBeAg—the presence of the hepatitis B "e" antigen helps to determine a patient's potential to infect others. It suggests that a patient has a high viral load and the virus is actively replicated, and thus that a patient is highly infectious.
3. anti-HBe—seroconversion from HBeAg to anti-HBe suggests that a patient's disease is resolving.
4. anti-HBs—seroconversion from HBsAg to anti-HBs also suggests that a patient's disease is abating and immunity is being established.

### Interpretation of the Hepatitis B Panel

| Test | Results | Interpretation |
|---|---|---|
| HBsAg<br>anti-HBc<br>anti-HBs | Negative<br>Negative<br>Negative | Susceptible |
| HBsAg<br>anti-HBc<br>anti-HBs | Negative<br>Positive<br>Positive | Immune due to natural infection |
| HBsAg<br>anti-HBc<br>anti-HBs | Negative<br>Negative<br>Positive | Immune due to hepatitis B vaccination |
| HBsAg<br>anti-HBc<br>anti-HBc IgM<br>anti-HBs | Positive<br>Positive<br>Positive<br>Negative | Acutely infected |
| HBsAg<br>anti-HBc<br>anti-HBc IgM<br>anti-HBs | Positive<br>Positive<br>Negative<br>Negative | Chronically infected |
| HBsAg<br>anti-HBc<br>anti-HBs | Negative<br>Positive<br>Negative | Four interpretations possible:<br>1. May be recovering from acute HBV infection<br>2. May be distantly immune and test is not sensitive enough to detect very low level of anti-HBs in serum<br>3. May be susceptible with a false-positive anti-HBc<br>4. May be an undetectable form of HBsAg present in the serum and the person is actually a carrier |

anti-HBc, hepatitis B core antibody; anti-HBc IgM, IgM antibody against HBc; anti-HBs, hepatitis B surface antibody; HBV, hepatitis B virus; HBsAg, hepatitis B surface antigen.
*Source:* Reprinted with permission from *Sexually Transmitted Infections Hepatitis B and C: The Ob/Gyn's Role. APGO Educational Series on Women's Health Issues.* 2002:1–17.

# INFECTIOUS DISEASES

## HEPATITIS C
### Fast Facts

- Hepatitis C is now the leading indication for liver transplantation in many U.S. medical centers.
- Approximately 50% of hepatitis C cases result from IV drug use.
- Risk of sexual transmission in a discordant monogamous couple is 5% over 10–20 years.
- 85–90% of infected patients are unable to clear the virus and are chronically infected.
- No guidelines for hepatitis C and pregnancy exist.
  - Perinatal transmission probably 5–6% of cases but higher in human immunodeficiency virus (HIV)–positive women.
  - Breastfeeding is not an established risk factor.
  - Pregnant women cannot be treated with alpha interferon or ribavirin.

### Screening and Evaluation

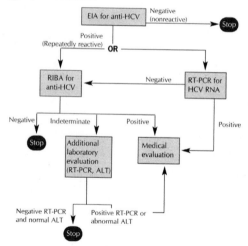

Hepatitis C virus (HCV) infection testing algorithm for asymptomatic persons.
*Source:* Reprinted with permission from Sexually Transmitted Infections Hepatitis B and C: The Ob/Gyn's Role. *APGO Educational Series on Women's Health Issues.* 2002: 1–17.

## Tests for Hepatitis C Virus (HCV) Infection

| Test/Type | Application | Comments |
|---|---|---|
| **Hepatitis C Virus Antibody (anti-HCV)** | | |
| EIA (enzyme immunoassay) | Indicates past or present infection, but does not differentiate between acute, chronic, and resolved infection in low-prevalence populations | Sensitivity >97% <br> EIA alone has low positive predictive value |
| Supplemental assay—i.e., recombinant immunoblot assay (RIBA) | All positive EIA results should be verified with a supplemental assay | |
| **HCV RNA** | | |
| Qualitative tests[a,b] <br> Reverse transcriptase polymerase chain reaction (RT-PCR) amplification of HCV RNA by in-house or commercial assays (e.g., Amplicor HCV) | Detect presence of circulating HCV RNA <br> Monitor patients on antiviral therapy | Detect virus as early as 1–2 wks after exposure <br> Detection of HCV RNA during course of infection might be intermittent; a single negative RT-PCR is not conclusive <br> False-positive and false-negative results might occur |
| Quantitative tests[a,b] <br> RT-PCR amplification of HCV RNA by in-house or commercial assays (e.g., Amplicor HCV Monitor) <br> Branched-chain DNA (bDNA) assays (e.g., Quantiplex HCV RNA Assay) | Determine concentration of HCV RNA <br> Might be useful for assessing the likelihood of response to antiviral therapy | Less sensitive than qualitative RT-PCR <br> Should not be used to exclude the diagnosis of HCV infection or to determine treatment endpoint |
| Genotype[a,b] <br> Several methodologies available (e.g., hybridization, sequencing) | Group isolates of HCV based on genetic differences into 6 genotypes and >90 subtypes <br> With new therapies, length of treatment might vary based on genotype | Genotype 1 (subtypes 1a and 1b) most common in the United States and associated with lower response to antiviral therapy |

*(continued)*

# INFECTIOUS DISEASES

## Tests for Hepatitis C Virus (HCV) Infection *(continued)*

| Test/Type | Application | Comments |
|---|---|---|
| **Hepatitis C Virus Antibody (anti-HCV)** | | |
| Serotype[a] | | |
| EIA based on immunoreactivity to synthetic peptides (e.g., Murex HCV Serotyping 1-6 Assay) | No clinical utility | Cannot distinguish between subtypes |
| | | Dual infections often observed |

[a]Currently not FDA approved; lacks standardization.
[b]Samples require special handling (e.g., serum must be separated within 2–4 hrs of collection and stored frozen from −20° C to −70° C; frozen samples should be shipped on dry ice).
*Source:* Reprinted with permission from Sexually Transmitted Infections Hepatitis B and C: The Ob/Gyn's Role. *APGO Educational Series on Women's Health Issues.* 2002:1–17.

## Interpretation of Hepatitis C (HCV) Tests

| Test Results | Infection Status |
|---|---|
| EIA positive, supplemental test positive[a] | HCV infected |
| EIA positive, supplemental test negative | Uninfected (unless abnormal ALT levels) |
| EIA negative | Uninfected |
| EIA positive, supplemental test indeterminate | Patient is in process of seroconversion or is chronically infected with HCV; otherwise false-positive result |

[a]The present RIBA supplemental test detects four viral antigens. If at least two antigens are identified, the test is considered positive. If only one is detected, the result is deemed indeterminate.
ALT, alanine aminotransferase; ELISA, enzyme-linked immunosorbent assay; PCR, polymerase chain reaction; RIBA, recombinant immunoblot assay.
*Source:* Reprinted with permission from Sexually Transmitted Infections Hepatitis B and C: The Ob/Gyn's Role. *APGO Educational Series on Women's Health Issues.* 2002:1–17.

# MANAGEMENT OF TUBERCULOSIS IN PREGNANCY

## Fast Facts

- Total number of cases of tuberculosis in 1999 (17,500).
- Pregnancy has no effect on tuberculin sensitivity.

## Mantoux Test

- 0.1 mL of purified protein derivative tuberculin (5 Tuberculin Units)
- Place intradermal
- Read after 48–72 hours
- Positive test

## Centers for Disease Control and Prevention Recommendations for Test Interpretation

| PPD Size | Considered Positive |
|---|---|
| ≥5 mm | Patients with known or suspected HIV infection |
| | Patients with recent close contact with an active case |
| | Patients with clinical or radiographic evidence of tuberculosis |
| ≥10 mm | Intravenous drug abusers known to be HIV negative |
| | Residents of healthcare institutions, shelters, and prisons |
| | Healthcare workers |
| | Immigrants from high-prevalence countries |
| | Certain minorities (Latinas, African Americans, Native Americans) |
| | Patients with diabetes mellitus |
| | Patients with renal failure |
| | Patients with previous gastrectomy or intestinal bypass |
| | Patients with certain hematologic and reticuloendothelial diseases |
| | Immunosuppressed patients (including those taking chronic steroids or immunosuppressive drugs) |
| | Silicosis patients |
| | Malnourished patients (10% below ideal body weight) |
| | Chronic alcoholic patients |
| ≥15 mm | All others (low-risk patients) |

PPD, purified protein derivative; HIV, human immunodeficiency virus.
*Source:* Reprinted with permission from Miller KS, Miller JM Jr. Tuberculosis in pregnancy: interactions, diagnosis, and management. *Clin Obstet Gynecol.* 1996, 39:126. Used with permission of Lippincott-Raven Publishers, Philadelphia. Adapted from Centers for Disease Control and Prevention. Screening for tuberculosis infection in high risk populations. *MMWR Recomm Rep.* 1995;4:(RR-11):24.

# INFECTIOUS DISEASES

## Bacillus of Calmette and Guerin (BCG)

- Vaccination used in many foreign countries to control tuberculosis.
- Purified protein derivative sensitivity after bacillus of Calmette and Guerin is variable.
- Positive tuberculin test should be evaluated as for other patients.

## Evaluation

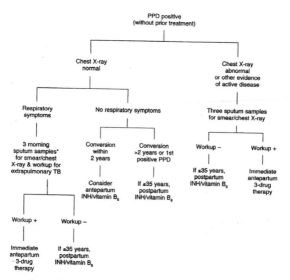

*Note:* Some providers may advocate four-drug therapy. For morning sputum examples, induced sputa may be necessary in patients unable to cough. PPD, purified protein derivative test; INH, isoniazid.

*Source:* Reprinted with permission from Riley L. Pneumonia and tuberculosis during pregnancy. *Infect Dis Clin North Am* 1997;11:119–133.

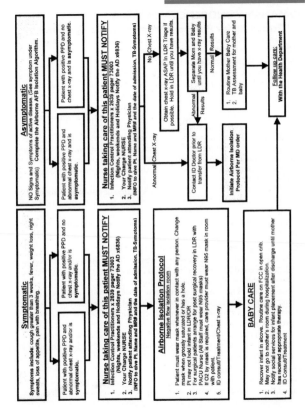

**Symptomatic**

Symptoms include: cough greater than 3 weeks, fever, weight loss, night sweats, loss of appetite, pain with breathing

Patient with positive PPD and abnormal chest x-ray and/or is symptomatic.

Patient with positive PPD and no chest x-ray and/or is symptomatic.

**Asymptomatic**

NO Signs and Symptoms of active disease. (See symptom under Symptomatic) Complete the Airborne AFB Isolation Algorithm.

Patient with positive PPD and abnormal chest x-ray and is asymptomatic.

Patient with positive PPD and chest x-ray and is asymptomatic.

**Nurse taking care of this patient MUST NOTIFY**
1. Infection Control Practitioners x 2639 pager 73003
   (Nights, weekends and Holidays Notify the AD x6836)
2. Your Charge NURSE
3. Notify patient attending Physician
   (INFO to give Pt. Name and MRR and the date of admission, TB-Symptoms)

**Nurse taking care of this patient MUST NOTIFY**
1. Infection Control Practitioners x 2639 pager 73003
   (Nights, weekends and Holidays Notify the AD x6836)
2. Your Charge NURSE
3. Notify patient attending Physician
   (INFO to give Pt. Name and MRR and the date of admission, TB-Symptoms)

No Chest X-ray

Obtain chest x-ray in LDR Triage if possible. Hold in LDR until you have results.

Abnormal Chest X-ray

Contact ID Doctor prior to transfer from LDR

Initiate Airborne Isolation Protocol Per MD order

Abnormal Results → Separate Mom and Baby until you have x-ray results.

Normal Results

1. Routine Mother Baby Care
2. TB Assessment for mother and baby

Follow up care:
**With the Health Department**

**Airborne Isolation Protocol**
Negative flow isolation room
1. Patient must wear mask whenever in contact with any person. Change mask when grossly saturated or has a hole.
2. Pt may not hold infant in LDR/OR
3. For surgical patients arrange for post surgical recovery in LDR with PACU Nurse (All Staff must wear N95 masks)
4. If O2 by mask is required, care provider must wear N95 mask in room with patient.
5. ID consult/Treatment/Chest x-ray

**BABY CARE**
1. Recover infant in alcove. Routine care on FCC in open crib.
2. May not go to mother's room during hospitalization.
3. Notify social services for infant placement after discharge until mother has received appropriate therapy.
4. ID Consult/Treatment

*Source:* From Pulmonary Tuberculosis Control Plan, Inova Fairfax Hospital, Fairfax, VA.

# INFECTIOUS DISEASES

## HUMAN IMMUNODEFICIENCY VIRUS

### HIV Screening for Pregnant Women and Their Infants

*Source:* Revised Recommendations for HIV Testing of Adults, Adolescents, and Pregnant Women in Health-Care Settings. *MMWR*. September 22, 2006;55(RR-14):1–17.

#### Universal Opt-Out Screening

- All pregnant women in the United States should be screened for HIV infection.
- Screening should occur after a woman is notified that HIV screening is recommended for all pregnant patients and that she will receive an HIV test as part of the routine panel of prenatal tests unless she declines (opt-out screening).
- HIV testing must be voluntary and free from coercion. No woman should be tested without her knowledge.
- Pregnant women should receive oral or written information that includes an explanation of HIV infection, a description of interventions that can reduce HIV transmission from mother to infant, and the meanings of positive and negative test results and should be offered an opportunity to ask questions and to decline testing.
- No additional process or written documentation of informed consent beyond what is required for other routine prenatal tests should be required for HIV testing.
- If a patient declines an HIV test, this decision should be documented in the medical record.

#### Addressing Reasons for Declining Testing

- Providers should discuss and address reasons for declining an HIV test (e.g., lack of perceived risk; fear of the disease; and concerns regarding partner violence or potential stigma or discrimination).
- Women who decline an HIV test because they have had a previous negative test result should be informed of the importance of retesting during each pregnancy.
- Logistical reasons for not testing (e.g., scheduling) should be resolved.
- Certain women who initially decline an HIV test might accept at a later date, especially if their concerns are discussed. Certain women will continue to decline testing, and their decisions should be respected and documented in the medical record.

#### Timing of HIV Testing

- To promote informed and timely therapeutic decisions, healthcare providers should test women for HIV as early as possible during each pregnancy. Women who decline the test early in prenatal care should be encouraged to be tested at a subsequent visit.
- A second HIV test during the third trimester, preferably <36 weeks of gestation, is cost-effective even in areas of low HIV prevalence and may be considered for

all pregnant women. A second HIV test during the third trimester is recommended for women who meet one or more of the following criteria:

- Women who receive healthcare in jurisdictions with elevated incidence of HIV or AIDS among women aged 15–45 years. In 2004, these jurisdictions included Alabama, Connecticut, Delaware, the District of Columbia, Florida, Georgia, Illinois, Louisiana, Maryland, Massachusetts, Mississippi, Nevada, New Jersey, New York, North Carolina, Pennsylvania, Puerto Rico, Rhode Island, South Carolina, Tennessee, Texas, and Virginia.
- Women who receive healthcare in facilities in which prenatal screening identifies at least one HIV-infected pregnant woman per 1000 women screened.
- Women who are known to be at high risk for acquiring HIV (e.g., injection-drug users and their sex partners, women who exchange sex for money or drugs, women who are sex partners of HIV-infected persons, and women who have had a new or more than one sex partner during this pregnancy).
- Women who have signs or symptoms consistent with acute HIV infection. When acute retroviral syndrome is a possibility, a plasma RNA test should be used in conjunction with an HIV antibody test to diagnose acute HIV infection.

## Rapid Testing during Labor

- Any woman with undocumented HIV status at the time of labor should be screened with a rapid HIV test unless she declines (opt-out screening).
- Reasons for declining a rapid test should be explored (see Addressing Reasons for Declining Testing).
- Immediate initiation of appropriate antiretroviral prophylaxis should be recommended to women on the basis of a reactive rapid test result without waiting for the results of a confirmatory test.

## Postpartum/Newborn Testing

- When a woman's HIV status is still unknown at the time of delivery, she should be screened immediately postpartum with a rapid HIV test unless she declines (opt-out screening).
- When the mother's HIV status is unknown postpartum, rapid testing of the newborn as soon as possible after birth is recommended so antiretroviral prophylaxis can be offered to HIV-exposed infants. Women should be informed that identifying HIV antibodies in the newborn indicates that the mother is infected.
- For infants whose HIV exposure status is unknown and who are in foster care, the person legally authorized to provide consent should be informed that rapid HIV testing is recommended for infants whose biologic mothers have not been tested.
- The benefits of neonatal antiretroviral prophylaxis are best realized when it is initiated <12 hours after birth.

# INFECTIOUS DISEASES

## Confirmatory Testing

- Whenever possible, uncertainties regarding laboratory test results indicating HIV infection status should be resolved before final decisions are made regarding reproductive options, antiretroviral therapy, cesarean delivery, or other interventions.
- If the confirmatory test result is not available before delivery, immediate initiation of appropriate antiretroviral prophylaxis should be recommended to any pregnant patient whose HIV screening test result is reactive to reduce the risk for perinatal transmission.

| Risk Factor | Possible Preventative Intervention |
|---|---|
| Antepartum risk factors | |
| Advanced HIV disease | |
| • Low CD4 count | Antiretroviral therapy |
| • High plasma viral load | |
| Intrapartum risk factors | |
| Prolonged rupture of membranes | Scheduled C/S, avoiding artificial rupture of membranes |
| Vaginal delivery | Scheduled C/S |
| Increased exposure to maternal blood | Scheduled C/S, avoiding fetal scalp electrodes, scalp sampling, and episiotomy |
| Postpartum risk factors | |
| Breastfeeding | Avoiding breastfeeding |

C/S, cesarean section; HIV, human immunodeficiency virus.

# INFECTIOUS DISEASES

## Prevention of Opportunistic Infections in Pregnancy

| Pathogen | Indication | Recommendation |
|---|---|---|
| *P. carinii* | CD4 <200 | TMP-SMX 160/800 mg/day |
| Toxoplasmosis | Anti-toxoplasma IgG and CD4 <100 | TMP-SMX 160/800 mg/day |
| Mycobacterium avium complex | CD4 <50 | Azithromycin 1200 mg/wk |
| *S. pneumoniae* | All patients with CD4 >200 | Pneumovax |
| Hepatitis B | Anti-HBc negative | HBV vaccine series |
| Influenza | All patients | Influenza vaccine |

Anti-HBc, antibody to hepatitis B core antigen; CD4, cluster of differentiation 4; HBV, hepatitis B virus; TMP-SMX, Trimethoprim-sulfamethoxazole.

*Source:* Reprinted with permission from Cotter AM, O'Sullivan MJ. Update on managing HIV in pregnancy. *Cont OB/GYN.* 2004;Nov:57–72. *Cont OB/GYN* is a copyrighted publication of Advanstar Communications Inc. All rights reserved.

# INFECTIOUS DISEASES

## Clinical Scenarios and Recommendations for the Use of Antiretroviral Drugs to Reduce Perinatal Human Immunodeficiency Virus Type 1 (HIV-1) Transmission

| Scenario #1 | Scenario #2 |
|---|---|
| HIV-1-infected pregnant women who have not received prior antiretroviral therapy. | HIV-1-infected women receiving antiretroviral therapy during the current pregnancy. |

**Scenario #1**

HIV-1-infected pregnant women who have not received prior antiretroviral therapy.

- Pregnant women with HIV-1 infection must receive standard clinical, immunologic, and virologic evaluation. Recommendations for initiation and choice of antiretroviral therapy should be based on the same parameters used for persons who are not pregnant, although the known and unknown risks and benefits of such therapy during pregnancy must be considered and discussed.

- The three-part ZDV chemoprophylaxis regimen, initiated after the first trimester, is recommended for all pregnant women with HIV-1 infection regardless of antenatal HIV RNA copy number to reduce the risk for perinatal transmission.

- The combination of ZDV chemoprophylaxis with additional antiretroviral drugs for treatment of HIV-1 infection is recommended for infected women whose clinical, immunologic, or virologic status requires treatment or who have HIV-1 RNA over 1000 copies/mL regardless of clinical or immunologic, status, and can be considered for women with HIV-1 RNA <1000 copies/mL.

- Women who are in the first trimester of pregnancy may consider delaying initiation of therapy until after 10–12 wks gestation.

**Scenario #2**

HIV-1-infected women receiving antiretroviral therapy during the current pregnancy.

- HIV-1 infected women receiving antiretroviral therapy in whom pregnancy is identified after the first trimester should continue therapy. ZDV should be a component of the antenatal antiretroviral treatment regimen after the first trimester whenever possible, although this may not always be feasible.

- For women receiving antiretroviral therapy in whom pregnancy is recognized during the first trimester, the woman should be counseled regarding the benefits and potential risks of antiretroviral administration during this period, and continuation of therapy should be considered. If therapy is discontinued during the first trimester, all drugs should be stopped and reintroduced simultaneously to avoid the development of drug resistance.

- Regardless of the antepartum antiretroviral regimen, ZDV administration is recommended during the intrapartum period and for the newborn.

*(continued)*

| Scenario #3 | Scenario #4 |
|---|---|

**HIV-1-infected women in labor who have had no prior therapy.**

- Several effective regimens are available. These include:

  1. Intrapartum intravenous ZDV followed by 6 wks of ZDV for the newborn;

  2. Oral ZDV and 3TC during labor, followed by one wk of oral ZDV/3TC for the newborn;

  3. A single dose nevirapine at the onset of labor followed by a single dose of nevirapine for the newborn at age 48 hrs; and

  4. The single-dose maternal/infant nevirapine regimen combined with intrapartum intravenous ZDV and 6 wk ZDV for the newborn.

- If single-dose nevirapine is given to the mother, alone or in combination with ZDV, consideration should be given to adding maternal ZDV/3TC starting as soon as possible (intrapartum or immediately postpartum) and continuing for 3–7 days, which may reduce development of nevirapine resistance.

- In the immediate postpartum period, the woman should have appropriate assessments (e.g., CD4+ count and HIV-1 RNA copy number) to determine whether antiretroviral therapy is recommended for her own health.

**Infants born to mothers who have received no antiretroviral therapy during pregnancy or intrapartum.**

- The 6-wk neonatal ZDV component of the ZDV chemoprophylactic regimen should be discussed with the mother and offered for the newborn.

- ZDV should be initiated as soon as possible after delivery—preferably within 6–12 hrs of birth.

- Some clinicians may choose to use ZDV in combination with other antiretroviral drugs, particularly if the mother is known or suspected to have ZDV-resistant virus. However, the efficacy of this approach for prevention of transmission has not been proven in clinical trials, and appropriate dosing regimens for neonates are incompletely defined for many drugs.

- In the immediate postpartum period, the woman should undergo appropriate assessments (e.g., CD4+ count and HIV-1 RNA copy number) to determine if antiretroviral therapy is required for her own health. The infant should undergo early diagnostic testing so that if HIV-infected, treatment can be initiated as soon as possible.

*Note:* Discussion of treatment options and recommendations should be noncoercive, and the final decision regarding the use of antiretroviral drugs is the responsibility of the woman. A decision to not accept treatment with ZDV or other drugs should not result in punitive action or denial of care. Use of ZDV should not be denied to a woman who wishes to minimize exposure of the fetus to other antiretroviral drugs and who therefore chooses to receive only ZDV during pregnancy to reduce the risk for perinatal transmission. HIV-1, human immunodeficiency virus-1; RNA, ribonucleic acid; ZDV, zidovudine.

*Source:* Reprinted with permission from Public Health Service Task Force. Recommendations for Use of Antiretroviral Drugs in Pregnant HIV-1-Infected Women for Maternal Health and Interventions to Reduce Perinatal HIV-1 Transmission in the United States. October 12, 2006, pg. 45. Accessed at http://www.aidsinfo.nih.gov/Guidelines/GuidelineDetail.aspx?MenuItem=Guidelines&Search=Off&GuidelineID=9&ClassID=2.

# INFECTIOUS DISEASES

## Comparison of Intrapartum/Postpartum Regimens for HIV-1–Infected Women in Labor Who Have Had No Prior Antiretroviral Therapy (Scenario #3)

| Drug Regimen | Source of Evidence | Maternal Regimen | Infant Postpartum |
|---|---|---|---|
| ZDV | Epidemiologic data, United States; compared to no ZDV treatment | 2 mg/kg intravenous bolus, followed by continuous infusion of 1 mg/kg/hr until delivery | 2 mg/kg orally every 6 hrs for 6 wks[a] |
| ZDV/3TC | Clinical trial, Africa; compared to placebo | ZDV 600 mg orally at onset of labor, followed by 300 mg orally every 3 hrs until delivery AND 3TC 150 mg orally at onset of labor, followed by 150 mg orally every 12 hrs until delivery | ZDV 4 mg/kg orally every 12 hrs AND 3TC 2 mg/kg orally every 12 hrs for 7 days |
| Nevirapine | Clinical trial, Africa; compared to oral ZDV given intrapartum and for 1 wk to the infant | Single 200 mg oral dose at onset of labor Consider adding intrapartum ZDV/3TC and 3–7 days of ZDV/3TC postpartum to reduce nevirapine resistance | Single 2 mg/kg oral dose at age 48–72 hrs[b] |
| ZDV-Nevirapine | Theoretical | ZDV 2 mg/kg intravenous bolus, followed by continuous infusion of 1 mg/kg/hr until delivery AND Nevirapine single 200 dose oral mg at onset of labor Consider adding intrapartum ZDV/3TC and 3–7 days of ZDV/3TC postpartum to reduce nevirapine resistance | ZDV 2 mg/kg orally every 6 hrs for 6 wks AND Nevirapine single 2 mg/kg oral dose at age 48–72 hrs[b] |

| Data on Transmission | Advantages | Disadvantages |
|---|---|---|
| Transmission 10% with ZDV compared to 27% with no ZDV treatment, a 62% reduction (95% CI, 19–82%) | Has been standard recommendation | Requires intravenous administration and availability of ZDV intravenous formulation<br><br>Adherence to 6-wk infant regimen<br><br>Reversible, mild anemia with 6-wk infant ZDV regimen |
| Transmission at 6 wks 9% with ZDV-3TC vs. 15% with placebo, a 42% reduction | Oral regimen<br><br>Adherence easier than 6 wks of ZDV | Requires administration of two drugs |
| Transmission at 6 wks 12% with nevirapine compared to 21% with ZDV, a 47% reduction (95% CI[a], 20–64%) | Inexpensive<br><br>Oral regimen<br><br>Simple, easy to administer<br><br>Can give directly observed treatment | Unknown efficacy if mother has nevirapine-resistant virus<br><br>Nevirapine resistance mutations have been detected postpartum in some women and in infants who became infected despite prophylaxis |
| No data | Potential benefit if maternal virus is resistant to either nevirapine or ZDV<br><br>Synergistic inhibition of HIV replication with combination *in vitro* | Requires intravenous administration and availability of ZDV intravenous formulation<br><br>Adherence to 6-wk infant ZDV regimen<br><br>Unknown if additive efficacy with combination<br><br>Nevirapine resistance mutations have been detected postpartum in some women and in infants who became infected despite prophylaxis |

CI, confidence interval; 3TC, lamivudine; ZDV, zidovudine.

[a]ZDV dosing for infants <35 wks gestation at birth is 1.5 mg/kg/dose intravenously, or 2.0 mg/kg/dose orally, every 12 hrs, advancing to every 8 hrs at 2 wks of age if ≥30 wks gestation at birth or at 4 wks of age if <30 wks gestation at birth.

[b]If the mother received nevirapine less than 1 hr prior to delivery, the infant should be given 2 mg/kg oral nevirapine as soon as possible after birth and again at 48–72 hrs.

*Source:* Reprinted with permission from Public Health Service Task Force. Recommendations for Use of Antiretroviral Drugs in Pregnant HIV-1-Infected Women for Maternal Health and Interventions to Reduce Perinatal HIV-1 Transmission in the United States. October 12, 2006, pg. 46. Accessed at http://www.aidsinfo.nih.gov/Guidelines/GuidelineDetail.aspx?MenuItem=Guidelines&Search=Off&GuidelineID=9&ClassID=2.

# INFECTIOUS DISEASES

## Mother-to-Child Transmission of HIV, According to Antenatal Antiretroviral Therapy Regimen

| Maternal Antiretroviral Therapy | Transmission Rate (%) |
|---|---|
| **Data from WITS** | |
| None | 20.0 |
| Zidovudine monotherapy | 10.4 |
| Dual-drug therapy | 3.8 |
| HAART | 1.2 |
| **Data from PACTG 367** | |
| None | 18.5 |
| Single agent | 5.1 |
| 2 NRTIs | 1.4 |
| ≥3 Agents | 1.3 |
|    NRTIs only | 3.4 |
|    +NNRTI (no PI) | 1.5 |
|    +PI | 1.1 |

WITS denotes Women and Infants Transmission Study. Dual-drug therapy denotes mostly therapy with dual nucleoside reverse-transcriptase inhibitors (NRTI) but may include nonnucleoside reverse-transcriptase inhibitors (NNRTI) or protease inhibitors (PI). HAART denotes highly active antiretroviral therapy, defined as three or more drugs including at least one NNRTI or PI. PACTG 367 denotes Pediatric AIDS Clinical Trials Group Protocol 367.

Data from Cooper ER et al. Combination antiretroviral strategies for the treatment of pregnant HIV-1 infected women and prevention of perinatal HIV-1 transmission. *J Acquir Immune Defic Syndr.* 2002;29:484–494; and Shapiro D et al. Mother to child HIV transmission risk. Presented at the 11th Conference on Retroviruses and Opportunistic Infections, San Francisco, February 8–11, 2004.

*Source:* Reprinted with permission from Riley, Laura E. and Sigal Yawetz. Case 32-2005: A 34-Year-Old HIV-Positive Woman Who Desired to Become Pregnant. *N Engl J Med.* 2005;353(16):1725–1732. Copyright © 2005 Massachusetts Medical Society. All rights reserved.

## Drugs Used to Prevent Mother-to-Child Transmission of HIV

| Drug Category | Drug Names | Selected Adverse Effects in Pregnancy | Recommended Monitoring |
|---|---|---|---|
| Nucleoside or nucleotide reverse-transcriptase inhibitors | Zidovudine Lamivudine Stavudine Didanosine Abacavir | Anemia[a]; mitochondrial toxic effects (lactic acidosis, pancreatitis, hepatosteatosis) in mother and possibly fetus; neuropathy; hypersensitivity | Complete blood counts and hemoglobin levels; monitoring for mitochondrial toxic effects (measurement of electrolytes and liver enzymes) |
| | Tenofovir | Possible effect on fetal bone metabolism | |
| Nonnucleoside reverse-transcriptase inhibitors | Efavirenz Nevirapine | Neural malformations Hepatotoxic effects (especially with CD4 T cells >250/mm$^3$), rash | Avoid in pregnancy Aminotransferase levels (every 2 wks initially, then monthly) |
| Protease inhibitors | Amprenavir Atazanavir Indinavir Lopinavir Nelfinavir Ritonavir Saquinavir | Hyperglycemia, gestational diabetes, possible increase in preterm births, hepatitis | Glucose levels (standard 1-hr glucose loading test early in pregnancy and repeated in third trimester) |

[a]Anemia is a side effect caused only by zidovudine, whereas the other effects listed are associated with the drug class.

A complete list of side effects may be found in the guidelines published by the Department of Health and Human Services.

Data from Lorenzi P et al. Antiretroviral therapies in pregnancy. *AIDS* 1998;12:F241–F247; the European Collaborative Study and the Swiss Mother and Child HIV Cohort Study. Combination antiretroviral therapy and duration of pregnancy. *AIDS*. 2000;14:2913–2920; and Tuomala RE et al. Antiretroviral therapy during pregnancy and risk of an adverse outcome. *N Engl J Med.* 2002;346:1863–1870.

# INFECTIOUS DISEASES

## Clinical Scenarios and Recommendations Regarding Mode of Delivery to Reduce Perinatal Human Immunodeficiency Virus Type 1 (HIV-1) Transmission

| Mode of Delivery Clinical Scenario | Recommendations |
| --- | --- |
| **Scenario A** | |
| HIV-1–infected women presenting late in pregnancy (after about 36 wks of gestation), known to be HIV-1–infected but not receiving antiretroviral therapy, and who have HIV-1 RNA level and lymphocyte subsets pending but unlikely to be available before delivery. | Therapy options should be discussed in detail. The woman should be started on antiretroviral therapy including at least the PACTG 076 ZDV regimen. The woman should be counseled that scheduled cesarean section is likely to reduce the risk of transmission to her infant. She should also be informed of the increased risks to her of cesarean section, including increased rates of postoperative infection, anesthesia risks, and other surgical risks.<br><br>If cesarean section is chosen, the procedure should be scheduled at 38 wks of gestation based on the best available clinical information. When scheduled cesarean section is performed, the woman should receive continuous intravenous ZDV infusion beginning 3 hrs before surgery and her infant should receive 6 wks of ZDV therapy after birth. Options for continuing or initiating combination antiretroviral therapy after delivery should be discussed with the woman as soon as her viral load and lymphocyte subset results are available. |
| **Scenario B** | |
| HIV-1–infected women who initiated prenatal care early in the third trimester, are receiving highly active combinational antiretroviral therapy, and have an initial virologic response, but have HIV-1 RNA levels that remain substantially over 1000 copies/mL at 36 wks of gestation. | The current combination antiretroviral regimen should be continued as the HIV-1 RNA level is dropping appropriately. The woman should be counseled that although she is responding to the antiretroviral therapy, it is unlikely that her HIV-1 RNA level will fall below 1000 copies/mL before delivery. Therefore, scheduled cesarean section may provide additional benefit in preventing intrapartum transmission of HIV-1. She should also be informed of the increased risks to her of cesarean section, including increased rates of postoperative infection, anesthesia risks, and surgical risks.<br><br>If she chooses scheduled cesarean section, it should be performed at 38 wks gestation according to the best available dating parameters, and intravenous ZDV should be begun 3 hrs before surgery. Other antiretroviral medications should be continued on schedule as much as possible before and after surgery. The infant should receive oral ZDV for 6 wks after birth. The importance of adhering to therapy after delivery for her own health should be emphasized. |

| Mode of Delivery Clinical Scenario | Recommendations |
|---|---|
| **Scenario C**<br>HIV-1–infected women on highly active combination antiretroviral therapy with an undetectable HIV-1 RNA level at 36 wks of gestation. | The woman should be counseled that her risk of perinatal transmission of HIV-1 with a persistently undetectable HIV-1 RNA level is low, probably 2% or less, even with vaginal delivery. There is currently no information to evaluate whether performing a scheduled cesarean section will lower her risk further.<br>Cesarean section has an increased risk of complications for the woman compared to vaginal delivery, and these risks must be balanced against the uncertain benefit of cesarean section in this case. |
| **Scenario D**<br>HIV-1–infected women who have elected scheduled cesarean section but present in early labor or shortly after rupture of membranes. | Intravenous ZDV should be started immediately since the woman is in labor or has ruptured membranes. If labor is progressing rapidly, the woman should be allowed to deliver vaginally. If cervical dilatation is minimal and a long period of labor is anticipated, some clinicians may choose to administer the loading dose of intravenous ZDV and proceed with cesarean section to minimize the duration of membrane rupture and avoid vaginal delivery. Others might begin Pitocin augmentation to enhance contractions and potentially expedite delivery.<br>If the woman is allowed to labor, scalp electrodes and other invasive monitoring and operative delivery should be avoided if possible. The infant should be treated with 6 wks of ZDV therapy after birth. |

PACTG, Pediatric AIDS Clinical Trials Group; RNA, ribonucleic acid; ZDV, zidovudine.
*Source:* Reprinted with permission from Public Health Service Task Force. Recommendations for Use of Antiretroviral Drugs in Pregnant HIV-1-Infected Women for Maternal Health and Interventions to Reduce Perinatal HIV-1 Transmission in the United States. October 12, 2006, pg. 48. Accessed at http://www.aidsinfo.nih.gov/Guidelines/GuidelineDetail.aspx?MenuItem=Guidelines&Search=Off&GuidelineID=9&ClassID=2.

# INFECTIOUS DISEASES

## HERPES SIMPLEX VIRUS

### Fast Facts

- 45 million adolescent and adult Americans are infected with HSV
  - Only 5–15% of infected individuals report recognition of infection
- 80% of infected infants are born to mothers with no reported history of HSV infection
  - $^1/_3$ to ∫ of neonatal HSV infections are from HSV-1
  - Infant mortality has been decreasing
    - ⇨ 30% for disseminated disease
    - ⇨ 4% for CNS disease
    - ⇨ 20% of survivors have neurologic long-term sequelae
  - Risk of vertical transmission from mother to fetus
    - ⇨ 30-60% if primary genital HSV infection at time of delivery
    - ⇨ 3% if recurrent genital lesion at time of delivery
    - ⇨ 2/10,000 if history of HSV but no prodrome or lesions
    - ⇨ "Very low" if non-genital HSV lesion in patient with history of HSV

### CDC Recommendations for HSV

- Persons who have genital herpes should be educated concerning the natural history of the disease, with emphasis on the potential for recurrent episodes, asymptomatic viral shedding, and the attendant risks of sexual transmission.
- Persons experiencing a first episode of genital herpes should be advised that suppressive therapy is available and is effective in preventing symptomatic recurrent episodes and that episodic therapy sometimes is useful in shortening the duration of recurrent episodes.
- All persons with genital HSV infection should be encouraged to inform their current sex partners that they have genital herpes and to inform future partners before initiating a sexual relationship.
- Sexual transmission of HSV can occur during asymptomatic periods. Asymptomatic viral shedding is more frequent in genital HSV-2 infection than genital HSV-1 infection and is most frequent during the first 12 months after acquiring HSV-2.
- All persons with genital herpes should remain abstinent from sexual activity with uninfected partners when lesions or prodromal symptoms are present.
- The risk of HSV-2 sexual transmission can be decreased by the daily use of valacyclovir by the infected person.
- Recent studies indicate that latex condoms, when used consistently and correctly, might reduce the risk for genital herpes transmission.
- Sex partners of infected persons should be advised that they might be infected even if they have no symptoms. Type-specific serologic testing of asymptomatic

partners of persons with genital herpes is recommended to deter- mine whether risk for HSV acquisition exists.

- The risk for neonatal HSV infection should be explained to all persons, including men. Pregnant women and women of childbearing age who have genital herpes should inform their providers who care for them during pregnancy and those who will care for their newborn infant. Pregnant women who are not infected with HSV-2 should be advised to avoid intercourse during the third trimester with men who have genital herpes. Similarly, pregnant women who are not infected with HSV-1 should be counseled to avoid genital exposure to HSV-1 during the third trimester (e.g., oral sex with a partner with oral herpes and vaginal intercourse with a partner with genital HSV-1 infection).
- Asymptomatic persons diagnosed with HSV-2 infection by type-specific serologic testing should receive the same counseling messages as persons with symptomatic infection. In addition, such persons should be taught about the clinical manifestations of genital herpes.

*Source*: Centers for Disease Control and Prevention. Sexually Transmitted Diseases Treatment Guidelines, 2006. *MMWR*. 2006;55(RR-11):1–100.

## ACOG Recommendations for HSV Infections in Pregnancy

The following recommendations and conclusions are based on limited or inconsistent scientific evidence (Level B):

- Women with active recurrent genital herpes should be offered suppressive viral therapy at or beyond 36 weeks of gestation.
- Cesarean delivery is indicated in women with active genital lesions or prodromal symptoms, such as vulvar pain or burning at delivery, because these symptoms may indicate an impending outbreak.

The following recommendations and conclusions are based primarily on consensus and expert opinion (Level C):

- In women with premature rupture of membranes, there is no consensus on the gestational age at which the risks of prematurity outweigh the risks of HSV.
- Cesarean delivery is not recommended for women with a history of HSV infection but no active genital disease during labor.
- Routine antepartum genital HSV cultures in asymptomatic patients with recurrent disease are not recommended.
- Routine HSV screening of pregnant women is not recommended.

*Source*: ACOG Practice Bulletin, Management of Herpes in Pregnancy, Number 82, June 2007.

# INFECTIOUS DISEASES

## Therapeutic Management of Genital Herpes[a]

| Agent | Dose and Schedule[b] | Efficacy | Advantages and Disadvantages Relative to Other Agents |
|---|---|---|---|
| **First episode of genital herpes** | | | |
| Acyclovir | 200 mg orally 5 times/day for 7–10 days or 400 mg orally 3 times/day for 7–10 days | 2-day decrease in time to resolution of signs and symptoms; 4-day decrease in time to healing of lesions; 7-day decrease in duration of viral shedding | Less expensive, smaller tablets; liquid formulation available; less convenient treatment schedule |
| Valacyclovir | 1.0 g orally twice daily for 7–10 days | No difference in efficacy as compared with acyclovir for first episode | More convenient treatment schedule; more expensive; larger caplets; no liquid formulation |
| Famciclovir | 250 mg orally 3 times/day for 7–10 days | No difference in efficacy as compared with acyclovir for first episode | More convenient treatment schedule; smaller tablets; more expensive; no liquid formulation |
| **Recurrent genital herpes, episodic treatment[c]** | | | |
| Acyclovir | 400 mg orally 3 times/day for 5 days or 800 mg orally twice daily for 5 days or 800 mg orally 3 times/day for 2 days | 1.1-Day decrease in time to resolution of signs and symptoms; 1.2-day decrease in time to healing of lesions; 2.0-day decrease in duration of viral shedding | Same as for first episode |
| Valacyclovir | 500 mg orally twice daily for 3 or 5 days or 1.0 g orally once daily for 5 days | No difference in efficacy as compared with acyclovir for episodic treatment | Same as for first episode |
| Famciclovir | 125 mg orally twice daily for 5 days or 1000 mg twice daily for 1 day | No difference in efficacy as compared with acyclovir for episodic treatment | Same as for first episode |

| Agent | Dose and Schedule[b] | Efficacy | Advantages and Disadvantages Relative to Other Agents |
|---|---|---|---|
| Suppressive therapy[d] | | | |
| Acyclovir | 400 mg orally twice daily | 71% of recipients recurrence-free after 4 mos; 80–94% reduction in no. of days with subclinical shedding | Same as for first episode |
| Valacyclovir | 500 mg orally once daily or 1.0 g once daily | 69% of recipients recurrence-free after 4 mos; 81% reduction in no. of days with subclinical shedding | Same as for first episode |
| Famciclovir | 250 mg orally twice daily | 78% of recipients recurrence-free after 4 mos; 87% reduction in no. of days with subclinical shedding | Same as for first episode |

[a]Data were modified from Sexually Transmitted Diseases Treatment Guidelines 2006. Allergic and other adverse reactions to acyclovir, valacyclovir, and famciclovir are rare.

[b]For the first episode of genital herpes, the range of duration of therapy reflects differences in the durations of treatment in the original clinical studies. If the shorter course of therapy is prescribed initially, the patient should be reevaluated toward the end of treatment, and therapy should be continued if new lesions continue to form, if complications develop, or if systemic signs and symptoms have not abated. Episodic therapy should be started within 24 hrs after the onset of a recurrence, or as soon as possible thereafter.

[c]The recommendations for episodic treatment in HIV-infected persons are as follows: acyclovir, 200 mg five times per day for 5–10 days or 400 mg three times per day for 5–10 days; valacyclovir, 1000 mg twice daily for 5–10 days; or famciclovir, 500 mg twice daily for 5–10 days.

[d]The recommendations for suppressive therapy in HIV-infected persons are as follows: acyclovir, 400–800 mg 2 or 3 times per day; valacyclovir, 500 mg twice daily; or famciclovir, 500 mg twice daily.

# INFECTIOUS DISEASES

## VARICELLA
### Fast Facts

- 0.4–0.7/1000 pregnancies complicated by maternal chickenpox.
- 25% of maternal infections result in evidence of fetal infection.
- First trimester maternal varicella results in <2.5–3% risk of congenital varicella syndrome (skin scarring, limb hypoplasia, CNS, eye abnormalities).
- Avoid delivery if possible during 7 day window because of increased risk of neonatal death.
  - 2 days before onset of maternal rash, 5 days after onset of rash
  - 11–21 days between exposure and rash (mean 15 days)
  - If delivery occurs during this window, the infant should receive varicella zoster immune globulin and acyclovir
- IV acyclovir can be used for severe maternal infections.
  - 10–30% of pregnant varicella patients develop varicella pneumonia
    ⇨ 40% mortality rate
- No fetal risk in cases of maternal herpes zoster (shingles).
- Immunize if non-immune preconception or postpartum.
- Breastfeeding should be avoided and the woman should be isolated from her infant with a new varicella infection.
- Breastfeeding is okay if an immunocompetent woman develops zoster as long as the lesion is not on the breast and does not contact the infant.

*Source:* ACOG Education Bulletin Number 258. Breastfeeding: Maternal and Infant Aspects. *Obstet Gynecol.* 2000;96:1–16; ACOG practice bulletin. Perinatal viral and parasitic infections. Number 20, September 2000.

## Management

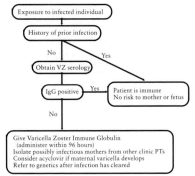

## RUBELLA

### Fast Facts

- Infection can be communicated 7 days before and 4 days after appearance of rash.
- Rash occurs 2–3 weeks following exposure.
  - Usually lasts 3 days "3-day measles"
- Rate of fetal infection depends on stage of gestation.
  - <11 weeks, 90% risk of congenital infection; 11–12 weeks, 33%; 13–14 weeks, 11%; 15–16 weeks, 24%; >16 weeks, 0%.
- Risk of fetal anomalies also dependent on gestational age.
  - 1st trimester, 25%; 1st month → 50%; 2nd month → 25%; 3rd month → 10%
  - 2nd trimester, <1%; 16–20 weeks: sensory only; >20 weeks: no reported cases

### Management

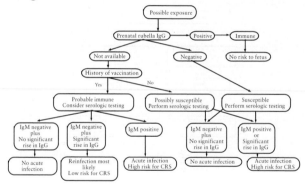

- *Post-exposure testing*
  - IgM and IgG drawn ASAP and paired IgG ASAP and in 4–5 weeks
- *Post-rash testing*
  - IgM and IgG drawn ASAP after rash and paired IgG ASAP after the rash and in 2–3 weeks.

*Source:* American College of Obstetricians and Gynecologists: Rubella and Pregnancy. Technical Bulletin 171. ACOG, Washington, DC © 1992. Reproduced with permission of the publisher, the American College of Obstetricians and Gynecologists.

# INFECTIOUS DISEASES

## TOXOPLASMOSIS
### Fast Facts

- $1/3$ of women have been exposed through ingestion of undercooked meat and contact with cat feces.
- Presence of IgG indicates immunity, IgM appears within 1 week and lasts for months.
- Increasing gestational age increases fetal infection rate but diminishes severity.
- Rate of fetal infection:
  - First trimester: 10–15%
  - Second trimester: 25%
  - Third trimester: 60%
- 55–85% of infants will develop sequelae including:
  - IUGR, microcephaly, chorioretinitis, intracranial calcifications, hearing loss, mental retardation, hepatosplenomegaly, ascites, fever, periventricular calcifications, ventriculomegaly, and seizures

*Source:* ACOG practice bulletin. Perinatal viral and parasitic infections. Number 20, September 2000.

### Management

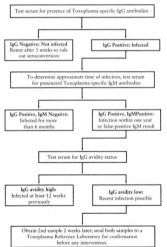

If IgM positive, refer to well-recognized reference lab. If acute infection suspected start spiramycin therapy. Amniocentesis at least 6 weeks after acute infection for *T. gondii* PCR testing. If intrauterine infection is established pyrimethamine, sulfonamides, and folinic acid are added.
*Source:* Singh S. Mother-to-child transmission and diagnosis of Toxoplasma gondii infection during pregnancy. *Indian Journal of Medical Microbiology.* 2003;21(2):69–76.

## CYTOMEGALOVIRUS
### Fast Facts

- 0.7–4% of pregnancies complicated by primary infections, up to 13.5% complicated by recurrent infections.
- Usually asymptomatic.
- 50–80% of mothers have been already infected.
- Cytomegalovirus (CMV) is the most common congenital infection occurring in 0.2–2.2% of all neonates.
  - Risk of malformations decrease with gestational age.
  - CMV tetrad: mental retardation, microcephaly, chorioretinitis, cerebral calcifications. Other complications include jaundice, petechiae, thrombocytopenia, hepatosplenomeglay, growth restriction, and nonimmune hydrops, hearing loss.
- Primary CMV infection: 30–40% risk of transmission, 10% with clinical signs of infection, 30% of severe infections die, and 80% of survivors have severe neurologic morbidity.
- Recurrent CMV infection: 0.15–2% risk of transmission infants are usually symptomatic. Most common sequelae is isolated hearing loss.
- Transmission via cervical secretions and breast milk is usually asymptomatic.

*Source:* ACOG practice bulletin. Perinatal viral and parasitic infections. Number 20, September 2000.

### Consequences of CMV in Pregnancy

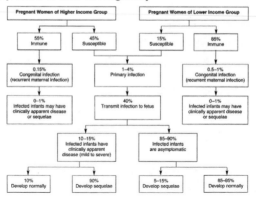

*Source:* Stagno S, Whitley RJ. Herpesvirus infections of pregnancy, Part I: Cytomegalovirus and Epstein-Barr virus infections. *N Engl J Med.* 1985;313(20):1270–1274. Copyright © 1985 Massachusetts Medical Society. All rights reserved.

# INFECTIOUS DISEASES

## Immunization during Pregnancy

| Viral Agent | Risk from Disease to Pregnant Woman | Risk from Disease to Fetus or Neonate | Type of Immunizing Agent | Risk from Immunizing Agent to Fetus | Indications for Immunization during Pregnancy | Dose Schedule | Comments |
|---|---|---|---|---|---|---|---|
| | | | Live Virus Vaccines | | | | |
| Measles | Significant morbidity, low mortality; not altered by pregnancy | Significant increase in abortion rate; may cause fetal malformations | Live attenuated virus vaccine | None confirmed | Contraindicated (see Immune Globulins) | Single dose SC, preferably as measles-mumps-rubella (MMR)a | Vaccination of susceptible women should be part of postpartum care |
| Mumps | Low morbidity and mortality; not altered by pregnancy | Probable increased rate of abortion in first trimester | Live attenuated virus vaccine | None confirmed | Contraindicated | Single dose SC, preferably as measles-mumps-rubella (MMR) | Vaccination of susceptible women should be part of postpartum care |
| Poliomyelitis | No increased incidence in pregnancy; but may be more severe if it does occur | Anoxic fetal damage reported; 50% mortality in neonatal cases | Live attenuated virus (oral polio vaccine (OPV)] and enhanced-potency inactivated virus (e-IPV) vaccine b | None confirmed | Not routinely recommended for women in United States, except persons at increased risk of exposure | Primary 2 doses of e-IPV SC at 4–8 wk intervals and a 3rd dose 6–12 mos after the second dose. Immediate protection: 1 dose OPV orally (in outbreak setting). | Vaccine indicated for susceptible pregnant women travelling in endemic areas or in other high-risk situations |
| Rubella | Low morbidity and mortality; not altered by pregnancy | High rate of abortion and congenital rubella syndrome | Live attenuated virus vaccine | None confirmed | Contraindicated | Single dose SC, preferably as measles-mumps-rubella (MMR) | Teratogenicity of vaccine is theoretic, not confirmed to date; vaccination of susceptible women should be part of postpartum care |
| Yellow fever | Significant morbidity and mortality; not altered by pregnancy | Unknown | Live attenuated virus vaccine | Unknown | Contraindicated except if exposure is unavoidable | Single dose SC | Postponement of travel preferable to vaccination, if pregnancy possible |

336

| | Effect on Pregnancy | Effect on Fetus/Newborn | Vaccine | Fetal Risk | Indications | Dose/Schedule | Comments |
|---|---|---|---|---|---|---|---|
| Varicella | Possible increase in severe pneumonia | Can cause congenital varicella in 2% of fetuses infected during the second trimester | Live attenuated virus vaccine | None confirmed | Contraindicated, but no adverse outcomes reported if given in pregnancy | Two doses needed with second dose given 4–8 wks after first dose. Should be strongly encouraged. | Teratogenicity of vaccine is theoretic, outcomes reported wks 4–8 not confirmed to date. Vaccination of susceptible women should be considered postpartum. |
| **Other** | | | | | | | |
| Influenza | Increase in morbidity and mortality during epidemic of new antigenic strain | Possible increased abortion rate; no malformations confirmed | Inactivated virus vaccine | None confirmed | Women with serious underlying diseases; public health authorities to be consulted for current recommendations | One dose IM every yr | — |
| Rabies | Near 100% fatality; not altered by pregnancy | Determined by maternal disease | Killed virus vaccine | Unknown | Indications for prophylaxis not altered by pregnancy; each case considered individually | Public health authorities to be consulted for indications, dosage and route of administration | — |
| Hepatitis B | Possible increased severity during third trimester | Possible increase in abortion rate and prematurity; neonatal hepatitis can occur; high risk of newborn carrier state | Recombinant vaccine | None reported | Pre- and post-exposure for women at risk of infection | Three- or four-dose series | Used with hepatitis B immune globulin for some exposures; exposed newborn needs vaccination as soon as possible |
| Hepatitis A | No increased risk during pregnancy | — | Inactivated virus | None reported | Pre-exposure and post-exposure for women at risk of infection; international travelers | Two-dose schedule 6 mos apart | — |

*(continued)*

| Viral Agent | Risk from Disease to Pregnant Woman | Risk from Disease to Fetus or Neonate | Type of Immunizing Agent | Risk from Immunizing Agent to Fetus | Indications for Immunization during Pregnancy | Dose Schedule | Comments |
|---|---|---|---|---|---|---|---|
| | | | **Inactivated Bacterial Vaccines** | | | | |
| Pneumococcus | No increased risk during pregnancy and no increase in severity of disease | Unknown | Polyvalent polysaccharide vaccine | No data available on use during pregnancy | Indications not altered by pregnancy; vaccine used only for high-risk individuals | In adults, 1 SC or IM dose only; consider repeat dose in 6 yrs for high-risk individuals | — |
| Meningococcus | Significant morbidity and mortality; not altered by pregnancy | Unknown, but depends on maternal illness | Quadrivalent polysaccharide vaccine | None reported | Indications not altered by pregnancy; vaccination recommended in unusual outbreak situations | One SC dose; public health authorities consulted | — |
| Typhoid | Significant morbidity and mortality; not altered by pregnancy | Unknown | Killed or live attenuated oral bacterial vaccine | None confirmed | Not recommended routinely except for close, continued exposure or travel to endemic areas | Killed: Primary: 2 injections SC at least 4 wks apart Booster: Single dose SC or ID (depending on type of product used) Booster: Schedule not yet determined | Oral vaccine preferred |
| Anthrax | Significant morbidity and mortality; not altered by pregnancy | Unknown, but depends on maternal illness | Preparation from cell-free filtrate of B anthracis; no dead or alive bacteria | None confirmed | Not routinely recommended unless pregnant women work directly with B anthracis, imported animal hides, potentially infected animals in high incidence area (not United States) or military personnel deployed to high-risk exposure areas | Six-dose primary vaccination SC, then annual booster vaccination | Teratogenicity of vaccine theoretical |

| | | | Toxoids | | | | |
|---|---|---|---|---|---|---|---|
| Tetanus-diphtheria | Severe morbidity; tetanus mortality 30%, diphtheria mortality 10%; unaltered by pregnancy | Neonatal tetanus mortality 60% | Combined tetanus-diphtheria toxoids (adult tetanus-diphtheria preferred; adult tetanus-diphtheria formulation) | None confirmed | Lack of primary series, or no booster within past 10 yrs | *Primary:* 2 doses IM at 1–2 mo interval with a 3rd dose 6–12 mos after the 2nd *Booster:* Single dose IM every 10 yrs, after completion of primary series | Updating of immune status should be part of antepartum care |
| | | | **Specific Immune Globulins** | | | | |
| Hepatitis B | Possible increased severity during third trimester | Possible increase in abortion rate and prematurity; neonatal hepatitis can occur, high risk of carriage in newborn | Hepatitis B immune globulin | None reported | Postexposure prophylaxis | Depends on exposure; consult Immunization Practices Advisory Committee recommendations (IM) | Usually given with HBV vaccine; exposed newborn needs immediate postexposure prophylaxis |
| Rabies | Near 100% fatality; not altered by pregnancy | Determined by maternal disease | Rabies immune globulin | None reported | Postexposure prophylaxis | Half dose at injury site, half dose in deltoid | Used in conjunction with rabies killed virus vaccine |
| Tetanus | Severe morbidity; mortality 21% | Neonatal tetanus mortality 60% | Tetanus immune globulin | None reported | Postexposure prophylaxis | One dose IM | Used in conjunction with tetanus toxoid |
| Varicella | Possible increase in severe varicella pneumonia | Can cause congenital varicella with increased mortality in neonatal period; very rarely causes congenital defects | Varicella-zoster immune globulin (obtained from American Red Cross) | None reported | Can be considered for healthy pregnant women exposed to varicella to protect against maternal, not congenital, infection | One dose IM within 96 hrs of exposure | Indicated also for newborns of mothers who developed varicella within 4 days prior to delivery or 2 days following delivery; approximately 90–95% of adults are immune to varicella; not indicated for prevention of congenital varicella *(continued)* |

### Immunization during Pregnancy (continued)

| Viral Agent | Risk from Disease to Pregnant Woman | Risk from Disease to Fetus or Neonate | Type of Immunizing Agent | Risk from Immunizing Agent to Fetus | Indications for Immunization during Pregnancy | Dose Schedule | Comments |
|---|---|---|---|---|---|---|---|
| **Standard Immune Globulins** | | | | | | | |
| Hepatitis A | Possible increased severity during third trimester | Probable increase in abortion rate and preterm birth; possible transmission to neonate at delivery if woman is incubating the virus or is acutely ill at that time | Standard immune globulin | None reported | Postexposure prophylaxis, but hepatitis A virus vaccine should be used with hepatitis A immune globulin | 0.03 mL/kg IM in one dose of immune globulin | Immune globulin should be given as soon as possible and within 2 wks of exposure; infants born to women who are incubating the virus or are acutely ill at delivery should receive one dose of 0.5 mL as soon as possible after birth |
| Cholera | Significant morbidity and mortality; more severe during third trimester | Increased risk of fetal death during third-trimester maternal illness | Killed bacterial vaccine | None confirmed | Indications not altered by pregnancy; vaccination recommended only in unusual outbreak situations | Single dose SC or IM depending on manufacturer's recommendations when indicated | |
| Plague | Significant morbidity and mortality; not altered by pregnancy | Determined by maternal disease | Killed bacterial vaccine | None reported | Selective vaccination of exposed persons | Public health authorities to be consulted for indications, dosage, and route of administration | |

ID, intradermally; IM, intramuscular; PO, orally; SC, subcutaneously.

[a] Two doses necessary for adequate vaccinations of students entering institutions of higher education, newly hired medical personnel, and international travelers.

[b] Inactivated polio vaccine recommended for nonimmunized adults at increased risk.

*Source:* Reprinted with permission from Center for Disease Control. *MMWR Recomm. Rep.* 51(RR-2):1–35. Available at www.cdc.gov/mmwr/ preview/mmwrhtm/nr5102al.htm. Retrieved October 11, 2002.

## VAGINITIS

### Diagnostic Tests Available for Vaginitis

| Test | Sensitivity (%) | Specificity (%) | Comment |
|---|---|---|---|
| Bacterial vaginosis | | | |
| pH >4.5 | 97 | 64 | |
| Amsel's criteria | 92 | 77 | Must meet 3 of 4 clinical criteria (pH >4.5, thin watery discharge, >20% clue cells, positive "whiff" test [amine odor present with addition of base]), but similar results achieved if 2 of 4 criteria met |
| Nugent criteria | | | Gram's stain morphology score (0–10) based on lactobacilli and other morphotypes; a score of 0–3 indicates normal flora, a score of 4–6 intermediate flora, and a score of 7–10 bacterial vaginosis; high interobserver reproducibility |
| Papanicolaou smear | 49 | 93 | |
| Point-of-care tests | | | |
| QuickVue Advance pH+ amines | 89 | 96 | Positive if pH >4.7 |
| QuickVue Advance G. vaginalis[a] | 91 | >95 | Tests for proline iminopeptidase activity in vaginal fluid; if used when pH >4.5, sensitivity is 95% and specificity is 99% |
| OSOM BV Blue[a] | 90 | >95 | Test for vaginal sialidase activity |
| Candida | | | |
| Wet mount | | | |
| Overall | 50 | 97 | |
| Growth of 3–4+ on culture | 85 | | C. albicans a commensal agent in 10–25% of women |
| Growth of 1+ on culture | 23 | | |
| pH ≥4.5 | | | pH may be elevated if mixed infection with bacterial vaginosis or T. vaginalis present |
| Papanicolaou smear | 25 | 72 | |

*(continued)*

## Diagnostic Tests Available for Vaginitis *(continued)*

| Test | Sensitivity (%) | Specificity (%) | Comment |
|---|---|---|---|
| *T. vaginalis* | | | |
| Wet mount | 45–60 | 95 | Increased visibility of microorganisms with a higher burden of infection |
| Culture | 85–90 | >95 | |
| pH >4.5 | 56 | 50 | |
| Papanicolaou smear | 92 | 61 | False positive rate, 8% for standard Pap test and 4% for liquid-based cytologic test |
| Point-of-care test | | | |
| OSOM | 83 | 98.8 | Requires 10 mins to perform; tests for *T. vaginalis* antigens |

[a]Proline iminopeptidase and sialidase are enzymes produced by many bacteria associated with bacterial vaginosis.

## Treatment Recommendations for Acute Vaginitis[a]

| Disease | Drug | Dose | Cost[b] |
|---------|------|------|---------|
| Bacterial vaginosis[c] | Metronidazole (Flagyl) | 500 mg orally twice a day for 7 days[d] | $ |
| | 0.75% Metronidazole gel (Metrogel) | One 5-g application intravaginally daily for 5 days[e] | $$$ |
| | 2% Clindamycin cream (Cleocin vaginal) | One 5-g application intravaginally every night for 7 days | $$$ |
| | 2% Extended-release clindamycin cream (Clindesse)[f] | One application intravaginally[e] | $$ |
| | Clindamycin[g] | 300 mg orally twice daily for 7 days | $$$ |
| Vulvovaginal candidiasis, uncomplicated Intravaginal therapy[e] | 2% Butoconazole cream (Mycelex-3) | 5 g per day for 3 days[h] | $$ |
| | 2% Sustained-release butoconazole cream (Gynazole) | One 5-g dose | $$$ |
| | 1% Clotrimazole cream (Mycelex-7) | 5 g for 7–14 days[h] | $ |
| | Clotrimazole (Gyne-Lotrimin 3) | Two 100-mg vaginal tablets per day for 3 days | $ |
| | | One 100-mg vaginal tablet per day for 7 days | |
| | 2% Miconazole cream | 5 g per day for 7 days[h] | $$ |
| | Miconazole (Monistat-7) | One 100-mg vaginal suppository per day for 7 days[h] | $$ |
| | Miconazole (Monistat-3) | One 200-mg vaginal suppository per day for 3 days[h] | $$ |
| | Miconazole (Monistat-1 vaginal ovule) | One 1200-mg vaginal suppository[h] | $ |
| | 6.5% Tioconazole ointment (Monistat 1-day) | One 5-g dose[h] | $ |
| | 0.4% Terconazole cream (Terazol 7) | 5 g per day for 7 days | $$$ |
| | 0.8% Terconazole cream (Terazol 3) | 5 g per day for 3 days | $$ |
| | Terconazole vaginal | One 80-mg vaginal suppository per day for 3 days | $$$ |
| | Nystatin vaginal | One 100,000-U vaginal tablet per day for 14 days | $$$ |

*(continued)*

## Treatment Recommendations for Acute Vaginitis[a] *(continued)*

| Disease | Drug | Dose | Cost[b] |
|---|---|---|---|
| Oral therapy[c] | Fluconazole (Diflucan) | One 150-mg dose orally | $ |
| Vulvovaginal candidiasis, complicated[i] | | | |
| Intravaginal therapy[e] | Azole | 7–14 days | $$ |
| Oral therapy[j] | Fluconazole (Diflucan) | Two 150-mg doses orally 72 hrs apart | $$$ |
| Trichomoniasis | Metronidazole (Flagyl) | One 2-g dose orally | $ |
| | | 500 mg orally twice daily for 7 days | $ |
| | Tinidazole (Tindamax) | One 2-g dose orally[k] | $$ |

[a]Recommendations are based on the CDC 2006 Guidelines for Treatment of Vaginitis.

[b]A single dollar sign indicates a cost of less than $15, two dollar signs a cost of $15 to $29, and three dollar signs a cost of $30 or more.

[c]Oral therapy is recommended for pregnant women.

[d]Drug may cause gastrointestinal upset in 5–10% of patients; a disulfuram reaction is possible; alcohol should be avoided for 24 hrs after ingestion. In the absence of a clear indication for a particular type of therapy (e.g., for women who are pregnant), the patient's preference, the response to prior therapy, and cost should guide the choice of therapy.

[e]Vaginal treatments cause local vaginal irritation in 2–5% of patients.

[f]This agent is approved by the Food and Drug Administration but is not listed in the CDC 2006 Guidelines.

[g]This agent is listed as an alternative treatment in the CDC 2006 Guidelines.

[h]This agent is available over the counter.

[i]Complicated vulvovaginitis refers to disease in women who are pregnant, women who have uncontrolled diabetes, women who are immunocompromised, or women who have severe symptoms, non–*Candida albicans* candidiasis, or recurrent episodes (four or more per year).

[j]Oral therapy is not recommended for pregnant women.

[k]Drug may cause gastrointestinal upset in 2–5% of patients; disulfuram reaction is possible; alcohol should be avoided for 72 hrs after ingestion.

*Source:* Reprinted with permission from Eckert, Linda O. Acute Vulvovaginitis. Clinical Practice. *N Engl J Med.* 2006;355(12):1244–1252. Copyright © 2006 Massachusetts Medical Society. All rights reserved.

## URINARY TRACT INFECTIONS

### Fast Facts
- Common symptoms are dysuria, frequency, and lower abdominal pain.
- Most common organisms:
  - *E. coli*
  - *S. saprophyticus*
  - *Proteus mirabilis*
  - *Enterococcus* sp.

### Treatment Regimens for Uncomplicated Urinary Infections in Women and the Relative Cost of Each Regimen[a]

| Treatment Regimen | Cost |
|---|---|
| Single-dose treatment | |
|     Ampicillin, 2 g | $ |
|     Amoxicillin, 3 g | $ |
|     Nitrofurantoin, 200 mg | $ |
|     Trimethoprim-sulfamethoxazole, 320/1600 mg | $ |
| 3-Day course | |
|     Amoxicillin, 500 mg 3 times daily | $ |
|     Ampicillin, 250 mg 4 times daily | $ |
|     Cephalexin, 250 mg 4 times daily | $$$ |
|     Nitrofurantoin, 50 mg 4 times daily; 100 mg twice daily | $$ |
|     Trimethoprim-sulfamethoxazole, 160/800 mg twice daily | $$ |
|     Ciprofloxacin, 250 mg twice daily | $$$ |
|     Levofloxacin, 250 mg daily | $$$ |
| Other | |
|     Nitrofurantoin, 100 mg at bedtime for 7–14 days | $$$ |
|     Nitrofurantoin, 100 mg 4 times daily for 7–14 days | $$$$ |
| Treatment failures | |
|     Nitrofurantoin, 100 mg at bedtime for 21 days | $$$$ |
| Suppression for bacterial persistence or recurrence | |
|     Nitrofurantoin, 100 mg at bedtime for remainder of pregnancy | N/A |

$ ≤ $5; $$ > $5 ≤ $15; $$$ > $15 ≤ $30; $$$$ > $30.

[a]Based on generic average wholesale price (from Redbook Pharmacy's Fundamental Reference) per regimen when available.

*Source:* Reprinted with permission from Sheffield JS, Cunningham FG. Urinary tract infection in women. *Obstet Gynecol.* 2005;106(5,1):1085–1092.

# INFECTIOUS DISEASES

**Intravenous and Oral Regimens for the Treatment of Acute Uncomplicated Pyelonephritis and the Relative Cost per Day of Each Regimen[a]**

| Regimen | Cost |
| --- | --- |
| Outpatient regimens (10–14 days) | |
| Ciprofloxacin, 500 mg twice daily | $ |
| Ciprofloxacin-XR, 1000 mg once daily | $ |
| Gatifloxacin, 400 mg once daily | $ |
| Levofloxacin, 250 mg once daily | $ |
| Ofloxacin, 400 mg twice daily | $ |
| Amoxicillin-clavulanate, 875/125 mg twice daily | $ |
| Trimethoprim-sulfamethoxazole DS, 160/800 mg twice daily | $ |
| Intravenous regimens | |
| Ciprofloxacin, 400 mg every 12 hrs | $$$ |
| Levofloxacin, 500 mg once daily | $$ |
| Cefepime, 2 g every 8 hrs | $$$$ |
| Cefotetan, 2 g every 12 hrs | $$$ |
| Ticarcillin-clavulanate, 3.1 g every 6 hrs | $$$ |
| Trimethoprim-sulfamethoxazole, 2 mg/kg every 6 hrs | $$ |
| Ceftriaxone, 1–2 g every 12–24 hrs | $$$$ |
| Gentamicin, 3–5 mg/kg per day (once daily dosing acceptable) | $ |
| Ampicillin, 2 g every 6 hrs—for suspected enterococcus | $$ |
| Aztreonam, 2 g every 8 hrs | $$$$ |
| Cefotaxime, 1–2 g every 8 hrs | $$$ |

$ ≤ $20; $$ > $20 ≤ $60; $$$ > $60 ≤ $100; $$$$ > $100.
[a]Based on generic average wholesale price per day when available.
*Source:* Reprinted with permission from Sheffield JS, Cunningham FG. Urinary tract infection in women. *Obstet Gynecol.* 2005;106(5,1):1085–1092.

## URINARY TRACT INFECTIONS IN PREGNANCY
### Risk Factors

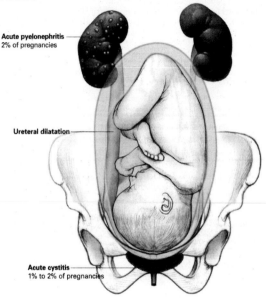

Acute pyelonephritis
2% of pregnancies

Ureteral dilatation

Acute cystitis
1% to 2% of pregnancies

**Mechanical changes** lead to urinary stasis and ureterovesical reflux. Beginning in the sixth week of gestation and peaking at 22–24 weeks, approximately 90% of pregnant women develop **ureteral dilation**, which remains until delivery. **Increased bladder volume** and **decreased bladder and ureteral tone** contribute to increased urinary stasis and ureterovesical reflux.

**Hormonal changes** lead to increased bacterial growth in the urine and possibly lowered resistance to bacteria. Up to 70% of pregnant women develop **glycosuria**, which encourages bacterial growth in the urine. **Increases in urinary progestins and estrogens** may lead to decreased ability of the lower urinary tract to resist invading bacteria.

*Source:* Reprinted with permission from Chen KT. UTI in pregnancy: 6 questions to guide therapy. *OBG Management.* 2004;Nov:36–53. Artist: Scott Bodell.

# INFECTIOUS DISEASES

## Fast Facts

- 5% of patients develop urinary tract infection or asymptomatic bacteruria.
- $^1/_3$ untreated patients develop pyelonephritis.
- Pyelonephritis in pregnancy is treated as an inpatient.
  - √ serum K$^+$ level on admission (may be hypokalemic)
- Initiate renal evaluation for multiple admissions or left-sided pyelonephritis.
  - Hydronephrosis usually occurs on the right because of uterine displacement.
- Consider suppression therapy for high-risk patients.

## Management of Asymptomatic Bacteriuria or Acute Cystitis in Pregnancy

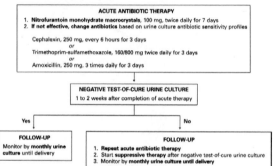

**ACUTE ANTIBIOTIC THERAPY**

1. **Nitrofurantoin monohydrate macrocrystals**, 100 mg, twice daily for 7 days
2. **If not effective, change antibiotics** based on urine culture antibiotic sensitivity profiles

Cephalexin, 250 mg, every 6 hours for 3 days
*or*
Trimethoprim-sulfamethoxazole, 160/800 mg twice daily for 3 days
*or*
Amoxicillin, 250 mg, 3 times daily for 3 days

**NEGATIVE TEST-OF-CURE URINE CULTURE**
1 to 2 weeks after completion of acute therapy

Yes

No

**FOLLOW-UP**
Monitor by **monthly urine culture** until delivery

**FOLLOW-UP**
1. **Repeat acute antibiotic therapy**
2. Start **suppressive therapy** after negative test-of-cure urine culture
3. Monitor by **monthly urine culture** until delivery

## Management of Acute Pyelonephritis in Pregnancy

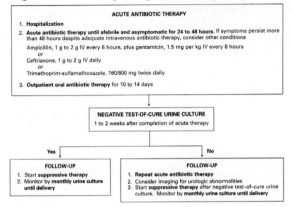

*Source:* Reprinted with permission from Chen KT. UTI in pregnancy: 6 questions to guide therapy. *OBG Management.* 2004;Nov:36–53.

# INFECTIOUS DISEASES

## SEXUALLY TRANSMITTED INFECTIONS

### Diagnostic Testing for STIs

| Infection | Diagnostic |
|---|---|
| Bacterial vaginosis | • Clinical criteria (3 of 4): vaginal pH >4.5, gray discharge, clue cells on wet mount, positive amine test (whiff test) <br> • Gram's stain of vaginal discharge |
| *Chlamydia trachomatis* | • Cervical swab: nucleic acid amplification (PCR), nucleic acid hybridization, enzyme immunoassay, direct fluorescent antibody, culture <br> • Urine: nucleic acid amplification (LCR) |
| Genital warts | • Clinical: raised papular, keratotic, or cauliform lesions; may also be flat <br> • Biopsy, if there is doubt <br> • Vesicular fluid or swab from ulcer: culture <br> • Type-specific serology |
| *Neisseria gonorrhoeae* | • Cervical swab: nucleic acid amplification (PCR), nucleic acid hybridization, enzyme immunoassay, culture, Gram's stain <br> • Urine: nucleic acid amplification (LCR) |
| Thichomonas | • Wet mount with motile trichomonads <br> • Vaginal swab: culture, polymerase chain reaction, antigen-based point of care test |
| Pubic lice | • Visual identification of lice or nits; magnifying glass may help |
| Syphilis | • Primary and secondary: darkfield microscopy of swab from lesions, serologic tests (nontreponemal[a] and treponemal[b]) |

LCR, ligase chain reaction; PCR, polymerase chain reaction.

[a]Nontreponemal tests: rapid plasma reagin (RPR) test, Venereal Disease Research Laboratory (VDRL).

[b]Treponemal tests: fluorescent treponemal antibody absorbed (FTA-ABS), microhemagglutination-*Treponema pallidum* (MHA-TP).

*Source:* Reprinted with permission from Gunter J. Sexually Transmitted Infections Update. *OB/GYN Special Edition.* 2005:19–24.

## 2006 CDC Guidelines for Treatment of STIs

| Disease | Recommended Regimens | Alternative Regimens | Pregnancy |
|---|---|---|---|
| Bacterial vaginosis | Metronidazole 500 mg PO bid × 7 days<br>Metronidazole 0.75% gel, 5 g per vagina qd × 5 days<br>Clindamycin cream 2%, 5 g per vagina qhs × 7 days | Clindamycin 300 mg PO bid × 7 days<br>Clindamycin ovules 100 g per vagina qhs × 3 days | Metronidazole 250 mg PO tid × 7 days<br>Clindamycin 300 mg PO bid × 7 days<br>Metronidazole 500 mg PO bid × 7 days |
| Chlamydial infections | Azithromycin 1 g PO × 1 days<br>Doxycycline 100 mg PO bid × 7 days | Erythromycin base 500 mg PO qid × 7 days<br>Erythromycin ethylsuccinate 800 mg PO qid × 7 days<br>Ofloxacin 300 mg PO bid × 7 days<br>Levofloxacin 500 mg PO qd × 7 days | Any erythromycin regimen<br>Amoxicillin 500 mg PO tid × 7 days<br>Azithromycin 1 g PO × 1 days |
| External genital warts | **Patient applied:**<br>Podofilox 0.5%<br>Imiquimod 5%<br>**Provider administered:**<br>Cryotherapy<br>Podophyllin resin 10–25%<br>TCA/BCA 80–90%<br>Surgical removal | Intralesional interferon<br>Laser ablation | Surgical removal |
| Gonorrhea (all regimens single dose) plus treat for chlamydia if not ruled out | Cefixime 400 mg PO<br>Ceftriaxone 125 mg IM<br>Ciprofloxacin 500 mg PO<br>Ofloxacin 400 mg PO<br>Levofloxacin 250 mg PO | Spectinomycin 2 g PO<br>Other single-dose cephalosporins<br>Other single-dose quinolones | Cefixime 400 mg PO<br><br>Ceftriaxone 125 mg IM<br><br>Spectinomycin 2 g PO |
| Internal genital warts | Cryotherapy with liquid nitrogen<br>TCA or BCA | Not applicable | Cryotherapy with liquid nitrogen<br>TCA or BCA |
| Trichomonas vaginalis | Metronidazole 2 g PO<br>Tinidazole 2 g PO | Metronidazole 500 mg PO bid × 7 days | Metronidazole 2 g PO |
| Pubic lice | Permethrin 1% cream rinse<br>Pyrethrins with piperonyl butoxide | Malathion 0.5% lotion applied for 8–12 hrs then washed off<br>Ivermectin 250 mcg/kg, repeat in 2 wks | Permethrin 1% cream rinse<br><br>Pyrethrins with piperonyl butoxide |

BCA, bichloroacetic acid; TCA, trichloroacetic acid.
*Source:* Adapted from *MMWR. Sexually Transmitted Diseases Treatment Guidelines, 2006.* August 4, 2006.

# INFECTIOUS DISEASES

## Ulcerative Lesions in Sexually Transmitted Diseases[a]

| Characteristic | Herpes | Syphilis | Chancroid | LGV | Granuloma Inguinale |
|---|---|---|---|---|---|
| Organism | Herpes simplex virus | *Treponema pallidum* | *Haemophilus ducreyi* | *Chlamydia trachomatis* | *Calymmatobacterium granulomatis* |
| Incubation | 3–7 days | 10–60 days | 2–6 days | 1–4 wks | 8–12 wks |
| Primary lesion | Vesicle | Papule | Papule/pustule | Papule/pustule/vesicle | Papule |
| Number | Multiple, coalescing | 1–2 | 1–5 | Single | Single or multiple |
| Pain | Yes | Rare | Often | No | Rare |
| Shape | Regular | Regular | Irregular | Regular | Regular |
| Margins | Flat | Raised | Red, undermined | Flat | Rolled, elevated |
| Depth | Superficial | Superficial | Excavated | Superficial | Elevated |
| Base | Red, smooth | Red, smooth | Yellow, gray | Variable | Red, rough |
| Induration | None | Firm | Rare, soft | None | Firm |
| Secretions | Serous | Serous | Purulent, hemorrhagic | Variable | Rare, hemorrhagic |
| Lymph nodes | Firm, tender | Firm, non-tender | Tender, suppurative | Tender, suppurative | Pseudoadenopathy |
| Duration | 5–10 days, recurrent | Weeks | Weeks | Days | Weeks |
| Diagnosis | Culture, PCR | Dark field, immunofluorescence, PCR | Culture, PCR | Culture, PCR | Giemsa staining |

LGV, lymphogranuloma venereum; PCR, polymerase chain reaction.

[a]Scabies, molluscum contagiosum, *Candida* species, and other dermatologic conditions (e.g., hidradenitis suppurativa) also may cause genital lesions. Boldfaced items are of particular help in making a differential diagnosis.

*Source:* Modified from Beckmann CR, Ling FW, Herbert WNP et al, eds. *Obstetrics and Gynecology.* 3rd ed. Baltimore: Williams & Wilkins, 1998:349.

## Recommended Regimens for Common Genital Ulcers: 2006 CDC Guidelines

| Disease | Recommended Regimens | | |
|---------|---------------------|---|---|
| Chancroid | Azithromycin 1 g PO × 1 dose | | |
| | Ceftriaxone 250 mg IM × 1 dose | | |
| | Ciprofloxacin 500 mg PO bid × 3 days[a] | | |
| | Erythromycin base 500 mg PO tid × 7 days | | |
| Genital HSV[b] | First episode (treat 7–10 days) | Recurrences (treat 5 days) | Suppressive therapy |
| | Acyclovir 400 mg PO tid | Acyclovir 400 mg PO tid | Acyclovir 400 mg PO bid |
| | Acyclovir 200 mg PO 5×/day | Acyclovir 200 mg PO 5×/day | Famciclovir 250 mg PO bid |
| | Famciclovir 250 mg PO tid | Acyclovir 800 mg PO | Valacyclovir 500 mg PO qd |
| | Valacyclovir 1 g PO bid | Famciclovir 125 mg PO bid | Valacyclovir 1 g PO qd |
| | | Valacyclovir 500 mg PO bid | |
| | | Valacyclovir 1 g PO qd | |
| Syphilis[b] | Primary, secondary, and early latent | | |
| | Benzathine penicillin G 2.4 million units IM × 1 dose | | |
| | Unknown duration | | |
| | Benzathine penicillin G 2.4 million units IM qwk × 3 doses | | |

CDC, Centers for Disease Control and Prevention; HSV, herpes simplex virus.
[a]Ciprofloxacin is not recommended during pregnancy.
[b]Treatment regimens for genital HSV and syphilis are the same during pregnancy.
*Source:* CDC. Sexually Transmitted Diseases Treatment Guidelines, 2006. *MMWR.* 2006;55(RR-11):1–100.

# INFECTIOUS DISEASES

## SYPHILIS

### Classification, Clinical Presentation, and Adverse Perinatal Effects of Syphilis

| Stage of Disease | Clinical Presentation | Frequency of Perinatal Transmission |
| --- | --- | --- |
| Primary | Painless chancre | 40–50% |
| Secondary | Generalized maculopapular rash | 40–50% |
| | Mucous patches | |
| | Condylomata lata | |
| Tertiary | Gumma formation | ≤10% |
| | Cardiac abnormalities | |
| | Central nervous system abnormalities | |
| Early latent | Asymptomatic | 40–50% |
| Late latent | Asymptomatic | ≤10% |

Source: Ling FW, Duff P, eds. *Obstetrics and Gynecology: Principles and Practice*. New York: McGraw-Hill, 2001:121.

## Oral Desensitization Protocol Used in 13 Pregnant Women with Allergies to Penicillin[a]

| Dose[b] | Penicillin V Suspension (U/mL) | Amount[c] | | Cumulative Dose (U) |
|---|---|---|---|---|
| | | mL | U | |
| 1 | 1000 | 0.1 | 100 | 100 |
| 2 | 1000 | 0.2 | 200 | 300 |
| 3 | 1000 | 0.4 | 400 | 700 |
| 4 | 1000 | 0.8 | 800 | 1500 |
| 5 | 1000 | 1.6 | 1600 | 3100 |
| 6 | 1000 | 3.2 | 3200 | 6300 |
| 7 | 1000 | 6.4 | 6400 | 12,700 |
| 8 | 10,000 | 1.2 | 12,000 | 24,700 |
| 9 | 10,000 | 2.4 | 24,000 | 48,700 |
| 10 | 10,000 | 4.8 | 48,000 | 96,700 |
| 11 | 80,000 | 1.0 | 80,000 | 176,700 |
| 12 | 80,000 | 2.0 | 160,000 | 336,700 |
| 13 | 80,000 | 4.0 | 320,000 | 656,700 |
| 14 | 80,000 | 8.0 | 640,000 | 1,296,700 |

[a]Observation period: 30 mins before parenteral administration of penicillin.
[b]Interval between doses, 15 mins; elapsed time, 3 hrs and 45 mins; cumulative dose, 13 million U.
[c]The specific amount of drug was diluted in approximately 30 mL of water and then given orally.
*Source:* Modified from Wendel GD Jr, Stark BJ, Jamison RB et al. Penicillin allergy and desensitization in serious infections during pregnancy. *N Engl J Med.* 1985;312:1230. Copyright © 1985 Massachusetts Medical Society. All rights reserved.

# INFECTIOUS DISEASES

## EXTERNAL GENITAL WARTS

### External Genital Wart Therapies

| Mode of Delivery | Treatment |
|---|---|
| **Applied by patient** | |
| Topical | Podofilox 0.5% solution or gel |
| | Imiquimod 5% cream |
| **Applied by a provider** | |
| Topical | Podophyllin resin (10–25%) |
| | Trichloroacetic acid (80–900) |
| | Bichloroacetic acid (80–90%) |
| Intralesional | Interferon |
| Surgical | Cryotherapy |
| | Manual excision |
| | Electrosurgical excision |
| | Laser vaporization |

*Source:* Reprinted with permission from Sexually Transmitted Infections Human Papillomavirus: The Ob/Gyn's Role. *APGO Educational Series on Women's Health Issues.* 2002:3–11.

### Comparison of Treatment Modalities

| Method | Cost | 4+ Disease | Pain/Rx | Pain/PO | Healing | Scar |
|---|---|---|---|---|---|---|
| Cryotherapy | Low | Possible | Moderate | Mild[b] | 4 days–4 wks | Little |
| Laser | High | Excellent | Great/none[a] | Mild[b] | 2–4 wks | Little[c] |
| Imiquimod | Low | Good | None | Mild/moderate | 2–3 wks | Rarely |
| Liquid nitrogen | Low | Poor | Some | Mild | 4 days–3 wks | Little |
| TCA/BCA | Low | Poor | Sharp | Some | 1–2 wks | Little |
| Podophyllin | Low | Poor | None | Some | 1–2 wks | Little |
| Cautery | Low | Possible | Great/none | Mild | 2–6 wks | Possible |
| Interferon | High | Possible | Some | None | None | None |

[a]If general or extensive local anesthesia used.

[b]Mild for small areas, can be very painful for large areas.

[c]If done expertly.

4+ Disease, severe or widespread; Pain/Rx, pain requiring prescription medication; Pain/PO, postoperative pain; TCA/BCA, trichloroacetic acid/bichloroacetic acid.

*Source:* Reprinted with permission from Sexually Transmitted Infections Human Papillomavirus: The Ob/Gyn's Role. *APGO Educational Series on Women's Health Issues.* 2002:3–11.

## Reported Clearance and Recurrence Rates for EGW Therapies

| Therapy | Range of Clearance Rates (%) | Rates of Recurrence (%) |
|---------|------------------------------|-------------------------|
| $CO_2$ laser | 27–82 | 7–72 |
| Cryotherapy | 68 | 38 |
| Imiquimod (female) | 72–84 | 5–19 |
| Interferon (intralesional) | 32–60 | 65–67 |
| Interferon (systemic) | 17–21 | Not reported |
| Podofilox | 45–88 | 33–60 |
| Podophyllin | 32–79 | 27–65 |
| TCA/BCA | 70–81 | Not reported |

TCA/BCA, trichloroacetic acid/bichloroacetic acid; EGW, external genital warts.

*Source:* Reprinted with permission from Sexually Transmitted Infections Human Papillomavirus: The Ob/Gyn's Role. *APGO Educational Series on Women's Health Issues.* 2002:3–11.

# INFECTIOUS DISEASES

## PELVIC INFLAMMATORY DISEASE AND SEXUALLY TRANSMITTED DISEASES

### Fast Facts

- Sequela of pelvic inflammatory diseases (PID): adhesions, hydrosalpinx, 10 × increase in ectopic, 4 × increase in pelvic pain
- Starts most often with cervical gonoccocal or *Chlamydia* leading to ascending infection
- 90% with lower abdominal pain
- 75% with mucopurulent cervical discharge
- 75% have ESR >15 mm/hour
- 50% have WBC >10,000 mm$^3$
- Have low threshold to treat as inpatient

### Diagnosis

**All three should be present**

1. History of lower abdominal pain and the presence of lower abdominal tenderness with or without evidence of rebound
2. Cervical motion tenderness
3. Adnexal tenderness (may be unilateral)

**Additional criteria that support a diagnosis of PID include:**

- Oral temperature >101° F (>38.3° C)
- Abnormal cervical or vaginal discharge
- Elevated erythrocyte sedimentation rate >15 mm/hour
- Elevated C-reactive protein
- Laboratory documentation of cervical infection with *N. gonorrhoeae* or *C. trachomatis*

**The definitive criteria for diagnosing PID in selected cases include:**

- Histopathologic evidence of endometritis on endometrial biopsy
- Transvaginal ultrasonography or other imaging techniques showing thickened fluid-filled tubes with or without free pelvic fluid or tubo-ovarian complex, and
- Laparoscopic abnormalities consistent with PID

## 2006 CDC Treatment Guidelines
### Outpatient

Recommended Regimen A

---

Levofloxacin 500 mg orally once daily for 14 days[a]

OR

Ofloxacin 400 mg orally twice daily for 14 days[a]

WITH OR WITHOUT

Metronidazole 500 mg orally twice a day for 14 days

---

[a]Quinolones should be used in persons with a history of recent foreign travel or partner's travel, infections acquired in California or Hawaii, or infections acquired in other areas with increased QRNG prevalence.

Oral ofloxacin has been investigated as a singe agent in two clinical trials and it is effective against both N. gonorrhoeae and C. trachomatis. Despite the results of these trials, lack of anaerobic coverage with ofloxacin is a concern; the addition of metronidazole to the treatment regimen provides this coverage. Levofloxacin is an effective ofloxacin and may be substituted. Azithromycin has been demonstrated in one randomized trial to be an effective regimen for acute PID. The addition of metronidazole should be considered as anaerobic organisms are suspected in the etiology of the majority of PID cases. Metronidazole will also treat BV, which frequently is associated with PID.

### Regimen B

---

Ceftriaxone 250 mg IM in single dose

PLUS

Doxycycline 100 mg orally twice a day for 14 days

WITH OR WITHOUT

Metronidazole 500 mg orally twice a day for 14 days

---

OR

---

Cefoxitin 2 g 1M in a single dose and Probenecid, 1 g orally administered concurrently in a single dose

PLUS

Doxycycline 100 mg orally twice a day for 14 days

WITH OR WITHOUT

Metronidazole 500 mg orally twice a day for 14 days

---

OR

---

Other parenteral third-generation cephalosporin (e.g., ceftriaxone or cefotaxime)

PLUS

Doxycycline 100 mg orally twice a day for 14 days

WITH OR WITHOUT

Metronidazole 500 mg orally twice a day for 14 days

---

# INFECTIOUS DISEASES

## Inpatient

### Recommended Parenteral Regimen A

Cefotetan 2 g IV every 12 hrs

OR

Cefoxitin 2 g IV every 6 hrs

PLUS

Doxycycline 100 mg orally or IV every 12 hrs

Because of the pain associated with infusion, doxycycline should be administered orally when possible, even when the patient is hospitalized. Oral and IV administration of doxycycline provide similar bioavailability.

Parenteral therapy may be discontinued 24 hrs after a patient improves clinically, and oral therapy with doxycycline (100 mg twice a day) should continue to complete 14 days of therapy. When tuboovarian abscess is present many healthcare providers use clindamycin or Metronidazole with doxycycline for continued therapy, rather than doxycycline alone, because it provides more effective anaerobic coverage.

Clinical data are limited regarding the use of other second- or third-generation cephalosporins (e.g., ceftizoxime, cefotaxime, and ceftriaxone), which also might be effective therapy for PID and may replace cefotetan or cefoxitin. However, these cephalosporins are less active than cefotetan or cefoxitin against anaerobic bacteria.

### Recommended Parenteral Regimen B

Clindamycin 900 mg IV every 8 hrs

OR

Gentamicin loading dose IV or IM (2 mg/kg of body weight), followed by a maintenance dose (1.5 mg/kg) every 8 hrs. Single daily dosing may be substituted.

The optimal choice of cephalosporin for Regimen B is unclear, although cefoxitin has better anaerobic coverage, ceftriaxone has better coverage against *N. gonorrhoeae*. Clinical trials have demonstrated that a single dose of cefoxitin is effective in obtaining short-term clinical response in women who have PID. However, the theoretical limitations in cefoxitin's coverage of anaerobes might require the addition of metronidazole to the treatment regimen. Metronidazole also will effectively treat BV, which is frequently associated with PID. No data has been published regarding the use of oral cephalosporins for the treatment of PID. Limited data suggest that the combination of oral metronidazole and doxycycline after primary parenteral therapy is safe and effective.

## Alternative Parenteral Regimens

Limited data support the use of other parenteral regimens, but the following three regimens have been investigated in at least one clinical trial and they have broad spectrum coverage.

Levofloxacin 500 mg IV once daily[a]

**WITH OR WITHOUT**

Metronidazole 500 mg IV every 8 hrs

**OR**

Ofloxacin 40 mg IV every 12 hrs

**WITH OR WITHOUT**

Metronidazole 300 mg IV every 8 hrs

**OR**

Ampicillin/Sulbactam 3 g IV every 6 hrs

**PLUS**

Doxycycline 100mg orally or IV every 12 hrs

[a]Quinolones should be used in persons with a history of recent foreign travel or partner's travel, infections acquired in California or Hawaii, or infections acquired in other areas with increased QRNG prevalence.

IV ofloxacin has been investigated as a single agent; however, because of concerns regarding its spectrum, metronidazole may be included in the regimen. Levofloxacin is as effective as ofloxacin and may be substituted; its single daily dosing makes it advantageous from a compliance perspective. One trial demonstrated high short-term clinical cure rates with azithromycin, either alone for 1 wk (at least one IV dose followed by oral therapy) or with a 12-day course of metronidazole. Ampicillin/sulbactam plus doxycycline is effective coverage against *C. trachomatis, N. gonorrhoeae,* and anaerobes and for patients who have tubo-ovarian abscess.

## Criteria for Hospitalization

- Suspected pelvic or tubo-ovarian abscess
- Pregnancy (rare)
- Temperature >38° C
- Uncertain diagnosis
- Nausea and vomiting precluding oral medications
- Upper peritoneal signs
- Failure to respond to oral antibiotics in 48 hours
- Noncompliant patient

*Source:* MMWR Recommendations and Reports, Sexually Transmitted Diseases Treatment Guidelines, 2006. August 4, 2006;55(RR–11):1–94.

# INFECTIOUS DISEASES

## BACTERIAL ENDOCARDITIS PROPHYLAXIS

### Indications for Prophylaxis

| Negligible-risk category (no greater risk than the general population) |
| :--- |

Surgical repair of atrial septal defect, ventricular septal defect, or patent ductus arteriosus (without residua beyond 6 mos)

Previous coronary artery bypass graft surgery

Mitral valve prolapse without valvar regurgitation

Physiologic, functional, or innocent heart murmurs

Previous Kawasaki disease without valvar dysfunction

Previous rheumatic fever without valvar dysfunction

Cardiac pacemakers (intravascular and epicardial) and implanted defibrillators

| Moderate-risk category |
| :--- |

Most other congenital cardiac malformations (other than listed here)

Acquired valvar dysfunction (e.g., rheumatic heart disease)

Hypertrophic cardiomyopathy

Mitral valve prolapse with valvar regurgitation and/or thickened leaflets

| High-risk category |
| :--- |

Prosthetic cardiac valves, including bioprosthetic and homograft valves

Previous bacterial endocarditis

Complex cyanotic congenital heart disease (e.g., single ventricle states, transposition of the great arteries, tetralogy of Fallot)

Surgically constructed systemic pulmonary shunts or conduits

---

*Recommended:* Surgical operations involving intestinal mucosa, cystoscopy, urethral dilation.
*NOT Recommended:* Vaginal hysterectomy[a], vaginal delivery[a], Cesarean section, In uninfected tissue: urethral catheterization; uterine dilation and curettage, therapeutic abortion, sterilization procedures, insertion/removal of IUD.

[a]Treatment optional in high-risk patients.

## Antibiotics and Dosage

## SBE Prophylaxis

| High-risk patients |
| --- |
| Ampicillin 2.0 g intramuscularly (IM) or intravenously (IV) plus gentamicin 1.5 mg/kg (not to exceed 120 mg) within 30 mins of starting the procedure; 6 hrs later, ampicillin 1 g IM/IV or amoxicillin 1 g orally |
| High-risk patients allergic to ampicillin/amoxicillin |
| Vancomycin 1.0 g IV over 1–2 hrs plus gentamicin 1.5 mg/kg IV/IM (not to exceed 120 mg); complete injection infusion within 30 mins of starting the procedure |
| Moderate-risk patients |
| Amoxicillin 2.0 g orally 1 hr before procedure, or ampicillin 2.0 g IM/IV within 30 mins of starting the procedure |
| Moderate-risk patients allergic to ampicillin/amoxicillin |
| Vancomycin 1.0 g IV over 1–2 hrs; complete infusion within 30 mins of starting the procedure |

*Source:* Dajani AS, Taubert KA, Wilson W et al. Prevention of bacterial endocarditis: recommendations by the American Heart Association. *JAMA.* 1997;277(22):1794–1801. Reproduced with permission of the American Medical Association.

# INFECTIOUS DISEASES

## TETANUS PROPHYLAXIS

### Recommendations for Tetanus Prophylaxis in Routine Wound Management

| History of Absorbed Tetanus Toxoid | Clean, Minor Wounds | | All Other Wounds[a] | |
|---|---|---|---|---|
| | TD[b] | TIG | TD | TIG |
| Unknown or <3 doses | Yes | No | Yes | Yes |
| ≥3 doses[c] | No[d] | No | No[e] | No |

TD, tetanus and diphtheria; TIG, tetanus immune globulin.

[a]Such as, but not limited to, wounds contaminated with dirt, feces, soil, or saliva; puncture wounds; avulsions; and wounds resulting from missiles, crushing, burns, or frostbite.

[b]For children older than 7 years, the TD toxoids and acellular pertussis vaccines (DtaP) or the TD toxoids and whole-cell pertussis vaccines (DTP)—or pediatric TD toxoids, if pertussis vaccines contraindicated—is preferred to tetanus toxoid (TT) alone. For children aged 7 years or less, the TD toxoids for adults is preferred to TT alone.

[c]If only three doses of *fluid* toxoid have been received, a fourth dose of toxoid—preferably an adsorbed toxoid—should be administered.

[d]Yes, if >10 yrs have elapsed since the last dose.

[e]Yes, if >5 yrs have elapsed since the last dose. More frequent boosters are not needed and can accentuate side effects.

*Source:* Bardenheier B, Prevots DR, Khetsuriani N, Wharton M. Tetanus surveillance—United States, 1995–1997. *MMWR CDC Surveill Summ.* 1998;47(2):1–13.

## CANCER STATISTICS 2006

**Estimated New Cases***

| | | | **Males** | **Females** | | | |
|---|---|---|---|---|---|---|---|
| Prostate | 234,460 | 33% | | Breast | 212,920 | 31% |
| Lung and Bronchus | 92,700 | 13% | | Lung and Bronchus | 81,770 | 12% |
| Colon and Rectum | 72,800 | 10% | | Colon and Rectum | 75,810 | 11% |
| Urinary Bladder | 44,690 | 6% | | Uterine Corpus | 41,200 | 6% |
| Melanoma of the Skin | 34,260 | 5% | | Non-Hodgkin Lymphoma | 28,190 | 4% |
| Non-Hodgkin Lymphoma | 30,680 | 4% | | Melanoma of the Skin | 27,930 | 4% |
| Kidney and Renal Pelvis | 24,650 | 3% | | Thyroid | 22,590 | 3% |
| Oral Cavity and Pharynx | 20,180 | 3% | | Ovary | 20,180 | 3% |
| Leukemia | 20,000 | 3% | | Urinary Bladder | 16,730 | 2% |
| Pancreas | 17,150 | 2% | | Pancreas | 16,580 | 2% |
| **All Sites** | **720,280** | **100%** | | **All Sites** | **679,510** | **100%** |

**Estimated Deaths**

| | | | **Males** | **Females** | | | |
|---|---|---|---|---|---|---|---|
| Lung and Bronchus | 90,330 | 31% | | Lung and Bronchus | 72,130 | 26% |
| Colon and Rectum | 27,870 | 10% | | Breast | 40,970 | 15% |
| Prostate | 27,350 | 9% | | Colon and Rectum | 27,300 | 10% |
| Pancreas | 16,090 | 6% | | Pancreas | 16,210 | 6% |
| Leukemia | 12,470 | 4% | | Ovary | 15,310 | 6% |
| Liver and Intrahepatic Bile Duct | 10,840 | 4% | | Leukemia | 9,810 | 4% |
| Esophagus | 10,730 | 4% | | Non-Hodgkin Lymphoma | 8,840 | 3% |
| Non-Hodgkin Lymphoma | 10,000 | 3% | | Uterine Corpus | 7,350 | 3% |
| Urinary Bladder | 8,990 | 3% | | Multiple Myeloma | 5,630 | 2% |
| Kidney and Renal Pelvis | 8,130 | 3% | | Brain and Other Nervous System | 5,560 | 2% |
| **All Sites** | **291,270** | **100%** | | **All Sites** | **273,560** | **100%** |

Ten leading cancer types for the estimated new cancer cases and deaths, by sex, United States, 2006. *Excludes basal and squamous cell skin cancers and *in situ* carcinoma except urinary bladder. Estimates are rounded to the nearest 10.
*Note:* Percentage may not total 100% due to rounding.
*Source:* Reprinted with permission from Jemal A, Siegel R, Ward E et al. Cancer statistics, 2006. *CA Cancer J Clin.* 2006;56:106–130.

# GYN-ONCOLOGY

## ENDOMETRIAL HYPERPLASIA

### Fast Facts

- Precursor to endometrial carcinoma
- Associated with unopposed estrogen stimulation of uterine endometrium
- Usually presents with abnormal uterine bleeding
- Risk of progression related to presence/absence of atypia

### Risk Factors

- Polycystic ovary syndrome with irregular or absent menses
- Obesity
- Early menarche/late menopause
- Unopposed estrogen therapy

### Pathologic Classification of Endometrial Hyperplasia

| Classification | Description |
| --- | --- |
| Simple | Benign proliferation of endometrial glands that are irregular and perhaps dilated but do not display back-to-back crowding or cellular atypia |
| Complex | Proliferation of endometrial glands with irregular outlines, architectural complexity, and back-to-back crowding but no atypia |
| Atypical | Varying degrees of nuclear atypia and loss of polarity. Found in both simple and complex hyperplastic lesions |

### Regression, Persistence, and Progression Rates of Endometrial Hyperplasia

| Type | N | % Regression | % Persistence | % Progression |
| --- | --- | --- | --- | --- |
| Simple | 93 | 80 | 19 | 1 |
| Simple with atypia | 13 | 69 | 23 | 8 |
| Complex | 29 | 80 | 17 | 3 |
| Complex with atypia | 35 | 57 | 14 | 29 |
| All lesions with atypia | 48 | 58 | 19 | 23 |

Data from Kurman RJ et al. *Cancer.* 1985;56:403–412.
*Source:* Reprinted with permission from Childs AJ, Check WE, Hoskins WJ. Conservative Management of endometrial hyperplasia: new strategies and experimental options. *OBG Management.* 2003;Sept:15–26.

**Treatment**

- Does not desire child bearing
  - Hysterectomy
- Desires child bearing or does not desire hysterectomy
  - Simple or complex hyperplasia without atypia
    ⇨ Medroxyprogesterone acetate (MPA) 10 mg daily × 3–6 months.
    ⇨ Megace 20–40 mg/day continuously × 2–3 months.
    ⇨ MPA 10 mg daily × 14 days q month × 3–6 months.
    ⇨ Sample endometrium after treatment course. If continues to show hyperplasia without atypia, consider hysterectomy or continue biopsies q6–12 months.
  - Complex atypical hyperplasia with atypia
    ⇨ Megestrol 40 mg bid × 3 months.
    ⇨ MPA 10 mg daily for 3 months.
    ⇨ Sample endometrium 3–4 weeks after completion of 3 months of therapy.
    ⇨ Abandon therapy if progression or persistent hyperplasia after 12 months of therapy.
    ⇨ If regression occurs, continue on low dose progesterone therapy but will need endometrial biopsy every 6–12 months, indefinitely.
- Alternative options
  - DepoProvera IM
  - Progesterone vaginal gel
  - Mirena (levonorgestrel intrauterine device)

# GYN-ONCOLOGY

## ENDOMETRIAL CARCINOMA

### Fast Facts

- Most common malignancy of the female genital tract, with 40,000 cases in 2007.
  - Frequency: endometrial > ovarian > cervical
  - Number of deaths: ovarian > endometrial > cervical
- >7000 deaths yearly in United States
- Median age 60 years.
- 90% of women have symptomatic bleeding leading to relatively early diagnosis.
  - 72% Stage I
  - 12% Stage II
  - 13% Stage III
  - 3% Stage IV

### Risk Factors

| Factors Influencing Risk | Estimated Relative Risk |
|---|---|
| Older age | 2–3 |
| Residency in North America or Northern Europe | 3–18 |
| Higher level of education or income | 1.5–2 |
| White race | 2 |
| Nulliparity | 3 |
| History of infertility | 2–3 |
| Menstrual irregularities | 1.5 |
| Late age at natural menopause | 2–3 |
| Early age at menarche | 1.5–2 |
| Long-term use of high dosages of menopausal estrogens | 1 0–20 |
| Long-term use of high dosages of combination oral contraceptives | 0.3–0.5 |
| High cumulative doses of tamoxifen | 3–7 |
| Obesity | 2–5 |
| Stein-Leventhal disease or estrogen-producing tumor | >5 |
| History of diabetes, hypertension, gallbladder disease, or thyroid disease | 1.3–3 |
| Cigarette smoking | 0.5 |

Relative risks depend on the study and referent group employed.
*Source:* Reprinted with permission from Elsevier. Gershenson DM, McGuire WP, Gore M et al, eds. *Gynecologic Cancer: Controversies in Management.* Copyright 2004.

## Histologic Types

- Type I: estrogen dependent
  - Lower grade nuclei
  - Endometrioid histology
  - Good prognosis
- Type II: non-estrogen dependent
  - High grade nuclei
  - Serous/clear cell histology
  - p53 tumor suppressor mutation
  - Poorer prognosis

## Screening

- Routine screening of asymptomatic women not recommended

## Diagnosis

- Endometrial sample obtained by endometrial biopsy in office or dilation and curettage under anesthesia.
- Premenopausal patients with amenorrhea for >6–12 months and abnormal bleeding should have endometrial biopsy.
- Postmenopausal patients with irregular vaginal bleeding on hormone replacement therapy (HRT) or any vaginal bleeding if not on HRT should have endometrial biopsy.

## Preoperative Evaluation

- Complete history and physical exam including rectovaginal exam
- Chest x-ray
- Complete blood count, liver and renal function tests as indicated
- Computed tomography (CT) scan, barium enema, cancer antigen (CA)-125 evaluation, and bone scan only for suspected metastatic disease

# GYN-ONCOLOGY

## Staging/Treatment

| Stage I | Tumor confined to corpus uteri | |
|---|---|---|
| IA | Tumor limited to endometrium | Total hysterectomy, BSO, pelvic/para-aortic lymph node dissection, cytology |
| IB | Tumor invades less than one-half of myometrium | Total hysterectomy, BSO, pelvic/para-aortic lymph node dissection, cytology |
| IC | Tumor invades more than one-half of myometrium | Total hysterectomy, BSO, pelvic/para-aortic lymph node dissection, cytology + adjuvant pelvic XRT |
| **Stage II** | **Tumor invades cervix but does not extend beyond uterus** | |
| IIA | Endocervical gland involvement only | Total hysterectomy, BSO, pelvic/para-aortic lymph node dissection, cytology<br>Adjuvant pelvic XRT |
| IIB | Cervical stroma invasion | Total hysterectomy, BSO, pelvic/para-aortic lymph node dissection, cytology<br>Adjuvant pelvic XRT |
| **Stage III** | **Local and/or regional spread** | |
| IIIA | Tumor invades serosa, and/or adnexa, and/or positive peritoneal cytology | Total hysterectomy, BSO, pelvic/para-aortic lymph node dissection, cytology<br>Adjuvant chemotherapy |
| IIIB | Vaginal metastasis | Total hysterectomy, BSO, pelvic/para-aortic lymph node dissection, cytology<br>Adjuvant chemotherapy |
| IIIC | Metastasis to pelvis and/or para-aortic lymph nodes | Total hysterectomy, BSO, pelvic and para-aortic lymph node dissection, cytology.<br>Adjuvant chemotherapy |
| **Stage IVA** | **Tumor invades bladder and/or bowel mucosa** | Palliative XRT, chemotherapy |
| Stage IVB | Distant metastasis including intraabdominal and/or inguinal lymph nodes | Palliative XRT, chemotherapy |

BSO, bilateral salpingo-oophorectomy; XRT, radiation therapy.
*Source:* National Comprehensive Cancer Network guidelines, 2006.

## Notes about the Staging

*Histopathology—degree of differentiation*

Cases of carcinoma of the corpus should be grouped with regard to the degree of differentiation of the adenocarcinoma as follows:

G1: 5% or less of a nonsquamous or nonmorular solid growth pattern

G2: 6–50% of a nonsquamous or nonmorular solid growth pattern

G3: More than 50% of a nonsquamous or nonmorular solid growth pattern

## Frequency of Nodal Metastases

| Risk Factor | No. of Patients | Pelvic Nodes (%) | Aortic Nodes (%) |
|---|---|---|---|
| Grade | | | |
|   1 Well | 180 | 5 (3%) | 3 (2%) |
|   2 Moderate | 288 | 25 (9%) | 14 (5%) |
|   3 Poor | 153 | 28 (18%) | 17 (11%) |
| Myometrial invasion | | | |
|   Endometrial | 187 | 1 (1%) | 1 (1%) |
|   Superficial | 279 | 15 (5%) | 8 (3%) |
|   Middle | 116 | 7 (6%) | 1 (1%) |
|   Deep | 139 | 35 (25%) | 24 (17%) |

*Source:* Data from Creasman WT, Morrow CP, Bundy BN, et al. Surgical pathologic spread patterns of endometrial cancer. A Gynecologic Oncology Group Study. Cancer 1987;60:2035–2041.

## Follow-Up
- Five-year survival
  - Stage I = 81–91%
  - Stage II = 71–78%
  - Stage III = 52–60%
  - Stage IV = 14–17%

*Source:* Based on Federation of Gynecology and Obstetrics (FIGO) annual report. *Int J Gynaecol Obstet.* 2003; 83:79.

# GYN-ONCOLOGY

## CERVICAL DYSPLASIA

### Background

- Squamocolumnar junction migrates out on ectocervix and is exposed to decrease in vaginal pH causing squamous metaplasia (transformation zone).
- More exposure to carcinogens → increases cervical intraepithelial neoplasia (CIN) → increased chance of dysplasia.

### Incidence

- 1650/100,000
- Untreated CIN III: 20% develop into invasive carcinoma in 20 years
- Average age of CIN diagnosis = 28 years
- Average age of cervical CA diagnosis = 42 years

### Risk Factors Associated with Precancerous Changes and Cancer of the Cervix

---

- Human papillomavirus infection
- Multiple sexual partners
- Sexual activity begun at an early age
- Parity
- Human immunodeficiency virus (HIV)
- Immune status
- Smoking
- History of other sexually transmitted diseases (e.g., herpes simplex, chlamydia, and bacterial vaginosis)
- Oral contraceptive use
- Low socioeconomic status
- Poor diet (e.g., vitamin deficiency)
- Alcoholism

---

*Source:* Reprinted with permission from Advances in the screening, diagnosis, and treatment of cervical disease. *APGO Educational Series on Women's Health Issues.* 2002. pg. 1–6.

## Common Genital HPV Genotypes

| Lesions/Malignancies | HPV Genotypes | |
|---|---|---|
| | Common | Less Common |
| **Anogenital lesions** | | |
| Condyloma acuminata | 6 | 2, 11, 16, 30, 42, 43, 44, 54, 55, 61 |
| CIN, VIN, VAIN, PAIN, PIN | 16, 18, 31 | 6, 11, 30, 34, 35, 39, 45, 51, 52, 56 |
| | | 59, 61, 62, 64, 66, 67, 69 |
| **Malignancies** | | |
| Cervical cancer | 16, 18, 31, 45 | 6, 10, 11, 26, 33, 35, 39, 51, 52, 55, |
| | | 56, 58, 59, 66, 68 |
| Other anogenital cancers | 6, 16, 18 | 11, 31, 33 |

CIN, cervical intraepithelial neoplasm; HPV, human papillomavirus; PIN, penile intraepithelial neoplasia; PAIN, perianal intraepithelial neoplasia; VAIN, vaginal intraepithelial neoplasia; VIN, vulvar intraepithelial neoplasia.
*Source*: Sexually Transmitted Infections. Human Papillomavirus: The Ob/Gyn's Role. *APGO Educational Series on Women's Health Issues*. 2002. pg. 3.

## Pathophysiology

- Metaplasia progresses from columnar to squamous
- Transformation zone = squamous meets columnar
- Cervical canal = lower $^2/_3$ = squamous epithelium, similar to vagina
- Upper $^1/_3$ = columnar epithelium, similar to lining of lower uterine segment
- Junction is not static → moves up in cervical canal with age
- Critical metaplasia periods:
  1. Fetal life
  2. Early adolescence
  3. First pregnancy
     ⇨ *Both 2 & 3 have high cervical eversion and are susceptible to CIN and cervical CA development.

# GYN-ONCOLOGY

## Histology

- Cervical intraepithelial neoplasia—abnormal proliferation of overgrowth of basal cell layer at squamocolumnar junction of cervical epithelium
- Atypical squamous cells of undetermined significance (ASCUS). Papanicolaou (Pap)—15–20% will have significant lesion: high-grade squamous intraepithelial lesions or rarely cervical CA

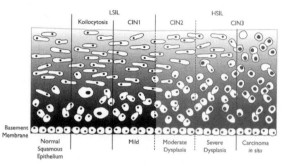

CIN, cervical intraepithelial neoplasia; CIN1, mild dysplasia; CIN2, moderate dysplasia; CIN3, severe dysplasia to carcinoma in situ (CIS); HGSIL or HSIL, high-grade squamous intraepithelial lesion; Koilocytosis, cell changes showing perinuclear vacuolization; LSIL, low-grade squamous intraepithelial lesion.
*Source:* Reprinted with permission from Advances in the screening, diagnosis, and treatment of cervical disease. *APGO Educational Series on Women's Health Issues.* 2002. pg. 1–6.

## Diagnosis

- Pap smear: provides cytologic diagnosis.
- Pap guidelines: see below.
- Colposcopic visualization—for low- and high-grade squamous intraepithelial lesion, atypical glandular cells of undetermined significance, ASCUS-H (H indicates that high grade cannot be ruled out) or recurrent ASCUS.
- Use 10 × magnification and 5% acetic acid.
- Biopsy abnormal areas.
- Colposcopy satisfactory if:
  - Transformation zone seen
  - Entire lesion seen
  - Endocervical curettage (ECC) without dysplasia

## Cervical Cytology Screening Guideline Recommendations

| Timing | ACS | ACOG | USPSTF |
|---|---|---|---|
| Initiate screening | 3 yrs after initiating sexual intercourse and before age 21 | 3 yrs after initiating sexual intercourse and before age 21 | 3 yrs after initiating sexual intercourse and before age 21 |
| Up to age 30 | Annual screening with conventional Pap or every 2 yrs with liquid Pap | Annually | Every 3 yrs following 2–3 consecutive normal results |
| Older than age 30 | Every 2–3 yrs[a,b] or screening every 3 yrs when adding HPV DNA testing to conventional or liquid Pap | Every 3 yrs following 3 consecutive normal results[b] | Every 3 yrs following 2–3 consecutive normal results |
| Cease screening | Age 70 following 3 consecutive, adequate negative Pap tests within the past 10 yrs[b] | No upper age limit recommended | Age 65 following recent adequate normal Pap results |
| Total hysterectomy | Screening not indicated.[b] Women with a history of CIN 2 or 3 should continue screening until 3 consecutive negative Pap test results within the past 10 yrs | Screening not indicated.[b] Women with a history of CIN 2 or 3 should continue screening until 3 consecutive negative Pap test results within the past 10 yrs | Screening not indicated |

ACS, American Cancer Society; ACOG, American College of Obstetricians and Gynecologists; CIN, cervical intraepithelial neoplasia; DNA, deoxyribonucleic acid; HPV, human papillomavirus; Pap, Papanicolaou; USPSTF, U.S. Preventive Services Task Force.

[a]Assuming women have had 3 consecutive satisfactory/normal results.

[b]Assuming no additional high-risk factors (e.g., history of in utero diethylstilbestrol exposure, are HIV+, or are immunocompromised).

*Source:* Reprinted with permission from Gold MA. Current cervical cancer screening guidelines and impact of prophylactic HPV vaccines. *Supplement to OBG Management.* 2006;July:S11–S17.

# GYN-ONCOLOGY

## Management

- See flow charts from the American Society for Colposcopy and Cervical Pathology.

## Risk of Progression

| Papanicolaou Diagnosis | Regress to Normal (95% CI) | Progress to/ Persist as HSIL in 24 mos (95% CI) | Progress to Invasive Cancer in 24 mos (95% CI) |
|---|---|---|---|
| ASCUS | 68.19% (57.51, 78.86) | 7.13% (0.8, 13.5) | 0.25% (0, 2.25) |
| LSIL | 47.39% (35.92, 58.86) | 20.81% (6.08, 35.55) | 0.15% (0, 0.71) |
| HSIL | 35.03% (16.57, 53.49) | 23.37% (12.82, 32.92) | 1.44% (0, 3.95) |

ASCUS, atypical squamous cells of undetermined significance; CI, confidence interval; HSIL, high-grade squamous intraepithelial lesion; LSIL, low-grade squamous intraepithelial lesion.

| | Within 2 yrs | Within 5 yrs | Within 10 yrs |
|---|---|---|---|
| **Progression** | | | |
| Mild to moderate or worse | 11.1% | 20.4% | 28.8% |
| Mild to severe or worse | 2.1% | 5.5% | 9.9% |
| Moderate to severe or worse | 16.3% | 25.1% | 32.0% |
| **Regression** | | | |
| Mild to first normal Pap | 44.3% | 74.0% | 87.7% |
| Moderate to first normal Pap | 33.0% | 63.1% | 82.9% |
| Mild to second normal Pap | 8.7% | 39.1% | 62.2% |
| Moderate to second normal Pap | 6.9% | 29.0% | 53.7% |

Pap, Papanicolaou.
*Source:* Reprinted with permission from Advances in the screening, diagnosis, and treatment of cervical disease. *APGO Educational Series on Women's Health Issues.* 2002. pg. 7.

### Definitions of Terms Utilized in the Consensus Guidelines

*Colposcopy* is the examination of the cervix, vagina, and, in some instances the vulva, with the colposcope after the application of a 3-5% acetic acid solution coupled with obtaining colposcopically-directed biopsies of all lesions suspected of representing neoplasia.

*Endocervical sampling* includes obtaining a specimen for either histological evaluation using an endocervical curette or a cytobrush or for cytological evaluation using a cytobrush.

*Endocervical assessment* is the process of evaluating the endocervical canal for the presence of neoplasia using either a colposcope or endocervical sampling.

*Diagnostic excisional procedure* is the process of obtaining a specimen from the transformation zone and endocervical canal for histological evaluation and includes laser conization, cold-knife conization, loop electrosurgical excision (i.e., LEEP), and loop electrosurgical conization.

*Satisfactory colposcopy* indicates that the entire squamocolumnar junction and the margin of any visible lesion can be visualized with the colposcope.

*Endometrial sampling* includes obtaining a specimen for histological evaluation using an endometrial biopsy or a "dilatation and curettage" or hysteroscopy.

ASCCP

2002. Copyright American Society for Colposcopy and Cervical Pathology

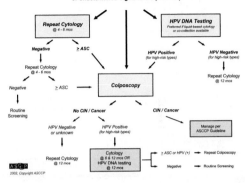

**Management of Women with Atypical Squamous Cells
of Undetermined Significance (ASC-US)**

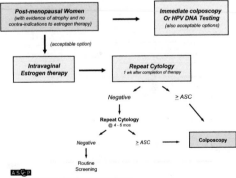

**Management of Women with Atypical Squamous Cells
of Undetermined Significance (ASC-US) In Special Circumstances**

*Source*: Reprinted from the *Journal of Lower Genital Tract Disease* Vol. 6 Issue 2, with the permission of ASCCP © American Society for Colposcopy and Cervical Pathology 2002. No copies of the algorithms may be made without the prior consent of ASCCP.

# GYN-ONCOLOGY

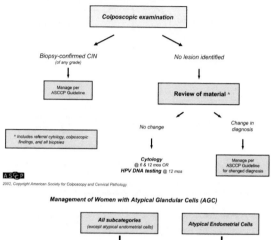

*Management of Women with Atypical Squamous Cells: Cannot Exclude High-grade SIL (ASC - H)*

Colposcopic examination

Biopsy-confirmed CIN *(of any grade)* → Manage per ASCCP Guideline

No lesion identified → Review of material ^

^ Includes referral cytology, colposcopic findings, and all biopsies

No change → Cytology @ 6 & 12 mos OR HPV DNA testing @ 12 mos

Change in diagnosis → Manage per ASCCP Guideline for changed diagnosis

ASCCP

2002, Copyright American Society for Colposcopy and Cervical Pathology

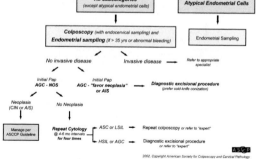

*Management of Women with Atypical Glandular Cells (AGC)*

All subcategories *(except atypical endometrial cells)*

Atypical Endometrial Cells

Colposcopy (with endocervical sampling) and Endometrial sampling (if > 35 yrs or abnormal bleeding)

Endometrial Sampling

No invasive disease

Invasive disease → Refer to appropriate specialist

Initial Pap AGC - NOS

Initial Pap AGC - "favor neoplasia" or AIS → Diagnostic excisional procedure (prefer cold-knife conization)

Neoplasia (CIN or AIS) → Manage per ASCCP Guideline

No Neoplasia → Repeat Cytology @ 4-6 mo intervals for four times

— ASC or LSIL → Repeat colposcopy or refer to "expert"

— HSIL or AGC → Diagnostic excisional procedure or refer to "expert"

ASCCP

2002, Copyright American Society for Colposcopy and Cervical Pathology

*Source*: Reprinted from the *Journal of Lower Genital Tract Disease* Vol. 6 Issue 2, with the permission of ASCCP © American Society for Colposcopy and Cervical Pathology 2002. No copies of the algorithms may be made without the prior consent of ASCCP.

*Management of Women with Low-grade
Squamous Intraepithelial Lesions (LSIL) \**

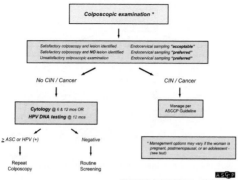

*Management of Women with Low-grade Squamous Intraepithelial Lesions
In Special Circumstances*

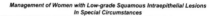

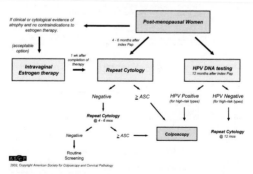

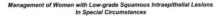

*Management of Women with Low-grade Squamous Intraepithelial Lesions
In Special Circumstances*

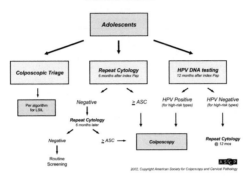

*Source*: Reprinted from the *Journal of Lower Genital Tract Disease* Vol. 6 Issue 2, with the permission of ASCCP © American Society for Colposcopy and Cervical Pathology 2002. No copies of the algorithms may be made without the prior consent of ASCCP.

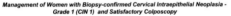

*Management of Women with Biopsy-confirmed Cervical Intraepithelial Neoplasia -
Grade 1 (CIN 1) and Satisfactory Colposcopy*

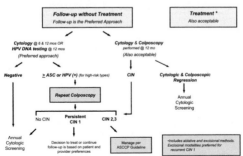

*Source*: Reprinted from the *Journal of Lower Genital Tract Disease* Vol. 7 Issue 3, with the permission of ASCCP © American Society for Colposcopy and Cervical Pathology 2003. No copies of the algorithms may be made without the prior consent of ASCCP.

*Management of Women with High-grade Squamous Intraepithelial Lesions (HSIL) \**

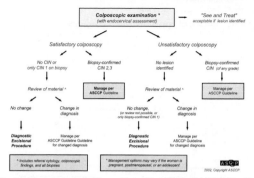

*Source*: Reprinted from the *Journal of Lower Genital Tract Disease* Vol. 6 Issue 2, with the permission of ASCCP © American Society for Colposcopy and Cervical Pathology 2002. No copies of the algorithms may be made without the prior consent of ASCCP.

*Management of Women with Biopsy-confirmed Cervical Intraepithelial Neoplasia - Grade 2 and 3 (CIN 2,3) \**

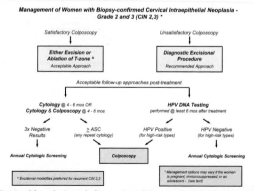

*Source*: Reprinted from the *Journal of Lower Genital Tract Disease* Vol. 7 Issue 3, with the permission of ASCCP © American Society for Colposcopy and Cervical Pathology 2003. No copies of the algorithms may be made without the prior consent of ASCCP.

# GYN-ONCOLOGY

## Management in Pregnancy

- ECC not recommended
- Biopsy areas suspicious for invasion

## Algorithm of Abnormal Pap Smear and Pregnancy

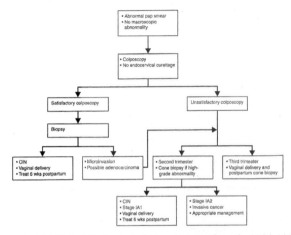

*Source:* Berek JS, Hacker NF, eds. *Practical Gynecologic Oncology.* 4th ed. Philadelphia (PA): Lippincott Williams & Wilkins; 2005, pg. 380. Reproduced with the permission of the publisher.

## CERVICAL CANCER

### Fast Facts
- Incidence in United States has declined by $^1/_3$ over the past 20 years.
  - 10,370 new cases in 2006
  - 3710 deaths in 2006
- Worldwide, cervical cancer is second only to breast cancer.
  - 75% of cases are in developing countries.

### Risk Factors
- Young age at first coitus
- Multiple sexual partners
- High parity
- History of other sexually transmitted diseases
- Smoking
- Human papillomavirus (HPV) infection
  - Most important risk factor.
  - 40–60% sexually active adults have evidence of HPV infection.
  - HPV DNA is present in 90% of preinvasive and invasive lesions.
  - HPV transcriptional activity identified in cervical neoplasia.
  - HPV oncogenes can mediate malignant transformation in transgenic mice.
  - Subtypes determine clinical disease.
    ⇨ <2% clinical manifestation of warts, abnormal Paps, or cervical CA
    ⇨ HPV 6,11→ 90% of benign warts (prominent acanthosis and parakeratosis)
    ⇨ HPV 16,18→ associated with 70% of cervical cancer cases
    ⇨ HPV quadrivalent vaccine (Gardasil, Merck) now available to protect against HPV 6/11/16/18
      ❖ Recommended for 9- to 26-year-old females

### Symptoms
- Vaginal discharge, abnormal bleeding (pre- or postmenopausal), postcoital bleeding, pelvic pain/mass

### Histology
- Squamous cell cancer (90%)
  - Large cell, small cell, and verrucous
- Adenocarcinoma (~10%)
  - Endocervical, endometrioid, clear cell, adenoid cystic, adenoma malignum
  - Increasing incidence observed
- Mixed carcinoma
  - Adenosquamous, glassy cell

# GYN-ONCOLOGY

## Diagnosis

- Screening Pap—Procedure identifies preinvasive and invasive neoplasia, scraping superficial cells from squamocolumnar junction and endocervix.
- Colposcopy—This is a direct biopsy. Use 3–5% acetic acid on cervix. Green filter accentuates vascular pattern. Adequate colpo-entire transformation zone is visualized. Acetowhite changes—acetic acid reacts with nuclei so more cellular areas reflect white.
- Cone biopsy/loop electrosurgical excision procedure—Procedure allows adequate evaluation if colposcopy is inadequate.

## Workup

- Complete history and physical, including rectovaginal exam. Palpate right-upper quadrant, inguinal, and supraclavicular to assess for metastatic disease.
- To establish extent of disease: colposcopy, conization, ECC, hysteroscopy, cystoscopy, proctoscopy, intravenous pyelogram, radiographic examination of lungs and bones (approved as tests for FIGO staging).
- CT scan and magnetic resonance imaging (MRI) for retroperitoneal and upper abdominal disease (results will not affect FIGO staging).
- Complete blood count, renal and liver function tests.

## Cervical Cancer Staging/Treatment
## Clinically Staged

| Stage I | Carcinoma strictly confined to the cervix | |
|---|---|---|
| IA | Invasive carcinoma diagnosed only by microscopy | |
| IA1 | Measured stromal invasion ≤3 mm in depth ≤7 mm in horizontal spread | Conization is possible |
| | | Simple hysterectomy more commonly accepted |
| IA2 | Measured stromal invasion >3 mm not more than 5 mm in depth and ≤7 mm in horizontal spread | Modified radical hysterectomy with lymphadenectomy vs. primary chemoradiotherapy vs. radical trachelectomy as an option |
| IB | Clinically visible lesion confined to cervix or microscopic lesion greater than above | |
| IB1 | Clinically visible lesion ≤4 cm in greatest dimension | Radical hysterectomy with lymphadenectomy + chemoradiotherapy |
| | | Primary chemoradiotherapy |
| | | Radical trachelectomy possible option |
| IB2 | Clinically visible lesion >4 cm in greatest dimension (i.e., "bulky" disease) | Primary chemoradiotherapy |
| | | Radical hysterectomy with lymphadenectomy + chemoradiotherapy |
| Stage II | Invades beyond uterus but not to the pelvic wall or to the lower third of vagina | Primary chemoradiotherapy |
| | | Radical hysterectomy with lymphadenectomy + chemoradiotherapy |
| IIA | Tumor without parametrial invasion | |
| IIB | Tumor with parametrial invasion | Primary chemoradiotherapy |
| Stage III | Extends to pelvic wall and/or lower third of vagina and/or causes hydronephrosis or non-functioning kidney | Primary chemoradiotherapy |
| IIIA | Tumor involves lower third of vagina, no extension to pelvic wall | |
| IIIB | Extends to pelvic wall and/or causes hydronephrosis or non-functioning kidney | |
| Stage IVA | Tumor invades mucosa of bladder or rectum and/or extends beyond the true pelvis | Primary chemoradiotherapy |
| Stage IVB | Distant metastasis | Systemic chemotherapy + radiotherapy |

## Treatment Specifics
## Radical Trachelectomy

■ Indication: Desire for future childbearing + any of the following: Stage IA1 without extensive lymphovascular space invasion, Stage IA2 disease, Stage IB1 ≤2 cm diameter—no involvement of upper endocervix on MRI or intraop frozen section, no metastasis to lymph nodes.

# GYN-ONCOLOGY

- Procedure: Cervix and parametria resected with placement of cerclage. Can be performed transvaginally, transabdominally, or combined with laparoscopic pelvic, para-aortic lymphadenectomy.
  ⇨ Complications: Vascular and urinary tract trauma. 10–17% planned procedures are abandoned due to extensive disease found at time of surgery
- Survival: 97% recurrence-free survival, 98% overall survival. 20% risk of preterm delivery. 50% rate of vaginal delivery.

## Radical Hysterectomy
- Indication: Ib, IIa
- Procedure: Excision of uterus, upper $1/3$ vagina, uterosacral ligaments, parametria pelvic node dissection, dissection of uterine artery to origin on hypogastric, and ovaries can be preserved.
- Complications: Most common is bladder dysfunction.
  ⇨ Fistula in 0–3%
- Survival: 90% at 5 years, 75% for stage I.

## Radiation Therapy (XRT)
- External beam and intracavitary radium.
  ⇨ Small bowel tolerates 4000–5000 rads.
  ⇨ External beam can deliver only 4000–5000 rads, but can give 6000 in intracavitary sources.
  ⇨ Point A: 2 cm superior and 2 cm lateral to external os. This area is parametrial tissues.
  ⇨ Point B: 3 cm lateral to point A. This area is pelvic nodes.
  ❖ Survival: 90% at 5 years for stage I.

## Follow-Up
- Recurrent cervical cancer
  - Symptoms: Weight loss, leg edema, vaginal discharge, symptoms of ureteral obstruction (pain, uremia).
    ⇨ 95% post-therapy ureteral obstructions are recurrent disease. Can place stent.
  - 75% occur in first 2 years following treatment. Most recurrences are local.
  - Central recurrences may be treated with pelvic exenteration.
    ⇨ Operative mortality is 5%.
    ❖ Survival: 30% at 5 years.
- Survival (following appropriate treatment) at 5 years
  - Stage Ia= 95%
  - Stages Ib & IIa= 80–90%
  - Stage IIb= 65%
  - Stage III= 40%
  - Stage IV= <20%

## Management of Cervical Cancer in Pregnancy

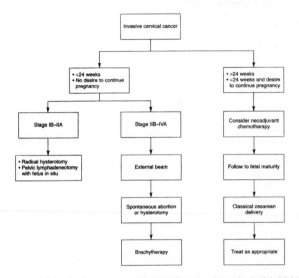

*Source:* Berek JS, Hacker NF, eds. *Practical Gynecologic Oncology.* 4th ed. Philadelphia (PA): Lippincott Williams & Wilkins; 2005, pg. 380. Reproduced with the permission of the publisher.

# GYN-ONCOLOGY

## EPITHELIAL OVARIAN CANCER

### Definition/Background
- Second most common gynecologic malignancy.
- Most common cause of death from gynecologic malignancy.
  - Ovarian cancer patients usually die secondary to bowel obstruction.
- No reliable screening test available.
- Median age 60–64 years.

### Incidence
- 1.4/100,000
- 20,000 deaths/year

### Risk Factors
- Nulliparity
- History of breast or colon cancer
- Hereditary non-polyposis colorectal cancer/Lynch syndrome II (12% risk of ovarian cancer)
- Family history of breast, colon, or ovarian cancer
- Uninterrupted and long period of ovulatory cycles

### Protective Factors
- Multiparity
- Oral contraceptive use
- Prior breastfeeding (lactational amenorrhea and anovulation)
- Anovulatory disorders

### Symptoms/Signs
- Abdominal discomfort, upper abdominal fullness, early satiety, fatigue, urinary frequency, dyspnea
- Pelvic mass, bilateral irregularity, solid or fixed mass, ascites or nodular cul-de-sac

### Histopathology
- Epithelial (59%)
  - Serous cystadenocarcinoma (46%)
    ⇨ Bilateral presentation w/psammoma bodies
  - Mucinous (36%)
  - Undifferentiated (15%)
  - Endometrioid (8%)
  - Clear cell (3%)
    ⇨ Hobnail appearance on pathology
      ❖ Clear cell cancers may be associated with worse prognosis
  - Brenner's (2%)
  - Squamous (<1%)

## Pretreatment Evaluation

- Complete history and physical examination including pelvic and rectovaginal examination, CT scan, ultrasound. Tumor markers CA-125, carcinoembryonic antigen (CEA)
  - Refer to gyn-oncologist: CA-125 >200 U/mL in premenopausal women, CA-125 >35 U/mL in postmenopausal women, ascites, or family history of breast or ovarian cancer in a first degree relative. (ACOG Committee opinion 2002)

## Management

- CA-125 elevated in 80% of non-mucinous advanced ovarian tumors.
  - Doubling of CA-125 level in a cancer patient during follow-up requires further investigation.
- Adjuvant therapy involves intravenous carboplatin/paclitaxel vs. intraperitoneal cisplatin/paclitaxel chemotherapy improves survival in advanced ovarian cancer s/p optimal cytoreductive surgery (*New Engl J Med.* 2006).

## 5-Year Survival

- Stage I = 65–89%
- Stage II = 64–79%
- Stage III = 29–49%
- Stage IV = 13%

# GYN-ONCOLOGY

## Ovarian Cancer Staging/Treatment

| Stage I | Tumor limited to ovaries | |
|---|---|---|
| IA | Limited to one ovary | Staging procedure: TAH, BSO, omentectomy, lymph node sampling, biopsies |
| IB | Limited to both ovaries | |
| IC | IA or IB + positive surface growth or malignant ascites or positive washings or ruptured capsule at or prior to surgery | Staging procedure followed by intravenous carboplatin/paclitaxel 3 vs. 6 cycles |
| Stage II | Tumor involves one or both ovaries with pelvic extension | Cytoreductive surgery followed by intravenous carboplatin/paclitaxel × 3 vs. 6 cycles |
| IIA | Extension or metastases to uterus and/or tubes | |
| IIB | Extension to other pelvic organs | |
| IIC | IIA or IIB + positive surface growth or malignant ascites or positive washings or ruptured capsule at or prior to surgery | |
| Stage III | Tumor involving one or both ovaries with microscopic peritoneal implants outside the pelvis and/or positive nodes. Superficial liver mets = Stage III | Cytoreductive surgery followed by intravenous or intraperitoneal chemotherapy for all Stage III |
| IIIA | Limited to true pelvis with negative nodes but microscopic seeding or abdominal peritoneal surface | IP chemo should be considered for all optimally debulked patients with good performance status |
| IIIB | Tumor with abdominal peritoneal implants but none >2 cm nodes, negative | |
| IIIC | Abdominal implants >2 cm and/or positive retroperitoneal or inguinal nodes | |
| Stage IV | Tumor involving both ovaries with distant mets. Pleural effusion must be tapped for cytology. Parenchymal liver mets = Stage IV | Cytoreductive surgery followed by intravenous carboplatin/paclitaxel for 6 cycles vs. neoadjuvant carboplatin/paclitaxel followed by interval cytoreductive surgery for selected patients |

BSO, bilateral salpingo-oopherectomy; TAH, total abdominal hysterectomy.

# GERM CELL OVARIAN TUMORS
## Ovarian Germ Cell Tumors
### Fast Facts
- Derived from primordial germ cells.
- Account for 20–25% of ovarian neoplasms.
  - Only 5% of malignant ovarian neoplasms.
- Tumors grow rapidly but most present with Stage IA disease.
- Presents in 10–30-year-olds—represents 70% of ovarian tumors in this age group.
- Malignant ovarian germ cell tumors occur more often in Asians/African Americans than Caucasians (3:1).

### Signs & Symptoms
- Abdominal pain and mass—both symptoms seen in 85% of patients.
- Precocious puberty (if estrogen-secreting tumor).
- Symptoms similar to pregnancy (from human chorionic gonadotropin [hCG] production).
- Tumors tend to be large—16 cm.

### Tumor Types
- Benign: Mature cystic teratoma (dermoid cyst)
- Malignant:

| Type | % |
|------|------|
| Immature teratomas | 35.6 |
| Dysgerminomas | 32.8 |
| Endodermal sinus | 14.5 |
| Mixed germ cell tumors | 5.3 |
| Embryonal | 4.1 |
| Mature teratomas with malignant degeneration | 2.9 |
| Teratocarcinoma | 2.6 |
| Choriocarcinoma | 2.1 |

*Source:* Smith et al. *Obstet Gynecol.* 2006;107:1075–1085.

- Immature teratomas are the only malignant ovarian germ cell tumors that are histologically graded.
  - <1% of all teratomas
- Bilateral ovarian disease is most common in dysgerminomas.

### Dysgerminoma
- Derived from germ cells and exquisitely radiosensitive
- Tumor rarely produces hCG and ± pregnancy test in non-sexually active patient

# GYN-ONCOLOGY

- Pathology shows lymphocytic infiltration
- Treatment: unilateral salpingo-oophorectomy (USO) with close inspections of other ovary (15% bilateral)
- Recurrence: treated with chemotherapy with good success

## Endodermal Sinus Tumor

- Median age at diagnosis is 19 years
- Produces alpha-fetoprotein
- Pathology: invaginated papillary structure with central blood vessel called "Schiller-Duvall Body"
- Treatment: Surgery (USO) and chemotherapy (bleomycin, etoposide, cisplatin [BEP] ×3; 95% curative)
- Prognosis: very poor, if no chemotherapy, 85% recur

## Embryonal Carcinoma

- Derived from primordial germ cells
- Very rare; occurs during childhood
- Presents with precocious puberty or mass
- Secretes AFP and hCG
- Prognosis: poor

## Choriocarcinoma

- Gestational = characteristics similar to uterine choriocarcinoma
- Non-gestational = resistant to chemotherapy and XRT→ fatal
- Secretes hCG
- Pathology: Arias stella reaction, increased aromatism, increased pleomorphism, increased mitotic activity

## Gonadoblastoma

- Associated with abnormal karyotype (gonadal dysgenesis associated with presence of Y chromosome)
- Symptoms: primary amenorrhea, virilization, or genital developmental problems
- Dysgerminoma often coexists forming a mixed germ cell tumor
- Therapy: bilateral salpingo-oopherectomy
- Prognosis: good

## Immature Teratoma

- Malignant corollary of cystic teratoma
- Three germ cell layers
- Pathology: immature embryonic elements with neural elements
- Rare, never bilateral, occurs in first 2 decades of life
- Prognosis: poor, but depends on grade (level of neural elements) and presence of immature implants

## Tumor Markers in Germ Cell Cancer

| Histology | Tumor Marker | | |
|---|---|---|---|
| | AFP | hCG | LDH |
| Dysgerminoma | rare | rare | + |
| Endodermal sinus tumor (yolk sac) | ++ | − | + |
| Immature teratoma | ± | − | ± |
| Mixed germ cell tumor | ± | ± | ± |
| Choriocarcinoma | − | ++ | ± |
| Embryonal cancer | ± | + | ± |
| Polyembryoma | ± | + | − |

AFP, alpha-fetoprotein; hCG, human chorionic gonadotropin; LDH, lactate dehydrogenase.

### Screening
- Routine annual pelvic examination

### Diagnosis
- Surgery is necessary for diagnosis

### Pretreatment Workup
- Complete history and physical examination including pelvic exam
- Order AFP, HCG, lactate dehydrogenase, CA-125

### Treatment
- Consider fertility sparing surgery if Stage IA and desires fertility
- Adjuvant chemotherapy for all except Stage I dysgerminoma and well-differentiated Stage I immature teratoma

### Future Fertility
- Ovarian function recovers in most women who receive 3–4 cycles of standard dose chemotherapy and childbearing is often preserved.

# GYN-ONCOLOGY

## SEX CORD-STROMAL CELL OVARIAN TUMORS

### Background
- Accounts for 5–8% of all primary ovarian neoplasms
- Most produce steroid hormones

### Signs & Symptoms
- Granulosa cell:
  - Large, unilateral discrete mass with mean size 12 cm
  - Vaginal bleeding can be seen if estrogen secreting tumor
- Sertoli-Leydig cell:
  - Androgen production results in oligomenorrhea and virilization
  - Large, unilateral tumors with mean size of 16 cm
- Pure Sertoli cell tumors are estrogenic and may secrete renin causing hypertension and hypokalemia.
- Pure Leydig cell tumors are androgenic.

### Tumor Types

#### Granulosa-Stromal Cell Tumors
  - Granulosa cell: Call-Exner bodies
  - Most common stromal tumor
  - Symptoms: hormone disturbances, precocious puberty
  - Pathology: Call-Exner bodies (eosinophilic substrate with few degenerated nuclei), coffee bean nuclei, microfollicular pattern, granulosa and thecal cells
  - Secretes estrogen
  - Usually low grade and frequently associated with endometrial hyperplasia or carcinoma
  - Treatment: if young, USO; if menopausal total abdominal hysterectomy/bilateral salpingo-oophorectomy.
  - Recurrence or > Stage II: treat with chemotherapy or XRT
  - Prognosis = long term survival is good (75–90%)

#### Fibromas
- Most common sex cord stromal tumor

#### Sertoli-Stromal Cell Tumors
  - Sertoli-Leydig cell tumors
    ⇨ Testosterone-producing tumors
    ⇨ Symptoms: virilization
    ⇨ Treatment: fertility-sparing surgery for local disease
    ⇨ Prognosis: good if low grade
  - Gynandroblastoma
    ⇨ Display both granulosa and Leydig cell types and tumor characteristics

- Sex cord tumor with annular tubules
  ⇨ Mostly benign
  ⇨ Pathology: reinke crystals (crystalized testosterone)
- Steroid (lipid) cell tumor

## Screening
- Routine annual pelvic examination

## Diagnosis
- Surgery is necessary for diagnosis
- Same staging system as epithelial ovarian cancer

## Pretreatment Workup
- Complete history and physical examination including pelvic exam
- Endometrial biopsy in patient with vaginal bleeding (due to the association of granulosa cell tumors and endometrial hyperplasia)
- Inhibin used as a tumor marker in granulosa cell tumors to gauge response to treatment, testosterone, androstenedione

|                 | Inhibin | Testosterone | Androstenedione |
|-----------------|---------|--------------|-----------------|
| Thecoma-fibroma | –       | –            | –               |
| Granulosa cell  | +       | –            | –               |
| Gonadoblastoma  | ±       | ±            | ±               |
| Sertoli-Leydig  | ±       | +            | +               |

# GYN-ONCOLOGY

## VULVAR CANCER

### Background
- Fourth most common gynecologic malignancy (after uterine, ovarian, cervical).
- Comprises 5% of malignancies of female genital tract.
- Incidence of vulvar intraepithelial lesion has increased, but incidence of vulvar cancer has remained stable.

### Risk Factors
- Postmenopausal female
- Cigarette smoking
- Vulvar dystrophy (e.g., lichen sclerosis)
- Vulvar intraepithelial lesion
- Cervical intraepithelial lesion
- HPV
- Immunodeficiency syndromes
- Prior history of cervical cancer
- European ancestry

### Symptoms
- Pruritus
- Vulvar bleeding or discharge
  - Dysuria or enlarged lymph nodes are less frequently encountered and signs of more advanced disease.

### Clinical Manifestations
- Unifocal vulvar plaque, ulcer, mass (fleshy, nodular, or warty) on labia majora

### Diagnosis
- Biopsy of gross lesions to determine diagnosis and depth of stromal invasion.
- Take biopsy from center of lesion and include dermis or connective tissue to help assess depth.
- If no gross lesion visible but clinical suspicion is high, colposcopic vulvar examination using 5% acetic acid is indicated. Use copious amounts with prolonged contact with keratinized vulvar squamous epithelium.

### Tumor Types
- Squamous cell—90% of all vulvar malignancies with two subtypes
  - Keratinizing, differentiated, or simple type is more common. Occurs in older women. Not related to HPV.
  - Classic, warty, or Bowenoid type predominantly associated with HPV 16, 18, 33.
    ⇨ Occurs in younger women

- Melanoma is second most common—5% of all vulvar malignancies. Usually pigmented but amelanotic lesions can also occur.
- Basal cell carcinoma—2% of all vulvar malignancies.
  - Appearance of "rodent" ulcer with rolled edges and central ulceration
    ⇨ Can also be pigmented and pearly
- Sarcoma—1% of all vulvar malignancies.
- Extramammary Paget's disease—1% of all vulvar malignancies.

## Workup
- Complete physical exam including inguinal, supraclavicular and axillary nodes
- Colposcopy of cervix, vagina and vulva
- Imaging based on clinical findings

# GYN-ONCOLOGY

## Vulvar Cancer Staging/Treatment

| Stage IA | Tumor confined to vulva or perineum, <2 cm in greatest dimension, negative nodes, stromal invasion <1.0 mm | Deep radical excision |
|---|---|---|
| Stage IB | Tumor confined to vulva or perineum, <2 cm in greatest dimension, negative nodes, stromal invasion >1.0 mm | Treatment same for IB as II: If lateral lesion—radical local excision or deep radical excision with ipsilateral groin dissection or radical hemivulvectomy with en bloc ipsilateral inguinal-femoral lymphadenectomy. |
| Stage II | Tumor confined to the vulva and/or perineum, >2 cm in greatest dimension, negative nodes | Treatment same for IB as II: If midline lesion—Vulvectomy with en bloc bilateral groin dissection or bilateral groin dissection with radical vulvectomy (triple incision technique). |
| Stage III | Tumor of any size with adjacent spread to the lower urethra or anus and/or unilateral regional lymph node metastasis | Radical resection pre- or post-irradiation. Rarely exenterative surgery. |
| Stage IVA | Tumor invades any of the following: upper urethra, bladder or rectal mucosa, pelvic bone, or bilateral regional node metastasis | Radical resection pre- or post-irradiation. Rarely exenterative surgery. |
| Stage IVB | Any distant metastasis including pelvic lymph nodes | Radical resection pre- or post-irradiation. Rarely exenterative surgery. |

*Source:* FIGO Committee on Gynecologic Oncology. Gynecologic cancer—staging and guidelines. *Int J Gynaecol Obstet.* 2000;70(2):209–262.

## VAGINAL CANCER STAGING

| Primary Tumor (T) | | |
|---|---|---|
| TX | – | Primary tumor cannot be assessed |
| T0 | – | No evidence of primary tumor |
| Tis | – | Carcinoma *in situ* |
| T1 | I | Tumor confined to vagina |
| T2 | II | Tumor invades paravaginal tissue but not to pelvic wall |
| T3 | III | Tumor extends to pelvic wall |
| T4* | IVA | Tumor invades bladder and/or bowel mucosa and/or extends beyond the true |
| | | Pelvic (bullous edema is not sufficient to classify a tumor as T4) |
| | IVB | Distant metastasis |

*Note: If the bladder mucosa is not involved, the tumor is Stage III.

| Regional Lymph Nodes (N) | |
|---|---|
| NX | Regional lymph nodes cannot be assessed |
| N0 | No regional lymph node metastasis |
| N1 | Pelvic or inguinal lymph node metastasis |

| Distant Metastasis (M) | |
|---|---|
| MX | Distant metastasis cannot be assessed |
| M0 | No distant metastasis |
| M1 | Distant metastasis (including pelvic lymph node metastasis) |

| Stage Grouping | | | |
|---|---|---|---|
| 0 | Tis | N0 | M0 |
| I | T1 | N0 | M0 |
| II | T2 | N0 | M0 |
| III | T1 | N1 | M0 |
| | T2 | N1 | M0 |
| | T3 | N0 | M0 |
| | T3 | N1 | M0 |
| IVA | T4 | Any N | M0 |
| IVB | Any T | Any N | M1 |

# GYN-ONCOLOGY

## GESTATIONAL TROPHOBLASTIC DISEASE

### Features of Partial and Complete Hydatidiform Moles

| Feature | Partial Mole | Complete Mole |
|---|---|---|
| Karyotype | Most commonly 69,XXX or 69,XXY | Most commonly 46,XX or 46,XY |
| Pathology | | |
|    Fetus | Often present | Absent |
|    Amnion, fetal red blood cells | Usually present | Absent |
|    Villous edema | Variable; focal | Diffuse |
|    Trophoblastic proliferation | Focal, slight to moderate | Diffuses slight to severe |
| Clinical presentation | | |
|    Diagnosis | Missed abortion | Molar gestation |
|    Uterine size | Small for gestational age | 50% larger for gestational age |
|    Theca lutein cysts | Rare | 15–25% |
|    Medical complications | Rare | Less than 25% |
|    Postmolar malignant sequelae | <5% | 6–32% |

*Source:* Modified from Soper JT, Lewis JL Jr., Hammond CB. Gestational troboblastic disease. In: Hoskins WJ, Perez CA, Young RC, eds. *Principals and Practice of Gynecologic Oncology.* 2nd ed. Philadelphia (PA): Lippincott-Raven; 1997, pg.1040.

### Signs and Symptoms

- First trimester bleeding
- Size/date discrepancy
- Sudden increase in uterine size
- Passage of vesicles
- Hyperemesis gravidarum
- Early preeclampsia
- Thyrotoxicosis
- β-hCG greater than expected

## Scoring System for Gestational Trophoblastic Disease (Based on Prognostic Factors)

| Prognostic Factors | Score | | | |
|---|---|---|---|---|
| | 0 | 1 | 2 | 4 |
| Age (yrs) | <40 | ≤40 | — | — |
| Antecedent pregnancy | Mole | Abortion | Term | |
| Interval mos from index pregnancy | <4 | 4–<7 | 7–<13 | ≥13 |
| Pretreatment human chorionic gonadotropin (IU/L) | $<10^3$ | $10^3$–$<10^4$ | $10^4$–$<10^5$ | $≥10^6$ |
| Largest tumor (cm) (including uterus) | | 3–5 | ≥5 | — |
| Site of metastases | Lung | Spleen, kidney | Gastrointestinal, liver | Brain |
| Number of metastases | — | 1–4 | 5–8 | >8 |
| Previous failed chemotherapy | — | — | Single drug | 2 or more drugs |

Total score is obtained by adding the individual scores for each prognostic factor. 0–4 = low risk, 5–6 = intermediate risk, >7 = high risk

Format for reporting to International Federation of Gynecology and Obstetrics (FIGO) Annual Report: in order to stage and allot a risk factor score, a patient's diagnosis is allocated to a stage as represented by a Roman numeral, i.e., I, II, III, and IV. This is then separated by a colon from the sum of all the actual risk factor scores expressed in Arabic numbers, e.g., stage II:4, stage IV:9. This stage and score will be allotted for each patient.

*Source:* Berek JS, Hacker NF; eds. *Practical Gynecologic Oncology.* 4th ed. Philadelphia (PA): Lippincott Williams & Wilkins; 2005, pg. 613. Reproduced with the permission of the publisher.

Sites of metastases: lung (80%), vagina (30%), brain (10%), liver (10%). Prognostic score ≥7 is considered high risk and requires intensive combination chemotherapy.

## Post-Mole Surveillance

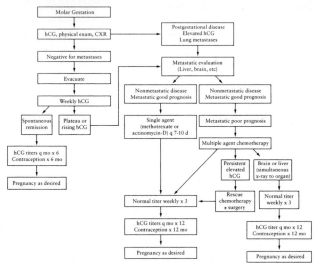

*Source:* DiSaia PJ, Creasman WT. Gestational trophoblastic neoplasia. In: *Clinical Gynecologic Oncology.* 4th ed. St. Louis: Mosby Year Book, 1993. Reproduced with the permission of the publisher.

## DENNIS SIEGLER'S* TOP TEN WAYS** TO SURVIVE GYN-ONCOLOGY (PRE-80 HOUR WORK WEEK)***

10. Do not become angry.

9. DO NOT BECOME ANGRY.

8. DO NOT BECOME ANGRY.

7. If angry, do not become frustrated.

6. If angry and frustrated, remember there is always another GOG form to complete+.

5. Remember that actual O.R. time = requested O.R. time × 2.

4. Chemotherapy admissions only seem to multiply like rabbits.

3. If all else fails, examine the patient.

2. PM rounds should be completed before AM rounds begin.

And the Number One way to survive Gyn-Onc:

1. Remember, it could be worse; you could be on Internal Medicine.

---

*Former Stanford Chief Resident.
**With apologies to David Letterman.
***Younger physicians may not get the joke... too bad.
+Yes, I know that these are now done electronically.

| Drug | Class | Cell Cycle | Mechanism of Action | Toxicities and Other Notes |
|------|-------|-----------|---------------------|----------------------------|
| Cisplatin | Platinate | G1 | Bifunctional alkylator (binds N7 of G&A); DNA intrastrand crosslinks and DNA adducts | Renal, ototoxicity, cortical blindness; amifostine (low dose IV 3×/wk reverses neurotoxicity—GOG 192), 5HT + dex (NCI); to limit neurotoxicity give Taxol 24 hrs and to limit myelo give Taxol first |
| Carboplatin | Platinate | Non-specific | Intrastrand DNA cross linking | Myelo (platelets)—nadir 3 wks, recovery 4–5 wks; hypersensitivity; to limit myelo, give Taxol first Calvert Formula: Total dose (mg) = Target AUC (mg/mL/min) × CrCl + (mL/min). CrCl calculated using the Cockcroft-Gault or Jelliffe formulas (the latter does not affect body surface area or body weight to adjust for body size) |
| Oxaliplatin | Platinate |  | DNA interstrand damage | Neurotoxicity, cold sensitivity, N&V |
| Paclitaxel | Taxane | M | Mitotic spindle poison | Hypersensitivity (2% with pre-meds); alopecia, myelo, reversible neurotoxicity; 3 hrs infusion; decrease neurotox |
| Docetaxel | Taxane | M | European Yew (Taxus baccata); promotes microtubule assembly and inhibits depolymerization of tubulin | Increase myelo (neutropenia) and less neurotoxicity than paclitaxel; fluid retention, diarrhea; no chromophore component, give over decreased dose with increased LFTs |
| Doxorubicin | Anthracycline | Late S; inhibits topo II in G2 | Strep peucetius; amino group sugar projects into minor groove (DNA and RNA affected) | Myelo; radiation recall; cardiomyopathy (free radicals) [<500 mg = 1%; 500–600 mg = 11%; >600 mg = 30%]; vesicant; 40% biliary excretion (decreased dose with increased LFTs) |
| Liposomal Doxorubicin | Anthracycline | Non-specific | Pegylation protects liposome from immune system; much longer plasma half-life (45 vs. 24 hrs); 4–16 × tumor-tissue concentration | PPE, stomatitis, alopecia (15%) |
| Topotecan | Topoisomerase inhibitor | S | Inhibits topo I | Severe myelo with 5-day regimen; N&V, stomatitis, asthenia, minimal alopecia; to limit toxicity give CDDP after topotecan |

| Drug | Class | Cell cycle | Mechanism | Toxicity / Notes |
|---|---|---|---|---|
| Etoposide | Topo-isomerase inhibitor | G2 | Inhibits topo II; stabilizes topo-II-DNA complex | Myelo (nadir 16 days, recovery 20–22 days); GI, severe hypotension with rapid infusion |
| Cyclophosphamide | Alkylator | Non-specific | DNA interstrand and intrastrand crosslinks; requires liver for activation | Hemorrhagic cystitis (acrolein binds to bladder epithelium; mesna protective); myelo (nadir 8–14 days, recovery 18–21 days), alopecia, SIADH, "busulfan lung," AML |
| Ifosfamide | Alkylator | Non-specific | Hydroxylation by P450 microsomal enzyme systems produces reactive 4-OH-IFEX metabolite and neurotoxin chloroacetaldehyde | Hemorrhagic cystitis (acrolein); encephalopathy (antidote = methylene blue); need adequate hydration pre and post (72 hrs); nephrotoxicity |
| Gemcitabine | Antimetabolite | S | Pro-drug; synthetic nucleoside analog; synergizes with CDDP and can reverse CDDP resistance | Myelo, fever; hemolytic uremic syndrome |
| Vincristine | Vinca alkaloid | M | Inhibits microtubule assembly | Peripheral neurotoxicity; jaw pain, vesicant |
| Vinblastine | Vinca alkaloid | M | Inhibits microtubule assembly | Myelo, mucositis, vesicant |
| Vinorelbine | Vinca alkaloid | M | Spindle poison | Myelo, fever, neurotoxicity, increased LFTs |
| Bleomycin | Antibiotic | G2 | Strep verticillus glycopeptide; copper-iron complexes (oxygen radicals, DNA scission) | Fever; pulmonary toxicity (pneumonitis); increased hydrolase diffuses bleo; liver, BM, GI, spleen; decreased hydrolase; skin and lung; total dose 400 mg; renal excretion |
| Hydroxyurea | Antimetabolite | Early S | Blocks ribonucleotide reductase catalytic subunit | Myelo, GI, maculo-papular rash, facial erythema, radiation recall |
| 5-Fluorouracil | Antimetabolite | Early S | Antifolate analog; reduces dihydrotetra | Ulcerative stomatitis, mucositis, myelo (nadir 9–14 days); acute cerebellar syndrome (neurotoxic metabolite fluoro-citrate); given IP as gloxuridine FUDR with CDDP for ovary (SWOG phase II); given IP with hyperthermia for pseudomyxoma peritonei |

*(continued)*

| Drug | Class | Cell Cycle | Mechanism of Action | Toxicities and Other Notes |
|------|-------|-----------|---------------------|----------------------------|
| Methotrexate | Antimetabolite | Early S | Antifolate analog; reduces dihydrofolate reductase | Ulcerative stomatitis, mucositis, glossitis, gingivitis, pharyngitis, severe hemorrhagic enteritis; hepatoxic; cleared by kidneys |
| Actinomycin-D | Antibiotic | GI | Strep parvulus; DNA base pair intercalation | Myelo (nadir 7–10 days); N&V, mucositis, diarrhea, radiation, recall; vesicant |
| Capecitabine (Xeloda) | Antimetabolite | S | Fluoropyrimidine pro-drug converted to 5-FU | PPE, diarrhea, N&V, increased bilirubin, drug is inactive until digestion |
| Hexamethylmelamine | Alkylator | Nonspecific | Unknown | GI, myelo, neurotoxicity |

5-FU, fluorouracil; 5HT, serotonin; AML, acute myeloid leukemia; AVC, ampulla of Vater cancer; BM, brain metastases; CDDP, cisplatin; CrCl, creatinine clearance; DNA, deoxyribonucleic acid; FUDR, floxuridine; GI, gastrointestinal; GOG, gynecologic oncology group; IFEX, ifosfamide; LFT, liver function test; N&V, nausea and vomiting; NCI, National Cancer Institute; PPE, palmar plantar erythrodysesthesia; RNA, ribonucleic acid; SIADH, syndrome of inappropriate antidiuretic hormone secretion; SWOG, Southwest Oncology Group.

## TREATMENT OF CHEMOTHERAPY EXTRAVASATION INJURY

| Class/Specific Agent | Local Antidote | Specific Procedure |
|---|---|---|
| **Alkylating Agents** | | |
| Cisplatin, mechlorethamine | $1/3$ or $1/6$ M sodium thiosulfate | Mix 4–8 mL 10% sodium thiosulfate U.S.P. with 6 ml of sterile water for injection, U.S.P. for a $1/3$ or $1/6$ M solution. Inject 2 mL into site for each mg of mechlorethamine or 100 mg of cisplatin extravasated. |
| Mitomycin-C | Dimethylsulfoxide (DMSO) 50–99% (w/v) | Apply 1.5 mL to the site every 6 hrs for 14 days. Allow to air-dry, do not cover. |
| **DNA intercalators** | | |
| Doxorubicin, daunorubicin, amsacrine | Cold compresses | Apply immediately for 30–60 mins, then alternate on/off every 15 mins for 1 day. |
| | Dimethylsulfoxide (DMSO) 50–99% (w/v) | Apply 1.5 mL to the site every 6 hrs for 14 days. Allow to air-dry, do not cover. |
| **Vinca alkaloids** | | |
| Vinblastine, vincristine | Warm compresses Hyaluronidase | Apply immediately for 30–60 mins, then alternate on/off every 15 mins for 1 day. Inject 150 U hyaluronidase (Wydase, others) into site. |
| **Epipodophyllotoxins** | | |
| Etoposide, teniposide | Warm compresses Hyaluronidase | Apply immediately for 30–60 mins, then alternate on/off every 15 mins for 1 day. Inject 150 U hyaluronidase (Wydase, others) into site. |

*Source:* Dorr RT. Pharmacologic management of vesicant chemotherapy extravasations. In: Dorr RT, Von Hoff DD, ed. *Cancer Chemotherapy Handbook,* 2nd ed. Norwalk, Conn.: Appleton & Lange, 1994. Reproduced with the permission of the publisher.

# GYN-ONCOLOGY

## BOWEL PREP (USUALLY FOR OVARIAN CANCER CASES)

### Teng Recipe
1. Golytely with 1–2 cups juice per liter, 4 liters PO (8 ounces q10minutes)
2. Kefzol 1 g IV 1 hour prior to operation
3. Fleets Enema night before and in AM
4. Clear liquids for dinner, NPO after midnight on day before surgery

### Chan/Husain Recipe
Ovarian cancer, endometrial, cervical cancer, or advanced laparoscopy
1. Fleets Phosphosoda
2. Kefzol 1g IV 1 hour prior to operation
3. Fleets enema night before and in AM
4. Clear liquid for dinner, NPO after midnight on day before surgery

## IV FLUID COMPOSITION

| | Na$^+$ | Cl$^-$ | K$^+$ | HCO$_3^-$ | Ca$^{+2}$ | Glucose |
|---|---|---|---|---|---|---|
| Extracellular fluid | 140 | 102 | 4.0 | 28 | 5.0 | |
| Normal saline | 154 | 154 | | | | |
| $^1/_2$ Normal saline | 77 | 77 | | | | |
| $^1/_4$ Normal saline | 34 | 34 | | | | |
| Lactated Ringers | 130 | 109 | 4.0 | 28 | 3.0 | |
| D5W | | | | | | 50 g |
| D10W | | | | | | 100 g |
| Peripheral parenteral nutrition | 47 | 40 | 13 | | | 100 g |
| Total parenteral nutrition | 25 | 30 | 44 | | | 250 g |
| D50 | | | | | | 500 g |

| | Amino Acids | Mg$^{+2}$ | PO$_4^{-3}$ | Acetate | Osm |
|---|---|---|---|---|---|
| Extracellular fluid | | | | | 290 |
| Normal saline | | | | | 308 |
| $^1/_2$ Normal saline | | | | | 154 |
| $^1/_4$ Normal saline | | | | | 78 |
| Lactated Ringers | | | | | 272 |
| D5W | | | | | 252 |
| D10W | | | | | 505 |
| Peripheral parenteral nutrition | 35 g | 3.0 | 3.5 | 52 | 500 |
| Total parenteral nutrition | 50 g | 5.0 | 15 | 99 | 190 |
| D50 | | | | | |

## BODY FLUID COMPOSITION

| | Na$^+$ | Cl$^-$ | K$^+$ | HCO$_3^-$ | Daily Production (mL) |
|---|---|---|---|---|---|
| Gastric juices | 60–100 | 100 | 10 | 0 | 1500–2000 |
| Duodenum | 130 | 90 | 5 | 0–10 | 300–2000 |
| Bile | 145 | 100 | 5 | 15–35 | 100–800 |
| Pancreatic juices | 140 | 75 | 5 | 70–115 | 100–800 |
| Ileum | 140 | 100 | 5 | 15–30 | 2000–3000 |

# GYN-ONCOLOGY

## STEROIDS

| Generic Name | Trade Name | Relative Potency Glucocorticoid and Anti-inflammatory | Mineralo-corticoid | Equivalent Doses (mg) | Starting Doses (mg) Moderate Illness | Severe Illness |
|---|---|---|---|---|---|---|
| **Short-acting** | | | | | | |
| Hydrocortisone (cortisol) | Cortef | 1 | 1 | 20 | 80–160 | |
| | Solu-Cortef | | | | | |
| Cortisone | | 0.8 | 0.8 | 25 | 100–200 | |
| Prednisone | Deltasone | 4 | 0.8 | 5 | 20–40 | 60–100 |
| | Meticorten | | | | | |
| Prednisolone | Delta-Cortef | 4 | 0.8 | 5 | 20–40 | 60–100 |
| | Meticorte-lone | | | | | |
| Methylpredniso-lone | Medrol | 5 | 0.5 | 4 | 16–32 | 48–80 |
| | Solu-Medrol | | | | | |
| **Intermediate-acting** | | | | | | |
| Triamcinolone | Aristocort | 5 | 0 | 4 | 16–32 | 48–80 |
| | Kenacort | | | | | |
| Paramethasone | Haldrone | 10 | 0 | 2 | 8–16 | 24–40 |
| **Long-acting** | | | | | | |
| Dexamethasone | Decadron | 25 | 0 | 0.75 | 3–6 | 9–15 |
| Betamethasone | Celestone | 25 | 0 | 0.6 | 2.4–4.8 | 7.2–12 |

*Source:* Klearman M, Pereira M. Arthritis and rheumatologic diseases. In: Dunagan WC, Ridner ML, eds. *Manual of Medical Therapeutics.* 27th ed. Boston: Little, Brown, 1992. Reproduced with the permission of the publisher.

## INVASIVE CARDIAC MONITORING

### Fast Facts

- Swan-Ganz catheter allows accurate measurement of hemodynamic parameters in acutely ill patient.
- Introduced into clinical practice in 1970.

### Indications

- Sepsis with refractory hypotension or oliguria
- Unexplained or refractory pulmonary edema, heart failure, or oliguria
- Severe PIH with pulmonary edema or oliguria
- Intraoperative or intrapartum cardiovascular decompensation
- Massive blood loss and volume loss or replacement
- Adult respiratory distress syndrome (ARDS)
- Shock of undefined etiology
- Some chronic conditions, particularly associated with labor or surgery
  - NYHA Class III or IV cardiac disease (structural or physiologic)
  - Peripartum or perioperative coronary artery disease (ischemia, infarction)

### Triple Lumen

*Distal port (red):* located in pulmonary artery. Attached to pressure transducer to provide continuous pulmonary artery pressure tracings and allow pulmonary capillary wedge pressure determination. Can also withdraw mixed venous blood from pulmonary artery.

*Proximal port (blue):* located in superior vena cava. Can be used in infused fluids and also used in cardiac output measurements.

*Thermistor:* a temperature sensor used in determination of cardiac output.

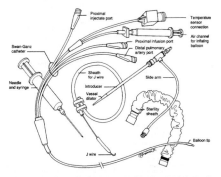

*Source:* Mabie WC. Critical care obstetrics. In: Gabbe SG, Niebyl JR, Simpson JL, eds. *Obstetrics: Normal and Problem Pregnancies.* 2nd ed. New York: Churchill Livingstone, 1991. Reproduced with the permission of the publisher.

# GYN-ONCOLOGY

## Wedge Pressure

A measurement of left ventricular preload. The pulmonary artery wedge pressure is obtained with a balloon-tipped catheter advanced into a branch of the pulmonary artery until the vessel is occluded, forming a free communication through the pulmonary capillaries and veins to the left atrium. A true wedge position is in the lung zone where both pulmonary artery and pulmonary venous pressures exceed alveolar pressure.

## Preload

Initial stretch of the myocardial fiber at end diastole. Clinically the right and left ventricular end-diastolic pressures are assessed by the central venous pressure and wedge pressure respectively.

## Afterload

Wall tension of the ventricle during ejection. Best reflected by systolic blood pressure.

## Contractility

The force of myocardial contractility when preload and afterload are held constant.

## Hemodynamic Therapy

|  | Decreased | Increased |
|---|---|---|
| **Preload** |  |  |
|  | Crystalloid | **Diuretics** |
|  | Colloid | Furosemide |
|  | Blood | Ethacrynic acid |
|  |  | Mannitol |
|  |  | **Venodilators** |
|  |  | Furosemide |
|  |  | Nitroglycerin |
|  |  | Morphine |
| **Afterload** |  |  |
|  | Volume | **Arterial dilators** |
|  | Inotropic support | Hydralazine |
|  | Vasopressors | Diazoxide |
|  | Norepinephrine |  |
|  | Phenylephrine | **Venous dilators** |
|  | Metaraminol | Nitroglycerin |
|  |  | **Mixed arteriovenous dilators** |
|  |  | Nitroprusside |
|  |  | Trimethaphan |
| **Contractility** |  |  |
|  | Dopamine |  |
|  | Dobutamine |  |
|  | Epinephrine |  |
|  | Calcium |  |
|  | Digitalis |  |

*Source:* Gomella LG, Braen GR, Olding MJ. Critical care. In: *Clinician's Pocket Reference: The Scut Monkey's Handbook.* 7th ed. Norwalk, Conn.: Appleton & Lange, 1993. Reproduced with the permission of the publisher.

## Derivation of Hemodynamic Parameters

| Mean arterial pressure | MAP | mm Hg | $\dfrac{\text{systolic pressure} + 2\,(\text{diastolic pressure})}{3}$ |
|---|---|---|---|
| Stroke volume | SV | mL/beat | CO/HR |
| Stroke index | SI | mL/beat/m² | SV/BSA |
| Cardiac index | CI | L/min/m² | CO/BSA |
| Pulmonary vascular resistance | PVR | dynes × sec × cm⁻⁵ | $\dfrac{\text{MPAP} - \text{PCWP}}{\text{CO}} \times 80$ |
| Systemic vascular resistance | SVR | dynes × sec × cm⁻⁵ | $\dfrac{\text{MAP} - \text{CVP}}{\text{CO}} \times 80$ |

BSA, body surface area; CI, cardiac index; HR, hemodynamic response; MAP, mean arterial pressure; MPAP, mean pulmonary artery pressure; PCWP, capillary wedge pressure; PVR, pulmonary vascular resistance; SI, stroke index; SV, stroke volume; SVR, systemic vascular resistance.

## Normal Hemodynamic Values

| Parameter | Nonpregnant | Trimester of Pregnancy | | |
|---|---|---|---|---|
| | | 1st | 2nd | 3rd |
| Heart beat (beats/min) | 60–100 | 81 | 84 | 84 |
| Central venous pressure (mm Hg) | 5–10 | | | |
| Pulmonary capillary wedge pressure (mm Hg) | 6–12 | | | |
| Mean arterial pressure (mm Hg) | 90–110 | 82 | 84 | 86 |
| Cardiac output (L/min) | 4.3–6.0 | 6.2 | 6.3 | 6.4 |
| Stroke volume (mL/beat) | 57–71 | 76 | 75 | 76 |
| Systemic vascular resistance (dynes × sec × cm⁻⁵) | 900–1400 | 1087 | 1093 | 1119 |
| Pulmonary vascular resistance (dynes × sec × cm⁻⁵) | <250 | | | |

*Source:* Adapted with permission from Clark SL, Cotton DB, Lee W, et al. Central hemodynamic assessment of normal term pregnancy. *Am J Obstet Gynecol.* 1989;161(6 Pt 1):1439–1442 and Rosenthal MH. Intrapartum intensive care management of the cardiac patient. *Clin Obstet Gynecol.* 1981;24(3):789–807.

# GYN-ONCOLOGY

## COAGULATION CASCADE
### Effects of Anticoagulants on the Coagulation Cascade

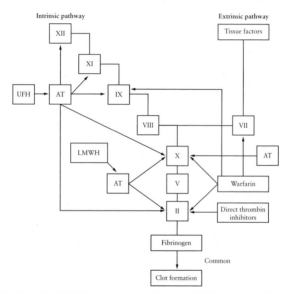

AT, antithrombin; LMWH, low molecular weight heparin; UFH, unfractionated heparin.
*Source:* Reprinted with permission from Haines ST. Update on the prevention of venous thromboembolism. *Am J Health-Syst Pharm.* 2004;7:S5–S11. © 2004, American Society of Health-System Pharmacists, Inc. All rights reserved.

## THROMBOEMBOLIC PHENOMENA
### Diagnostic Algorithm for Deep Vein Thrombosis

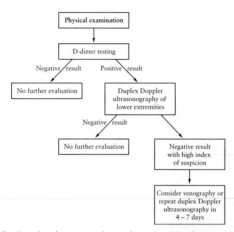

If the duplex Doppler ultrasonography results are positive, begin anticoagulation therapy with low molecular weight heparin or unfractionated heparin. If contraindications for anticoagulation exist, consider placement of an inferior vena caval filler. *Source:* Reprinted with permission from Krivak TC, Zorn KK. Venous thromboembolism in obstetrics and gynecology. *Obstet Gynecol.* 2007;109(3):761–777.

### Diagnostic Algorithm for Pulmonary Embolism

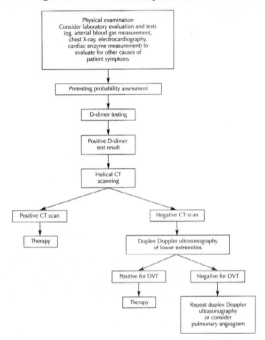

Therapy may consist of unfractionated heparin or low molecular weight heparin, as well as supportive care (supplemental oxygen). If the patient is unstable, thrombolytic therapy may be considered. If contraindication for coagulation exists, consider placement of inferior vena caval filter. If the D-dimer test result is negative and pretest probability is low, duplex Doppler ultrasonography of lower extremities would be considered. Withhold anticoagulation therapy if both test results are negative.

*Source:* Reprinted with permission from Krivak TC, Zorn KK. Venous thromboembolism in obstetrics and gynecology. *Obstet Gynecol.* 2007;109(3):761–777.

## Current Diagnosis of Venous Thromboembolism
### Recommendation 1

Validated clinical prediction rules should be used to estimate pretest probability of both deep vein thrombosis (DVT) and pulmonary embolism (see Wells Criteria tables). (*See pregnancy comment.)

### Wells Prediction Rule for Diagnosing Deep Vein Thrombosis: Predicting Pretest Probability

| Clinical Characteristic | Score |
|---|---|
| Active cancer (treatment ongoing, within previous 6 mos, or palliative) | 1 |
| Paralysis, paresis, or recent plaster immobilization of the lower extremities | 1 |
| Recently bedridden >3 days or major surgery within 12 wks requiring general or regional anesthesia | 1 |
| Localized tenderness along the distribution of the deep venous system | 1 |
| Entire leg swollen | 1 |
| Calf swelling 3 cm larger than asymptomatic side (measured 10 cm below tibial tuberosity) | 1 |
| Pitting edema confined to the symptomatic leg | 1 |
| Collateral superficial veins (nonvaricose) | 1 |
| Alternative diagnosis at least as likely as deep venous thrombosis | −2 |

*Note:* Clinical probability: low <0; intermediate 1–2; high >3. In patients with symptoms in both legs, the more symptomatic leg is used.
*Source:* Reprinted with permission from Wells PS, Anderson DR, Bormanis J et al. Value of assessment of pretest probability of deep-vein thrombosis in clinical management. *Lancet.* 2002;350:1795–1798. Copyright 2002, from Elsevier.

### Wells Prediction Rule for Diagnosing Pulmonary Embolism (PE): Predicting Pretest Probability of PE

| Clinical Characteristic | Score |
|---|---|
| Previous pulmonary embolism or deep vein thrombosis | +1.5 |
| Heart rate >100 beats per min | +1.5 |
| Recent surgery or immobilization | +1.5 |
| Clinical signs of deep vein thrombosis | +3 |
| Alternative diagnosis less likely than PE | +3 |
| Hemoptysis | +1 |
| Cancer | +1 |

Note: Clinical probability of pulmonary embolism: low 0–1; intermediate 2-6; high >7.
*Source:* Reprinted with permission from Chagnon I, Bounameaux H, Aujesky D et al. Comparison of two clinical prediction rules and implicit assessment among patients with suspected pulmonary embolism. *Am J Med.* 2002;113:269–275. Copyright 2002, from Elsevier.

*Note that pregnancy is not considered in either table because pregnancy was an exclusion criteria for the Wells' study. In discussing this with one of the consensus paper's authors, he felt that giving pregnancy a 1 point score would be reasonable. Absent other data, it would be reasonable to add one point in the second table for pregnancy.

# GYN-ONCOLOGY

## Recommendation 2

With a low pretest probability of DVT or pulmonary embolism, D-dimer testing is a probable first option, and if negative, indicates a low likelihood of venous thromboembolism (VTE). Caution: use in cancer patients has a 79% negative predictive value vs. 96% negative predictive value in non-cancer patients.

### Deep Vein Thrombosis Incidence Based on Prediction and D-Dimer Testing

| Pretest Prediction | D-Dimer Negative |
|---|---|
| Low | 0.5% |
| Medium | 3.5% |
| High | 21% |

## Recommendation 3

Ultrasound is recommended for patients with intermediate to high pretest probability of DVT in the lower extremities.

*Note:* Ultrasound is less sensitive in patients who have DVT limited to the calf. Venography may be required for patients who have a suspected calf vein DVT and a negative ultrasound.

## Recommendation 4

Patients with intermediate or high pretest probability of pulmonary embolism will require diagnostic imaging studies. Options include:
1. Ventilation-perfusion scan
2. Multi-detector helical CT
3. Pulmonary angiography

Note: Helical CT may lack sensitivity in certain cases. Further imaging studies are likely needed in patients who have a high pretest probability of pulmonary embolism and a negative CT scan (e.g., single or sequential ultrasound assessment of the lower extremities or pulmonary angiography).

*Source: Annals of Family Medicine. 5(1), January-February 2007.*

## Treatment

### Venous Thromboembolism and Pulmonary Embolism in Gynecology:

- Therapeutic IV unfractionated heparin (UFH) or low molecular weight heparin (LMWH) × 5 days while being converted to warfarin.
  - UFH: activated partial thromboplastin time 1.5–2 times the upper limit of normal.
  - LMWH: enoxaparin 1 mg/kg SC every 12 hours or dalteparin 120 units/kg. SC every 12 hours, maintain international normalized ratio at 2.5 (range 2–3).
  - LMWH is as effective and safe as UFH and is clearly superior because therapeutic dosing is more rapidly and dependably achieved.
  - If first VTE episode → treat with warfarin × 6 months.

- If positive DVT in the presence of malignancy → continue LMWH for the duration of an active malignancy (alternate = warfarin).
  - If second VTE episode → lifelong warfarin.
- If there is a contraindication for anticoagulant therapy → inferior vena cava filter.
  - Contraindications to anticoagulation
    ⇨ Active bleeding
    ⇨ History of heparin-induced thrombocytopenia
    ⇨ History of bleeding ulcer
    ⇨ History of anaphylaxis to heparins
    ⇨ Recent surgical procedure
- *Note:* Patients with extensive proximal DVT producing severe limb swelling and pain, or patients with massive pulmonary embolism producing shock or systemic hypoperfusion, may be candidates for emergent thrombolytic therapy or (in the case of DVT) thrombectomy.

## Venous Thromboembolism in Obstetrics

- IV or SC UFH or LMWH convert to warfarin postpartum.
  - UFH: activated partial thromboplastin time 1.5–2 × the upper limit of normal
  - LMWH: enoxaparin 30–80 mg SC bid, maintain international normalized ratio at 2.5 (range 2–3)
- Newly diagnosed without underlying thrombophilia or other risk factors should be treated with warfarin for 6 weeks–3 months postpartum for a total of at least 6 months.
- Thrombectomy only for emergent situations.
- Inferior vena cava filter if contraindication to anticoagulant therapy.
- $O_2$ titrate to keep $O_2$ sat >92.
- IV heparin: Stanford uses loading dose 80 units/kg rounded to nearest 100 units.
- Maintence 15 units/kg/hr rounded to nearest unit/hr to keep partial thrombo-plastin time 1.5–2 × normal.
- Coumadin started after 4–7 days on heparin.
  - Give 10 mg, 10 mg, 10 mg, 5 mg.
  - Follow prothrombin time (keep 1.5–2.0 × normal).

*Source:* Krivak TC, Zorn KK. Venous thromboembolism in obstetrics and gynecology. *Obstet Gynecol.* 2007;109(3):761–777.

# GYN-ONCOLOGY

## Stanford Hospital Guide for Preventing Venous Thromboembolism

| | |
|---|---|
| **Low risk** (<5% risk of DVT) | |
| -Patient <40 yrs old **and**<br>-Minor surgery **and**<br>-No additional risk factors | No specific prophylaxis; early mobilization |
| **Moderate risk** (10–20% risk of DVT) | |
| -Age 40–60 years old with no additional risk factors **or**<br>-Minor surgery in patients with additional risk factors | -UFH 5000 units SC q8hrs or<br>-LMWH (enoxaparin) 40mg SC qday<br>Add GCS or IPC |
| **High risk** (20–40% risk of DVT) | |
| -Surgery in patients >60 years old **or**<br>-Age 40–60 with additional risk factors | -UFH 5000 units SC q8hrs or<br>-LMWH (enoxaparin) 30mg SC bid<br>Add GCS or IPC if possible |
| **Highest risk** (40–80% risk of DVT) | |
| -Surgery in patient with multiple risk factors **or**<br>-Hip or knee arthroplasty **or**<br>-Hip fracture surgery **or**<br>-Major trauma **or**<br>-Spinal cord injury | -LMWH (enoxaparin) 30mg SC bid or<br>-Fondiparinux 2.5mg SC qday or<br>-Warfarin started day of surgery, target INR 2–3<br>Add GCS or IPC if possible<br>Consider extended (4 wks) out of hospital prophylaxis at discharge |

DVT, deep vein thrombosis; GCS, graduated compression stockings; INR, international normalized ratio; IPC, intermittent pneumatic compression; LMWH, low molecular weight heparin; UFH, unfractionated heparin.

## Venous Thromboembolism Prophylaxis - Inova Fairfax Hospital

The presence of one (1) high risk factor or two (2) or more other risk factors is an indication for VTE prophylaxis.

### VTE High Risk Factors

Trauma (abdomen, pelvis, hip and leg)
Major surgery (especially abdomen, pelvis, hip and leg)
Prior history of VTE (DVT or PE)
Malignancy

### Other VTE Risk Factors

Age > 40 yrs
Intensive care unit admission
Chronic lung disease
Respiratory failure
Pneumonia
Inflammatory disorders
Central line/venous catheter
Known thrombophilia
Active collagen vascular disorder
Serious infection
Prolonged immobility (>24 hrs)
Varicose veins
Nephrotic syndrome
Sickle cell disease
Pregnancy or estrogen use
Obesity
Congestive heart failure

### Anticoagulant Prophylaxis Exclusion Criteria

Active bleeding
Uncontrolled hypertension
Coagulopathy
Current anticoagulant treatment
Recent intraocular or intracranial surgery
Presence or history of heparin-induced thrombocytopenia (HIT)
Significant renal insufficiency
Epidural anesthesia or spinal tap within 24 h
Hypersensitivity to unfractionated heparin or low molecular weight heparin

### Standard Venous Thromboembolism Prophylaxis Options

Intermittent sequential pneumatic compression device (SCD)
Heparin 5000 units SC q8hrs
Lovenox 40 mg SC daily
    (Lovenox 30 mg subcutaneously daily for creatinine clearance <30 mL/min)

## Recommendations for Preoperative and Postoperative Anticoagulation in Patients Who Are Taking Oral Anticoagulants

| Indication | Before Surgery | After Surgery |
|---|---|---|
| Acute VTE | | — |
| Mo 1 | IV heparin[a] | IV heparin[a] |
| Mos 2 and 3 | No change[b] | IV heparin |
| Recurrent VTE[c] | No change[b] | SC heparin |
| Acute arterial embolism, mo 1 | IV heparin[d] | |
| Mechanical heart valve | No change[b] | SC heparin |
| Nonvalvular atrial fibrillation | No change[b] | SC heparin |

IV heparin, intravenous heparin at therapeutic doses; SC heparin, subcutaneous unfractionated or low-molecular-weight heparin in doses recommended for prophylaxis against venous thromboembolism (VTE) in high-risk patients.

[a]Insertion of a vena cava filter should be considered if acute VTE has occurred within 2 weeks or if the risk of bleeding during IV heparin therapy is high.

[b]If patients are hospitalized, SC heparin may be administered, but hospitalization is not recommended solely for this purpose.

[c]The term refers to the condition of patients whose last episode of VTE occurred more than 3 months before evaluation but who require long-term anticoagulation because of a high risk of recurrence.

[d]IV heparin should be administered after surgery only if the risk of bleeding is low.

*Source:* Modified from Kearon C, Hirsh J. Management of anticoagulation before and after elective surgery. *N Engl J Med.* 1997;336:1510. Copyright © 1997, Massachusetts Medical Society. All rights reserved.

## SEPSIS SYNDROME

### Definition

- Clinical syndrome of systemic toxicity (sepsis) related to infection which often leads to cardiovascular collapse

### Fast Facts

- 70–80% are the result of gram-negative bacteria.
- 70,000–300,000 cases annually.
- 30–50% of episodes associated with septic shock.
- Mortality rate approaches 30%.

### Diagnosis

#### Each of the Following Four:

- Clinical evidence to support a presumptive diagnosis of gram-negative infection, and evidence of deleterious systemic effects.
- Core temperature T >38.3° C (101° F) or unexplained hypothermia <35.6° C
- Tachycardia (>90 bpm) in absence of β-blockade and tachypnea (respiratory rate >20 or requiring mechanical ventilation)
- Hypotension (systolic blood pressure ≤90 mm Hg or drop in systolic blood pressure ≥40 mm Hg) in presence of adequate volume status and no antihypertensive agents.

  *or*

#### Evidence of Systemic Toxicity or Poor End-Organ Perfusion Defined by at Least Two of the Following:

- Unexplained metabolic acidosis (pH <7.3, a base deficit of >5, or increased plasma lactate)
- Arterial hypoxia ($PO_2$ ≤75 mm Hg or $PO_2/FiO_2$ ratio <250) in patient without overt pulmonary disease
- Acute renal failure (urinary output <30 cc/hour) for 1 hour despite acute volume loading and evidence of adequate intravascular volume
- Recent (within 24 hours) unexplained coagulation abnormalities (increased prothrombin time/partial thromboplastin time) or unexplained platelet depression (<100,000 or decrease of 50% from baseline)
- Mental status changes
- Elevated cardiac index (>4 L/min/m²) with low SVR (<800 dyne-second/cm⁵)

### Management

1. History and physical exam
2. Volume replacement
3. Blood/urine/sputum cultures
4. $O_2$, labs, x-rays (chest x-ray, kidney-ureter-bladder radiography, etc.)
5. Broad spectrum antibiotics
6. Consider transfer to intensive care unit for pressor support

# GYN-ONCOLOGY
## ABDOMINAL DEHISCENCE
### Predisposing Factors
- Inadequate closure
- Previous radiation
- Infection (cellulitis must be examined)
- Poor nutrition (albumin <3.0 g/dL)

### Signs and Symptoms
- Sudden wound discomfort or none at all
- Sensation of disruption by patient
- Appearance of copious, persistent serosanguineous wound drainage
- Prolonged paralytic ileus
  *These signs represent dehiscence until proven otherwise.*

### Management
- Semi-Fowler's position
- Cover bowels/wound with sterile, wet gauze pads
- Place nasogastric tube to decompress bowel
- Initiate broad spectrum antibiotic coverage
- Plan for surgical closure if operative candidate

## HEMORRHAGE

"Hypovolemia is a problem." —Teng, 1991

### Unsatisfactory Hemostasis

#### Signs and Symptoms

- Can be revealed or concealed
- Tachycardia, ectopy, chest pain
- Cold extremities
- Confusion secondary to hypoxia
- Abdominal distention
- Hemoperitoneum

  *Early recognition is crucial.*

#### Management

- Medical stabilization
- Surgical re-exploration

### Coagulopathy

#### Signs and Symptoms

- Unexplained bleeding from wound, IV sites, etc.
- Red top tube fails to clot
- Microangiopathic changes revealed on disseminated intravascular coagulation panel

#### Management

- Correction of underlying cause
- Sepsis, fetal demise, tissue necrosis, replacement of blood products

### Blood Products

| Component | Contents | Volume | Indication |
|-----------|----------|--------|------------|
| Packed red blood cells | Red cells with most plasma removed | 1 unit = 250–300 cc<br>1 unit raises Hct by 3% | Acute or chronic blood loss |
| Platelets | Platelets only | One pack = 50 cc<br>One pack raises platelets by 6K; six-pack is from 6 donors blood | Platelets <20 K in non-bleeding patient<br>Platelets <50 K in bleeding patient |
| Fresh frozen-plasma (FFP) | Fibrinogen, Factor II, VII, IX, X, XI, XII, XIII and heat labile V and VII, | 1 unit = 150–250 cc<br>11 g albumin<br>500 mg fibrinogen<br>0.7–1.0 units clotting factor | DIC, transfusion >10 units<br>Liver disease, IgG deficiency<br>1 unit raises fibrinogen by 10 mg/dL |
| Cryoprecipitated antihemophilic factor (Cryo) | Factors VIII, XIII, von Willebrand's, fibrinogen | 1 unit = 10 cc<br>250 mg fibrinogen<br>80 units factor VIII | Hemophilia A, von Willebrand's disease, fibrinogen deficiency |

# GYN-ONCOLOGY

## ACID/BASE DISTURBANCES

### Interpretation of Arterial Blood Gases

*Rule I:* A change in $PCO_2$ down or up of 10 mm Hg is associated with an increase or decrease of pH of 0.08 units.

*Rule II:* A pH change of 0.15 is equivalent to a base change of 10 mEq/L.

*Rule III:* The dose of bicarbonate (in mEq) required to fully correct a metabolic acidosis is:

$$\frac{\text{Base deficit (mEqL)} \times \text{patient weight (kg)}}{4}$$

*Rule IV:* If the alveolar ventilation increases, $PCO_2$ will decrease, if alveolar ventilation decreases, $PCO_2$ will increase.

*Source:* Gomella LG, Braen GR, Olding MJ. Blood gases and acid base disorders. In: *Clinician's Pocket Reference: The Scut Monkey's Handbook.* 7th ed. Norwalk, Conn.: Appleton & Lange, 1993. Reproduced with the permission of the publisher.

### Differential Diagnosis

|  | pH | HCO₃ | PCO₂ |
|---|---|---|---|
| Metabolic acidosis | ↓ | ↓↓ | ↓ |
| Metabolic alkalosis | ↑ | ↑↑ | ↑ |
| Respiratory acidosis | ↓ | ↑ | ↑↑ |
| Respiratory alkalosis | ↑ | ↓ | ↓↓ |

## Metabolic Acidosis

*Anion gap*

P araldehyde
L actate
U remia
M ethanol
S alicylates
E thylene glycol
E thanol
D iabetic ketoacidosis

*Non-anion gap*

D iarrhea, dilution
U reteral conduit
R enal tubular acidosis
H yperal
A cetazolamide, acid administration
M ultiple myeloma

*As in Durham, N.C. home of the*
**Duke Blue Devils!**

## Metabolic Alkalosis

*Chloride responsive*
(Urinary Chloride <10 mEq/L)

- Gastrointestinal losses (emesis, nasogastric)
- Diuretics
- Chronic hypercapnea
- Cystic fibrosis

*Chloride resistant*
(Urinary Chloride >10 mEq/L)

- Cushing's syndrome
- Conn's syndrome
- Exogenous steroids
- Barter's syndrome

# BREAST DISEASE

## BENIGN BREAST DISORDERS
### Common Benign Breast Disorders in Women

| Symptom or Finding | Possible Causes or Disorders |
|---|---|
| Breast pain | |
|   Cyclic pain | Hormonal stimulation of normal breast lobules before menses |
|   Noncyclic pain | Stretching of Cooper's ligaments |
| | Pressure from brassiere |
| | Fat necrosis from trauma |
| | Hidradenitis suppurativa |
| | Focal mastitis |
| | Periductal mastitis |
| | Cyst |
| | Mondor's disease (sclerosing periphlebitis of breast veins) |
| Nonbreast pain | |
|   Chest-wall pain | Tietze's syndrome (costochondritis) |
| | Localized lateral chest-wall pain |
| | Diffuse lateral chest-wall pain |
| | Radicular pain from cervical arthritis |
|   Non–chest-wall pain | Gallbladder disease |
| | Ischemic heart disease |
| Nipple discharge | |
|   Presence of galactorrhea | |
|     From multiple ducts bilaterally | Hyperprolactinemia from pituitary tumor, hypothyroidism, drugs[a] |
|   Absence of galactorrhea | |
|     From one duct—elicited or spontaneous and bloody, with occult blood, or serosanguineous | Intraductal papilloma <br> Ductal carcinoma *in situ* <br> Paget's disease of breast |
|     From multiple ducts—elicited and bloody or nonbloody, bilateral, black or clear | Fibrocystic changes <br> Ductal ectasia |
| Discrete solitary lump | |
|   Age <30 yrs | |
|     Firm, rubbery lump | Most common lesion: fibroadenoma |
|   Age 30–50 yrs | |
|     Firm, discrete lump | Most common lesions: fibroadenoma, cyst, fibrocystic changes, usual ductal hyperplasia, atypical ductal hyperplasia, atypical lobular hyperplasia[b] |
|   Age >50 yrs | |
|     Firm, discrete lump | Most common lesions: cyst, ductal carcinoma *in situ*, invasive cancer |
|   Diffuse lumpiness ("lumpy-bumpy") | |
|     Absence of discrete lump | Fibrocystic changes |

[a]Data on drugs with galactorrhea as an adverse effect are listed in standard textbooks.
[b]Usual ductal hyperplasia, atypical ductal hyperplasia, and atypical lobular hyperplasia may be detected incidentally in female patients undergoing biopsy of masses with other causes, such as fibroadenomas and fibrocystic changes.

*Source:* Reproduced with permission from Santen, Richard J. Benign breast disorders. *N Engl J Med.* 2005;353(3):275–285. Copyright © 2005 Massachusetts Medical Society. All rights reserved.

## BENIGN BREAST DISEASE AND RISK OF CANCER

### Benign Breast Disease and Relative Risks for Subsequent Invasive Breast Cancer

| Classification | Relative Risks |
|---|---|
| Nonproliferative lesions | 1.0 (no increase in risk) |
|     Cyst, micro or macro | |
|     Duct ectasia | |
|     Fibroadenoma | |
|     Papillary apocrine changes | |
|     Mild sclerosing adenosis | |
|     Fibrosis | |
|     Mastitis | |
|     Metaplasia, squamous or apocrine | |
|     Mild epithelial hyperplasia | |
| Proliferative lesions | 1.5–2.0 (slight increase in risk) |
|     Moderate or florid hyperplasia | |
|     Intraductal papilloma | |
|     Florid sclerosing adenosis | |
| Proliferative lesions with atypia | 4.0–5.0 (moderate increase in risk) |
|     Atypia hyperplasia, lobular or ductal | |
| Carcinoma *in situ* | 8.0–10.0 (high risk) |
|     Ductal carcinoma *in situ* | |
|     Lobular carcinoma *in situ* | |

*Source:* Modified from Hansen N, Morrow M. Breast disease. *Med Clin N Am.* 1998;82:208.

# BREAST DISEASE

## Classification of Benign Breast Lesions on Histologic Examination, According to the Relative Risk of Breast Cancer

| Risk | Proliferation | Histologic Findings |
|------|---------------|---------------------|
| No increase | Minimal | Fibrocystic changes (within the normal range ): cysts and ductal ectasia (72%), mild hyperplasia (40%), nonsclerosing adenosis (22%), and periductal fibrosis (16%[a]); simple fibroadenoma (15–23%); and miscellaneous (lobular hyperplasia, juvenile hypertrophy, and stromal hyperplasia) |
| | | Benign tumors: hamartoma, lipoma, phyllodes tumor,[b] solitary papilloma, neurofibroma, giant adenoma, and adenomyoepithelioma |
| | | Traumatic lesions: hematoma, fat necrosis, and lesions caused by penetration by a foreign body |
| | | Infections: granuloma and mastitis |
| | | Sarcoidosis |
| | | Metaplasia: squamous and apocrine |
| | | Diabetic mastopathy |
| Small increase (relative risk, 1.5–2.0) | Proliferative without atypia | Usual ductal hyperplasia, complex fibroadenoma (containing cysts >3 mm in diameter, sclerosing adenosis, epithelial calcifications, or papillary apocrine changes), papilloma or papillomatosis, radial scar, and blunt duct adenosis |
| Moderate increase (relative risk, >2.0) | Proliferative with atypia | Atypical ductal hyperplasia and atypical lobular hyperplasia |

[a]Percentages indicate the percentage of breasts examined at autopsy in which the lesion was found.
[b]Most phyllodes tumors are considered to be benign fibroepithelial tumors, but some have malignant clinical and histologic features.
*Source:* Reproduced with permission from Santen, Richard J. Benign breast disorders. *N Engl J Med.* 2005; 353(3):275–285. Copyright © 2005 Massachusetts Medical Society. All rights reserved.

## EVALUATION OF BREAST PROBLEMS
### How to Follow Up Clinical Breast Exam Findings

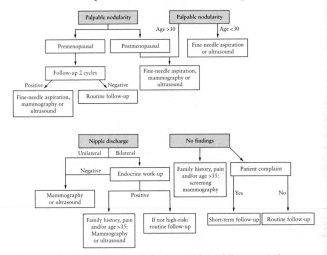

*Fibrocystic changes such as vague thickening, nodularity, fullness, cystic, lumpy, etc.
†Any persistent palpable nodularity requires tissue diagnosis.
*Source:* Reproduced with permission from Zylstra S, Greenwald L, Mondor M. Cutting the legal risk of breast cancer screening. *OBG Management.* 2005;Sept:54–59; with data from ProMutual Group. Managing risk in breast cancer. Cambridge, MA.

# BREAST DISEASE

## Algorithm for the Evaluation of Breast Discharge

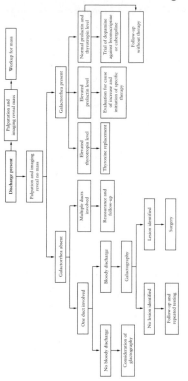

In the presence of the involvement of multiple ducts, if there is a spontaneous and persistent discharge of gross blood from a single duct, galactography should be considered.

*Source:* Reproduced with permission from Santen, Richard J. Benign breast disorders. *N Engl J Med.* 2005;353(3):275–285. Copyright © 2005 Massachusetts Medical Society. All rights reserved.

## Schematic Evaluation of Breast Masses In Premenopausal Women

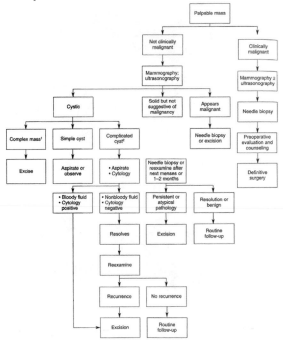

[1]Complex mass—a cystic mass with a solid component that may be malignant.
[2]Complicated cyst—usually multiple simple cysts or cysts with septations.
*Source:* Berek JS, Hacker NG, eds. *Practical Gynecologic Oncology.* 4th ed. Philadelphia: Lippincott Williams & Wilkins; 2005: pg. 640. Reproduced with the permission of the publisher.

# BREAST DISEASE

## Fine Needle Aspiration of a Breast Cyst

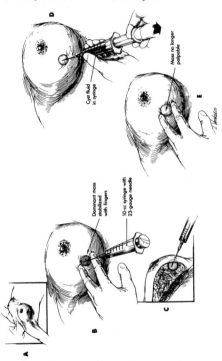

(A) The mass is palpated, and the skin is wiped with an alcohol sponge. (B, C) The needle penetrates the cyst without passing through the opposite wall. No local anesthesia is necessary. (D, E) Fluid is withdrawn until the mass disappears.

*Source:* Nichols DH. *Gynecologic and Obstetric Surgery.* Chicago: Mosby Year Book, 1993. Reproduced with the permission of the publisher.

## Fine Needle Aspiration of a Breast Lump

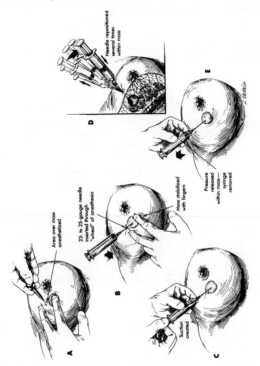

(A) After the mass is localized, local anesthesia (1% lidocaine without adrenalin) is applied. (B) The mass is stabilized, and the needle inserted. (C) Suction is created as the needle is withdrawn. (D) The needle is repositioned several times. (E) Suction is released as the needle is withdrawn.

*Source:* Nichols DH. *Gynecologic and Obstetric Surgery.* Chicago: Mosby Year Book, 1993. Reproduced with the permission of the publisher.

# BREAST DISEASE

## MASTALGIA

### Comparison of Mastalgia Therapies

| Treatment | Response Rate, % | Dose | Side Effects |
|---|---|---|---|
| Reassurance | 70–85 | | None |
| Well-fitted brassiere | 75 | | None |
| Caffeine reduction | 0; 60–65 | | Withdrawal headaches |
| Low-fat diet | 90 | <15% saturated fat | None |
| Evening primrose oil | 27–58 | 3 g/day or 1.5 g bid | Nausea, stool softening, indigestion, platelet inhibition, seizures |
| Danazol | 31–79 | Starting dose of 100 mg bid. After 2 mos wean to 100 mg daily. After 4 mos wean to 100 mg daily during the luteal phase (cycle days 14–28) | Nausea, depression, menstrual irregularity, decreased libido, weight gain, deepened voice, acne, headaches, thromboembolism, pseudotumor cerebri, hepatic adenoma |
| Bromocriptine | 20–70 | 1.25 mg/day hs, with 1.25-mg increments over 2 wks to 2.5 mg bid | Nausea, dizziness, headaches, fatigue, abdominal pain, anorexia, postural hypotension, visual disturbances, hallucination, gastrointestinal bleeding, seizures, stroke, myocardial infarction |
| Tamoxifen | 86–90 | 10 mg/day on cycle days 15–25 × 3 mos | Hot flashes, reduced bone mass, stroke, myocardial infarction, heart failure, pulmonary embolism |

bid, twice daily; hs, at bedtime.

*Source:* Reproduced with permission from Thompson KB, Keehbauch J. Evaluation and management of common breast complaints. *The Female Patient.* 2006;31:30.

# BREAST CANCER

## Fast Facts

- Leading site of cancer in women (see page 365) with a 12.6% lifetime risk.
- Leading cause of death from cancer in women 35–54 years old.
- Risk of death from breast cancer has remained constant at 3.6%.
  - More than 80% of patients live longer than 5 years.
- 80% of women with breast cancer have no known risk factor.

## Risk Factors

| Risk Factor | Relative Risk |
|---|---|
| Age (50 yrs vs. <50 yrs) | 6.5 |
| Family history of breast cancer | |
|     First-degree relative | 1.4–13.6 |
|     Second-degree relative | 1.5–1.8 |
| Age at menarche (<12 yrs vs. ≥14 yrs) | 1.2–1.5 |
| Age at menopause | |
|     (≥55 yrs vs. <55 yrs) | 1.5–2.0 |
| Age at first live birth | |
|     (<30 yrs vs. <20 yrs) | 1.3–2.2 |
| Benign breast disease | |
|     Breast biopsy (any histologic finding) | 1.5–1.8 |
|     Atypical hyperplasia | 4.0–4.4 |
| Hormone replacement therapy | 1.0–1.5 |

*Source:* Modified from Armstrong K, Eisen A, Weber B. Assessing the risk of breast cancer. *N Engl J Med.* 2000;342:566–567. Copyright © 2000 Massachusetts Medical Society. All rights reserved.

# BREAST DISEASE

## Relative Risks of Breast Cancer According to the Gail Model[a]

| Risk Factor | | Relative Risk |
|---|---|---|
| **Category A** | | |
| Age at menarche | | |
| ≥14 yrs | | 1.00 |
| 12–13 yrs | | 1.10 |
| <12 yrs | | 1.21 |
| **Category B** | | |
| No. of breast biopsies and woman's age | | |
| 0 | Any age | 1.00 |
| 1 | <50 yrs | 1.70 |
| | ≥50 yrs | 1.27 |
| ≥2 | <50 yrs | 2.88 |
| | ≥50 yrs | 1.62 |
| **Category C** | | |
| No. of first-degree relatives with breast cancer and woman's age at first live birth | | |
| 0 | <20 yrs | 1.00 |
| | 20–24 yrs | 1.24 |
| | 25–29 yrs or nulliparous | 1.55 |
| | ≥30 yrs | 1.93 |
| 1 | <20 yrs | 2.61 |
| | 20–24 yrs | 2.68 |
| | 25–29 yrs or nulliparous | 2.76 |
| | ≥30 yrs | 2.83 |
| ≥2 | <20 yrs | 6.80 |
| | 20–24 yrs | 5.78 |
| | 25–29 yrs or nulliparous | 4.91 |
| | ≥30 yrs | 4.17 |

[a]Composite risk scores for women <50 yrs and for those ≥50 yrs are derived by multiplying the appropriate relative risks from categories A, B, and C. These risk scores are then translated into 5-yr and lifetime risks by using adjusted population rates of breast cancer.

*Source:* Modified from Armstrong K, Eisen A, Weber B. Assessing the risk of breast cancer. *N Engl J Med.* 2000;342:566–567. Copyright © 2000 Massachusetts Medical Society. All rights reserved.

## Levels of Risk for Breast Cancer

**Average Risk**
- Presence of usual (i.e., not atypical) epithelial hyperplasia
- Gail model score of <1.7

**Elevated, or High, Risk**
- Cellular atypia
- 5-yr Gail risk 1.7%
- ≥2 affected second-degree premenopausal relatives
- Combined estrogen and progesterone hormone therapy for >10 yrs
- High mammographic breast density
- Family history of breast cancer plus adult-onset obesity

**Very High Risk**
- Personal history of invasive breast cancer, or ductal or lobular carcinoma *in situ*
- Breast irradiation before age 20 yrs
- BRCA1 or BRCA2 mutation
- ≥2 affected first-degree relatives with breast and/or ovarian cancer
- Atypia plus affected first-degree relative with breast and/or ovarian cancer

*Source:* Reproduced with permission from Storniolo AM. Section 3. Effective application of breast cancer risk assessment in clinical practice. *Cont OB/GYN.* 2006;July:10. *Cont OB/GYN* is a copyrighted publication of Advanstar Communications Inc. All rights reserved.

# BREAST DISEASE

## Characteristics, Advantages, and Limitations of the Gail, Claus, and BRCAPRO Risk-Assessment Tools

| Characteristics | Gail Model | Claus Model | BRCAPRO Model |
|---|---|---|---|
| Variables included | | | |
| Age | √ | √ | — |
| First-degree family history[a] | √ | √ | √ |
| Second-degree family history[b] | — | √ | √ |
| Age at onset in relatives | — | √ | — |
| Age at menarche | √ | — | — |
| Age at first live birth | √ | — | — |
| Number of breast biopsies | √ | — | — |
| Atypical hyperplasia | √ | — | — |
| Race and ethnicity[c] | — | — | √ |
| Advantages | • Accurately predicts number of expected cases of breast cancer in large clinical trials<br>• Incorporates risk factors other than family history | • Incorporates both first- and second-degree relative data, including paternal family history<br>• Incorporates age at diagnosis of affected relative | • Most comprehensive estimate of genetic mutation risk<br>• Highly sensitive |

| Characteristics | Gail Model | Claus Model | BRCAPRO Model |
|---|---|---|---|
| Disadvantages | • Not all relevant family history data are included<br>• May overestimate risk for young women<br>• Not validated for African-American, Hispanic, and other racial/ethnic groups<br>• May underestimate risk for women with BRCA mutations or with family history on paternal side<br>• Modest discriminatory accuracy in individual women | • Does not estimate risk for African-American or other nonwhite women<br>• Risk for relatives of very young patients may be underestimated<br>• Does not include all combinations of affected relatives | • Underestimates risk in women with family history unrelated to BRCA mutations<br>• Does not include factors other than family history and ethnicity<br>• Requires specific computer software and data entry that is time consuming<br>• Accuracy depends on knowing frequency of BRCA genes in population to which patient belongs |
| Definition of increased risk | Score of ≥1.7% | — | — |

[a]e.g., mother, sister(s), daughter(s).
[b]e.g., aunts, grandmothers.
[c]Including eastern European Jewish heritage.
*Source:* Reproduced with permission from Vogel VG. Section 2. Effective application of breast cancer risk assessment in clinical practice. *Cont OB/GYN.* 2006;July:7. *Cont OB/GYN* is a copyrighted publication of Advantar Communications Inc. All rights reserved.

## Biopsy Indications
• Cyst aspiration and fine needle aspiration are crucial in clinical evaluation of breast disease.
• Perform open biopsy if one of the following is present:
  ▪ Equivocal findings on aspiration
  ▪ Bloody cyst fluid
  ▪ Recurrence of cyst after 1–2 aspirations
  ▪ Bloody nipple discharge
  ▪ Nipple excoriation
  ▪ Skin edema or erythema suspicious of inflammatory breast carcinoma

# BREAST DISEASE

## Management
- Follow up, follow up, follow up.
- Mammography alone is not sufficient in palpable breast lump.
- Listen to the patient.
- See open biopsy indications.
- Choice of surgical therapy dependent on several factors.

## Prognosis
- Axillary node status is most important prognostic feature.
- Higher recurrence rates in 17β-estradiol receptor negative tumors.
- Deoxyribonucleic acid ploidy studies also predictive (aneuploid worse).

## Breast Cancer and Pregnancy
- 2% of cancers diagnosed in pregnancy.
- Pregnancy delays diagnosis, but no effect on prognosis.
- 1st trimester:
  - Mastectomy/axillary nodes.
  - Wide local excision and radiation contraindicated.
  - Pregnancy termination does not improve survival.
- 2nd trimester:
  - As above
- 3rd trimester:
  - Depends on maturity.
  - Consider observation until delivery.
- Chemotherapy probably safe in 2nd, 3rd trimester.

**Mammographic Detection of Breast Cancer**

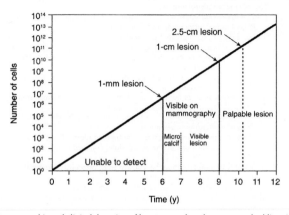

Mammographic and clinical detection of breast mass, based on average doubling time of 100 days. Micro calcif, microcalcification.
*Source:* Modified from Beckmann CRB, Ling FW, Barzansky BM, et al. *Obstetrics and Gynecology.* 2nd ed. Baltimore: Williams & Wilkins, 1995: pg. 240.

# BREAST DISEASE

## Breast Cancer Staging

TX      Primary tumor cannot be assessed

T0      No evidence of primary tumor

Tis     Carcinoma *in situ*; intraductal carcinoma, lobular carcinoma *in situ*, or
Paget's disease of the nipple with no tumor

T1      Tumor 2 cm or less in greatest dimension

             T1a    Tumor 0.5 cm but not more than 1 cm in greatest dimension

             T1b    Tumor more than 0.5 cm but not more than 1 cm in greatest
dimension

             T1c    Tumor more than 1 cm but not more than 2 cm in greatest
dimension

T2      Tumor more than 2 cm but not more than 5 cm in greatest dimension

T3      Tumor more than 5 cm in greatest dimension

T4      Tumor of any size with direct extension to chest wall or skin

             T4a    Extension to chest wall

             T4b    Edema (including peau d'orange) or ulceration of the skin of the
breast or satellite skin nodules confined to the same breast

             T4c    Both T4a and T4b

NX     Regional lymph nodes cannot be assessed (e.g., previously removed)

N0     No regional lymph node metastasis

N1     Metastasis to movable ipsilateral axillary lymph node(s)

N2     Metastasis to ipsilateral axillary lymph node(s), fixed to one another or other
structures

N3     Metastasis to ipsilateral mammary lymph node(s)

MX    Presence of distant metastasis cannot be assessed

M0    No evidence of distant metastasis

M1    Distant metastasis, including metastasis to ipsilateral supraclavicular lymph
node(s)

| Stage | Tumor Size | Lymph Node Metastasis | Distant Metastasis |
|-------|-----------|----------------------|-------------------|
| 0 | Tis | N0 | M0 |
| I | T1 | N0 | M0 |
| IIa | T0 | N1 | M0 |
| | T1 | N1 | M0 |
| | T2 | N0 | M0 |
| IIb | T2 | N1 | M0 |
| | T3 | N0 | M0 |
| IIIa | T0 | N2 | M0 |
| | T1 | N2 | M0 |
| | T2 | N2 | M0 |
| | T3 | N1, N2 | M0 |
| | T4 | Any N | M0 |
| | Any T | N3 | M0 |
| IV | Any T | Any N | M1 |

## Breast Cancer Treatment Guidelines

| Stage | Surgery | Adjuvant Treatment |
|---|---|---|
| Stage 0 | Total mastectomy vs. breast conservation therapy (includes lumpectomy and breast irradiation) | |
| Stage I | Total mastectomy vs. breast conservation therapy (includes lumpectomy and breast irradiation) ± sentinel node biopsy/axillary lymph-node dissection | Chemotherapy >1 cm ± Tamoxifen |
| Stage II | Modified radical mastectomy vs. breast conservation therapy (includes lumpectomy and breast irradiation)/axillary lymph node dissection | Chemotherapy ± Tamoxifen<br>Radiation therapy of the supraclavicular nodes ± chest wall, if mastectomy performed if ≥4 positive nodes |
| Stage III | Modified radical mastectomy vs. breast conservation therapy/axillary lymph node dissection | Chemotherapy ± neoadjuvant chemotherapy ± Tamoxifen<br>Radiation therapy of the supraclavicular nodes ± chest wall, if mastectomy performed<br>Radiation therapy of the breast (inflammatory breast cancer) |
| Stage IV | Surgery for local control | ± Chemotherapy ± Hormonal agents |

*Source:* Modified from Gemignani ML. Breast cancer. In: Barakat RR, Berers MW, Gershenson DM, Hoskins WJ, eds. *The Memorial Sloan-Kettering & MD Anderson Cancer Center Handbook of Gynecologic Oncology.* 2nd ed. London: Martin Dunitz Publishers; 2002. p. 297–319.

# BREAST DISEASE

## Breast Cancer Treatment Risks

| Complication | Risk Factors |
| --- | --- |
| Common (affecting >10% of patients) | |
| Pain or numbness in breast, chest wall, or axilla (10–25%) | Greater extent of surgery |
| Arm swelling or lymphedema (10–25%) | Greater extent of axillary surgery, obesity, weight gain, radiation therapy, infection |
| Restricted arm motion or weakness (8–10%) | Greater extent of surgery, radiation therapy, recent surgery |
| Reoperation after breast-implant reconstruction (20–34%) | Radiation therapy |
| Uncommon (affecting 1–10% of patients) | |
| Cellulitis | Radiation, seroma |
| Plexopathy or nerve damage | Higher dose of radiation or larger field |
| Contralateral breast cancer | Familial or hereditary breast cancer, younger age at diagnosis, higher dose of radiation or larger field |
| Increased risk of heart disease | Left-sided radiation with older techniques, anthracycline-based chemotherapy |
| Pneumonitis | Larger radiation field, older age, chemotherapy |
| Rib fracture | Higher dose of radiation or larger field |
| Rare (affecting <1% of patients) | |
| Second cancers other than breast cancer (angiosarcoma, sarcoma, cutaneous cancer, esophageal cancer) | Lymphedema, radiation therapy |
| Arterial insufficiency | Radiation therapy |
| Pulmonary fibrosis | Radiation therapy |

Broad estimates of incidence reflect different study methods and treatments. Patient surveys typically reveal more frequent symptoms than do chart reviews, although most cases are mild.
*Source:* Burnstein HJ, Winer EP. Primary care for survivors of breast cancer. *N Engl J Med.* 2000; 343(15):1086–1094. Copyright © 2000 Massachusetts Medical Society. All rights reserved.

### Breast Cancer Follow-Up

| Procedure | Frequency |
|---|---|
| History taking or elicitation of symptoms and examination | Every 3–6 mos for 3 yrs, then every 6–12 mos for 2 yrs, then annually |
| Breast self-examination | Monthly |
| Mammography | Annually |
| Pelvic examination | Annually |
| Routine laboratory testing (complete blood count, liver-function tests, automated blood chemical studies, measurement of tumor markers such as CEA, CA 15-3, CA 27-29) | Not recommended |
| Routine radiologic studies (bone scanning, computed tomography, ultrasonography of the liver, chest radiography, pelvic or transvaginal sonography) | Not recommended |
| Screening for other cancers (e.g., colon, ovarian) | According to recommended guidelines for the general population[a] |

[a]Women at risk for hereditary breast or ovarian cancer syndromes may merit additional surveillance for ovarian cancer, including pelvic ultrasonography and measurement of serum CA-125 levels, although the benefits of such surveillance are not known.

*Source:* Burnstein HJ, Winer EP. Primary care for survivors of breast cancer. *N Engl J Med.* 2000; 343(15):1086–1094. Copyright © 2000 Massachusetts Medical Society. All rights reserved.

# BREAST DISEASE

## Treatment of Hot Flashes in Breast Cancer Survivors

| Agent | Dose | Type of Drug and Comments |
|-------|------|---------------------------|
| Vitamin E | 800 IU daily | Marginal improvement in clinical outcome as compared with placebo. |
| Megestrol acetate | 20 mg twice daily or 500 mg IM every 2 wks | Progestin; 50–90% of patients report 50% decrease in frequency of hot flashes. Concern about the use of hormonal agent in survivors of breast cancer. |
| Fluoxetine | 20 mg twice daily or 500 mg IM every 2 wks | Selective serotonin-reuptake inhibitor; statistically significant reduction in frequency and intensity of hot flashes as compared with placebo. |
| Venlafaxine | 75 mg daily | Selective serotonin-reuptake inhibitor; statistically significant reduction in frequency and intensity of hot flashes as compared with placebo. |
| Paroxetine | 20 mg daily | Selective serotonin-reuptake inhibitor; 67% reduction in number of hot flashes, 75% reduction in intensity score. |
| Clonidine | Oral or patch, 0.1 mg daily | Antihypertensive; 10–20% reduction in symptoms as compared with placebo; substantial side effects. |
| Ergotamine and phenobarbital based preparations | Various | No benefit after 8 wks compared with placebo. |
| Raloxifene | 60 mg daily | Selective estrogen-receptor modulator; no difference in incidence of hot flashes compared with placebo. |
| Soy phytoestrogens | Daily tablets, each morning 50 mg of soy isoflavones | No improvement in hot flashes as compared with placebo. |

*Source:* Burnstein HJ, Winer EP. Primary care for survivors of breast cancer. *New Engl J Med.* 2000; 343(15):1086–1094.

## HOT FLASHES

### Incidence

- Overall incidence
  - Premenopausal: 25%
  - Late perimenopausal: 69%
  - Late postmenopausal: 39%

### Background

- Usually a sensation of heat, sweating, flushing, dizziness, palpitations, irritability, anxiety, and/or panic
- Classic hot flash (HF): head-to-toe sensation of heat, culminating in perspiration
- Large cross-cultural variability in prevalence

| %  | Culture |
|----|---------|
| 0  | Mayan women in Mexico |
| 18 | Chinese factory workers in Hong Kong |
| 70 | North American women (black women > white women) |
| 80 | Dutch women |

- Despite these vast differences, some trends are seen
  - HFs usually last 0.5–5.0 years (but may last up to 15 years); one study reported that among women who had experienced moderate to severe HFs, 58% persisted at 5 years, 12% at 8 years, and 10% at 15 years out.
  - Generally more severe in women who undergo surgical menopause; one study reported that 100% of patients undergoing surgical menopause had vasomotor symptoms, and 90% of them had continuing symptoms for 8.5 years. It is postulated that slower, continuous reductions on gonadal steroid levels result in downward regulation of hormone receptors in the hypothalamus in women undergoing natural (vs. surgical) menopause.
  - Recent finding challenges dogma that HFs cause sleep disturbances: no correlation between the HFs and sleep disturbance (Freedman and Roehrs, 2004).
  - HFs have been associated with a diminished sense of well-being (likely as a result of fatigue, irritability, poor concentration, anxiety-type symptoms).
  - Premenopausal/early perimenopausal women with symptoms may be more likely to report a ↓ sense of well-being than late perimenopausal and late postmenopausal women.
  - Some studies estimate that approximately 50% of breast cancer survivors list HF as their most prominent complaint.

# MENOPAUSE

## Etiology

- Speculative but believed to be related to estrogen withdrawal (not seen in 45,XO patients).
- Estrogen modulates the firing rate of thermosensitive neurons in the preoptic area of the hypothalamus in response to thermal stimulation in the rat.
- Responsiveness of arterioles to catecholamines is greater in women with HFs than in those without HFs. Estrogen enhances $\alpha_2$-adrenergic activity, and estrogen withdrawal may therefore lead to vasomotor flushes as a result of $\downarrow \alpha_2$-adrenergic activity.
- Women who experience HFs have a significantly smaller thermoneutral zone than women without HFs ($0.0°$ C vs. $0.4°$ C, respectively); small elevations in core body temperature have been shown to precede most HFs.
- Other causes: thyroid disease, epilepsy, infection, insulinoma, pheochromocytoma, carcinoid syndromes, leukemia, pancreatic tumors, autoimmune disorders, and mast-cell disorders.

## Evidence of the Efficacy of Nonestrogenic Prescription Drugs for the Treatment of Menopausal Hot Flashes from Randomized, Controlled Clinical Trials[a]

| Treatment | Oral Dose | Evidence of Benefit | Outcome[b] | Side Effects[c] |
|---|---|---|---|---|
| **Nonestrogen hormones** | | | | |
| Progestins | | | | |
| MPA | 20 mg daily | Yes | Improvement of 48% over placebo | Nausea, vomiting, constipation, somnolence, depression, breast tenderness, and uterine bleeding; concern about increased risks of venous thromboembolism, cardiovascular events, and breast cancer |
| Megestrol | 20 mg twice daily | Yes | Improvement of 47% over placebo in breast cancer survivors | |
| Tibolone[d] | 1.25–5.0 mg | Yes | Improvement of 35–50% over placebo | Headache, weight gain, and uterine bleeding; unknown effects on venous thromboembolic events, cardiovascular disease, and breast and uterine cancer |
| **Antidepressants** | | | | |
| SSRIs | | | | Extensive list of side effects[e] |
| Citalopram | 30 mg | No | No benefit over placebo | |
| Fluoxetine | 20 mg | Mixed | Improvement of 24% over placebo among breast cancer survivors | |
| | 30 mg | | No benefit among women without breast cancer | |

| Treatment | Oral Dose | Evidence of Benefit | Outcome[b] | Side Effects[c] |
|---|---|---|---|---|
| Paroxetine | 10–20 mg | Yes | Improvement of 30% over placebo among breast cancer survivors | |
| | 12.5–25 mg CR | | Improvement of 25% over placebo among women without breast cancer | |
| Sertraline | | No | No benefit over placebo among breast cancer survivors | |
| **SNRIs** | | | | |
| Venlafaxine | 75 or 150 mg | Mixed | Improvement of 34% over placebo among breast cancer survivors | Same side effects as for SSRIs, but minimal effect on cytochrome P-450 enzymes (only slightly inhibits conversion of tamoxifen to active metabolites); possible hypertension |
| | 75 mg ER | | No benefit over placebo among women without breast cancer | |
| **Gabapentin** | | | | |
| | 300 mg 3 times daily | Yes | Improvement of 31% over placebo among breast cancer survivors and 23% over placebo among women without breast cancer | Nausea, vomiting, somnolence, dizziness, rash, ataxia, fatigue, and leukopenia |
| **Alpha-blockers** | | | | |
| Clonidine | 0.1 mg transdermal | Mixed | Little or no benefit or improvement of 27% over placebo | Dry mouth, drowsiness, dizziness, hypotension, and rebound hypertension |
| Methyldopa | 375–1125 mg daily in divided doses | No | No benefit over placebo | |

[a]CR, controlled release; ER, extended release; MPA, medroxyprogesterone acetate; SNRI, serotonin–norepinephrine reuptake inhibitor; SSRI, selective serotonin-reuptake inhibitor.

[b]The hot-flash score was the main outcome of the majority of the clinical trials, measured as the number of hot flashes per day weighted by severity, reported as mild (1), moderate (2), or severe (3).

[c]Side effects were reported in clinical trials of the therapy or on the Epocrates Rx Web site.

[d]This drug is currently not available in the United States.

[e]Side effects of SSRIs include nausea, vomiting, diarrhea, insomnia, somnolence, anxiety, decreased libido, dry mouth, worsening depression, mania, suicidality, the serotonin syndrome, and the withdrawal syndrome. Paroxetine, and possibly other SSRIs, decrease the activity of cytochrome P-450 enzymes, thereby decreasing the production of active metabolites of tamoxifen, which may interfere with the anti–breast cancer effects of tamoxifen.

*Source:* Reproduced with permission from Grady D. Management of menopausal symptoms. *N Engl J Med.* 2006;355(22):2338–2347. Copyright © 2006 Massachusetts Medical Society. All rights reserved.

# MENOPAUSE

**Selected Estrogen and Progestin Preparations for the Treatment of Menopausal Vasomotor Symptoms[a]**
**(See also pages 473 and 474)**

| Preparation | Generic Name | Brand Name | Doses (mg/day) |
|---|---|---|---|
| **Estrogen[b]** | | | |
| Oral | Conjugated estrogens | Premarin | 0.3, 0.45, 0.625, 0.9, 1.25 |
| | 17β-Estradiol | Estrace | 0.5, 1.0, 2.0 |
| Transdermal | 17β-Estradiol | Alora | 0.025, 0.05, 0.075, 0.1 (patch applied twice weekly) |
| | | Climara | 0.025, 0.0375, 0.05, 0.075, 0.1 (patch applied weekly) |
| Vaginal | Estradiol acetate | Femring vaginal ring[c] | 0.05, 0.1 (inserted every 90 days) |
| **Progestogen** | | | |
| Oral | MPA | Provera | 2.5, 5.0, 10.0 |
| | Micronized progesterone | Prometrium | 100, 200 (in peanut oil) |
| Vaginal | Progesterone | Prochieve 4% | 45 |
| **Combination preparation** | | | |
| Oral sequential[d] | Conjugated estrogens and MPA | Premphase | 0.625 conjugated estrogens plus 5.0 MPA |
| Oral continuous[e] | Conjugated estrogens and MPA | Prempro | 0.625 conjugated estrogens plus 2.5 or 5.0 MPA; 0.45 conjugated estrogens plus 2.5 MPA; or 0.3 or 0.45 conjugated estrogens plus 1.5 MPA |
| Transdermal continuous[e] | 17β-Estradiol–norethindrone acetate | Activella | 1.0 estradiol plus 0.5 norethindrone |
| | 17β-Estradiol–levonorgestrel | Climara Pro | 0.045 estradiol plus 0.015 levonorgestrel (patch applied weekly) |
| | 17β-Estradiol–norethindrone acetate | CombiPatch | 0.05 estradiol plus 0.14 or 0.25 norethindrone (patch applied twice weekly) |

[a]MPA denotes medroxyprogesterone acetate.
[b]Estrogen should be avoided in women who have a history of or are at high risk for cardiovascular disease, breast cancer, uterine cancer, or venous thromboembolic events and in those with active liver disease. Hormone therapy can cause uterine bleeding, breast tenderness, and headache. Doses of estrogen that are approximately biologically equivalent include the following: 0.625 mg of Premarin, 1.0 mg of Estrace, and 0.05 mg of Alora, Climera, or Femring.
[c]Unlike other vaginal preparations listed in the previous table, Femring delivers a higher systemic level of estrogen and should be opposed by a progestin in women with a uterus.
[d]The first 14 pills contain estrogen and the subsequent pills (15–28) contain progestin with estrogen.
[e]Each pill or patch contains estrogen and progestin.
*Source:* Reproduced with permission from Grady D. Management of menopausal symptoms. *N Engl J Med.* 2006;355(22):2338–2347. Copyright © 2006 Massachusetts Medical Society. All rights reserved.

## Selected Estrogen Vaginal Preparations for the Treatment of Menopausal Vaginal Symptoms[a]

| Preparation | Generic Name | Brand Name | Dose |
|---|---|---|---|
| Vaginal cream | Conjugated estrogens | Premarin | 0.625 mg per 2 g cream: 2 g daily for 2 wks, then 1–2 g 2 to 3 times per wk |
| | 17β-Estradiol | Estrace | 0.1 mg per 2 g cream: 2 g daily for 2 wks, then 1–2 g 2 to 3 times per wk |
| Vaginal tablet | Estradiol hemihydrate | Vagifem | 0.025 mg per tablet: 1 tablet per day for 2 wks, then 1 tablet twice per wk |
| Vaginal ring | 17β-Estradiol | Estring | 0.0075 mg per day (inserted every 90 days) |

[a]Most products listed in the table for the treatment of menopausal hot flashes are also approved for the treatment of vaginal dryness. A vaginal moisturizer, Replens, has been found to be as effective for the treatment of vaginal symptoms as estrogen vaginal cream. Other vaginal moisturizers (such as Yes, K-Y Silk-E, and Astroglide Silken Secret) may also be effective but have not been studied in randomized trials.

*Source:* Reproduced with permission from Grady D. Management of menopausal symptoms. *N Engl J Med.* 2006;355(22):2338–2347. Copyright © 2006 Massachusetts Medical Society. All rights reserved.

# MENOPAUSE

## Hormone Therapy Decision-Making Flowchart

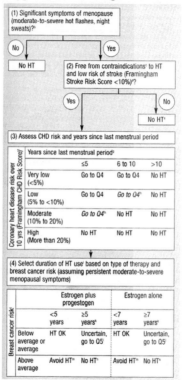

(1) Significant symptoms of menopause (moderate-to-severe hot flashes, night sweats)?ᵇ

No → No HT

Yes →

(2) Free from contraindicationsᶜ to HT and low risk of stroke (Framingham Stroke Risk Score <10%)ᵈ?

Yes →

No → No HTᵉ

(3) Assess CHD risk and years since last menstrual period

| Coronary heart disease risk over 10 yrs (Framingham CHD Risk Score)ᶠ | Years since last menstrual periodᵍ | | |
|---|---|---|---|
| | ≤5 | 6 to 10 | >10 |
| Very low (<5%) | Go to Q4 | Go to Q4 | No HT |
| Low (5% to <10%) | Go to Q4 | *Go to Q4*ʰ | No HT |
| Moderate (10% to 20%) | *Go to Q4*ʰ | No HT | No HT |
| High (More than 20%) | No HT | No HT | No HT |

(4) Select duration of HT useⁱ based on type of therapy and breast cancer risk (assuming persistent moderate-to-severe menopausal symptoms)

| Breast cancer riskᵏ | Estrogen plus progestogen | | Estrogen alone | |
|---|---|---|---|---|
| | <5 years | ≥5 yearsˡ | <7 years | ≥7 yearsˡ |
| Below average or average | HT OK | Uncertain, go to Q5ⁱ | HT OK | Uncertain, go to Q5ⁱ |
| Above average | Avoid HTᵐ | No HTⁿ | Avoid HTᵐ | No HTⁿ |

This treatment algorithm is provided only as a guideline for the appropriate use of hormonal therapies in postmenopausal women. The ultimate treatment decisions must be made between a patient and her healthcare professional. As health is unpredictable, the decision whether to start or stay on hormone therapy should be revisited on a regular basis.

aReassess each step at least once every 6–12 months (assuming patient's continued preference for hormone therapy).

bWomen who have vaginal dryness without moderate-to-severe vasomotor symptoms may be candidates for vaginal estrogen.

cTraditional contraindications: unexplained vaginal bleeding; active liver disease; history of venous thromboembolism due to pregnancy, oral contraceptive use, or unknown etiology; blood clotting disorder; history of breast or endometrial cancer; history of coronary heart disease, stroke, transient ischemic attack, or diabetes. For other contraindications, including high triglycerides (>400 mg/dL), active gallbladder disease, and history of venous thromboembolism due to past immobility, surgery, or bone fracture, oral hormone therapy should be avoided, but transdermal hormone therapy may be an option (see f below).

d10-year risk of stroke based on Framingham Stroke Risk Score (D'Agostino RB et al. *Stroke*. 1994;25:40–43).

eConsider selective serotonin reuptake inhibitor, gabapentin, clonidine, soy, or alternative.

f10-year risk of coronary heart disease, based on Framingham Coronary Heart Disease Risk Score (Available at www.nhlbi.nih.gov/about/framingham/riskabs.htm)

gWomen more than 10 years past menopause are not good candidates for starting (first use of) hormone therapy.

hAvoid oral hormone therapy. Transdermal hormone therapy may be an option because it has a less adverse effect on clotting factors, triglyceride levels, and inflammation factors than oral hormone therapy.

iHormone therapy should be continued only if moderate-to-severe menopausal symptoms persist. The recommended cut points for duration are based on results of the Women's Health Initiative estrogen-progestin and estrogen-alone trials, which lasted 5.6 and 7.1 years, respectively. For longer durations of hormone therapy use, the balance of benefits and risks is not known.

jAbove-average risk of breast cancer; one or more first-degree relatives with breast cancer; susceptibility genes such as *BRCA1* or *BRCA2*, or a personal history of breast biopsy demonstrating atypia.

kWomen with premature surgical menopause may take hormone therapy until average age at menopause (age 51 in the United States) and then follow flowchart for subsequent decision-making.

lTry to reduce hormone therapy doses. If progestin is taken daily, avoid extending duration. If progestogen is clinical or infrequent, avoid extending duration more than 1–2 years. For estrogen alone, avoid extending duration more than 2–3 years.

mIf menopausal symptoms are severe, estrogen plus progestin can be taken for 2–3 years maximum and estrogen alone for 4–5 years maximum.

nIf at high risk of osteoporotic fracture, consider bisphosphonate, raloxifene, or alternative.

oIncreased risk of osteoporosis; documented osteopenia, personal or family history of nontraumatic fracture, current smoking, or weight less than 125 lbs.

*Source:* Reproduced with permission from Simon JA, Archer DF, Manson JE et al. *Women, Hormones, and Therapy: New Observations from the Women's Health Initiative and the Nurses' Health Study.* Trevose, PA: Medical Education Group, 2007: pg.15.

# MENOPAUSE

## OSTEOPOROSIS

### Definition

- Low bone mass and microarchitectural deterioration with consequent ↑ bone fragility and susceptibility to fracture.
- Osteoporosis (OP) most frequently found in postmenopausal white women, although it can occur in any age group.
- Approximately 10–15% of women who take estrogen lose bone.
- Diagnosis: bone densitometry.

### Prevalence and Incidence

- 13–18% in women >50 years of age (Looker et al., 1997)
- >1.3 million osteoporotic fractures/year in the United States

Legend:
- Hip (n > 300 000)
- Other (n > 300 000)
- Wrist (n = 200 000)
- Vertebral (n = 700 000)

Annual incidence of osteoporotic fractures in the United States. Reproduced with permission from Ettinger MP. Aging bone and osteoporosis: strategies for preventing fractures in the elderly. *Arch Intern Med.* 2003;163(18):2237.

- 8 million women: OP (United States).
- 20 million women: osteopenia (United States).
- 250,000 hip fractures.
- Postmenopausal women lose approximately 3% cortical and 8% trabecular bone/year.

Proportion of population (%)

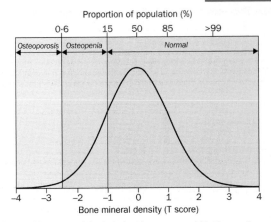

Distribution of bone mineral density in healthy women aged 30–40 years. Reproduced with permission from Kanis JA. Diagnosis of osteoporosis and assessment of fracture risk. *Lancet.* 2002;359(9321):1929.

## Screening

- Controversial but justified for the following reasons:
  - Common disease.
  - Associated with high morbidity, mortality, and cost.
  - Estimated cost of osteoporotic fracture in the United States for 1995 was $13.8 billion (Ray et al., 1997).
  - Accurate and safe diagnostic tests are available.
  - Effective treatments are available.
- Follicle stimulating hormone (FSH) stimulates the formation and function of osteoclasts in vitro and in vivo. High circulating FSH may cause hypogonadal bone loss (Sun, 2006).

# MENOPAUSE

## Factors That Increase the Likelihood of Developing Osteoporosis

- Current low bone mass
- Personal history of fracture after age 50
- History of fracture in a primary relative
- Being female
- Being thin and/or having a small frame
- Advanced age
- A family history of osteoporosis
- Estrogen deficiency as a result of menopause
- Especially early or surgically induced
- Abnormal absence of menstrual periods (amenorrhea)
- Anorexia nervosa
- Low lifetime calcium intake
- Vitamin D deficiency
- Use of certain medications, such as corticosteroids and anticonvulsants
- Presence of certain chronic medical conditions
- Low testosterone levels in men
- An inactive lifestyle
- Current cigarette smoking
- Excessive use of alcohol
- Being Caucasian or Asian

## Diagnosis

- Silent disease until complicated by stress fracture.
- Clinically, vertebral fracture can be suspected in patients with back pain, vertebral deformities by physical examination (kyphosis), or loss of height.
- After a hip fracture, nearly 1 in 6 patients aged 50–55 years and more than $1/2$ of those older than 90 years are discharged from the hospital to a nursing home (Walker-Bone et al., 2001).
- Standard x-rays do not detect OP until approximately 40% of bone mass is lost.
- Gold standard of bone mineral density (BMD): dual energy x-ray absorptiometry (DXA) of the spine and hip:
  - Assesses cortical and cancellous bone; BMD ↑ 3–6% in the 1st year of bisphosphonate therapy.
  - DXA can be used to monitor response to treatment.
  - DXA T score: number of standard deviations (SDs) above or below the average BMD for a healthy 30-year-old woman.
  - DXA Z score: number of SDs above or below the average BMD for age- and sex-method controls; a Z score below −1 indicates a value in the lowest 25% of the reference range (risk of fractures doubled).
- Note: Z scores rather than T scores should be used for healthy premenopausal women.
- Biochemical markers:
  - Assess cancellous bone only.
  - Provide monitoring information; subject to diurnal variation.
  - Change in markers seen as early as 1–3 months into therapy.
  - Some clinicians recommend checking markers at 3 months.

## Types of Bone Mineral Density Tests

| Test | Purpose |
|------|---------|
| DXA (Dual Energy X-ray Absorptiometry) | Measures spine, hip, or total body |
| pDXA (Peripheral Dual Energy X-ray Absorptiometry) | Measures wrist, heel, or finger |
| SXA (Single Energy X-ray Absorptiometry) | Measures wrist or heel |
| QUS (Quantitative Ultrasound) | Uses sound waves to measure density at heel, lower leg, or patella |
| QCT (Quantitative Computed Tomography) | Measures spine |
| PQCT (Peripheral Quantitative Computed Tomography) | Measures wrist |
| RA (Radiographic Absorptiometry) | X-ray of hand; bone mineral density compared to metal wedge |
| DPA (Dual Photon Absorptiometry) | Measures spine, hip, or total body |
| SPA (Single Photon Absorptiometry) | Measures wrist |

*Source:* Reproduced with permission from Stanford E. Prevention and management of osteoporosis and osteoporosis-related fractures. *OB/GYN Special Edition.* 2006:31.

## Bone Densiometry Testing Guidelines

| Organization | Criteria |
|--------------|----------|
| National Osteoporosis Foundation | • All women 65 and older regardless of risk factors <br> • Younger postmenopausal women with 1 or more risk factors other than being white, female, or postmenopausal <br> • Postmenopausal women who present with fractures to confirm diagnosis and determine disease severity |
| U.S. Preventive Services Task Force | • All women 65 yrs of age and older <br> • All women 60 or older who are at increased risk for osteoporotic fractures <br> • The Task Force makes no recommendation for or against routine osteoporosis screening in postmenopausal women younger than 60 yrs or women 60–64 yrs of age who are not at increased risk for osteoporotic fractures |
| International Society for Clinical Densitometry | • Women 65 yrs of age and older <br> • Postmenopausal women younger than 65 with risk factors <br> • Men aged 70 and older <br> • Adults with a fragility fracture <br> • Adults with a disease or condition associated with low bone mass or bone loss <br> • Adults taking medications associated with low bone mass or bone loss <br> • Anyone being considered for bone-conserving pharmacologic therapy <br> • Anyone being treated for bone conservation, to monitor treatment effect <br> • Anyone not receiving bone-conserving therapy in whom evidence of bone loss would lead to treatment |

*Note:* Per guidelines of the International Society for Clinical Densitometry, women discontinuing estrogen should be considered for bone density testing according to the indications listed above.
*Source:* Reproduced with permission from Goldstein SR. Osteopenia: when to intervene? *OBG Management.* 2006;Jan:45–55.

# MENOPAUSE

## Selection Criteria Suggested from the National Osteoporosis Foundation Practice Guidelines and Four Clinical Decision Rules for Bone Mineral Density Testing among Postmenopausal Women Considering Treatment[a]

| Guideline/Rule | Selection Cut Point | Scoring System |
|---|---|---|
| National Osteoporosis Foundation (NOF) | Score ≥1 | One point each for[b]<br>Age ≥65 yrs<br>Weight <57.6 kg<br>Personal history of fracture: minimal trauma fracture >40 yrs<br>Family history of fracture[c]<br>Current cigarette smoking |
| Simple Calculated Osteoporosis Risk Estimation (SCORE) | Score ≥6 | Points are given for<br>Race: 5 if not black<br>Rheumatoid arthritis: 4 if applicable<br>History of minimal trauma fracture after age 45 yrs<br>    4 for each fracture of the wrist,[d] hip, or rib, to a maximum of 12<br>Age: 3 times the first digit of age in yrs<br>Estrogen therapy: 1 if never used<br>Weight: −1 times weight in lbs divided by 10 and truncated to integer |
| Osteoporosis Risk Assessment Instrument (ORAI) | Score ≥9 | Points are given for<br>Age: 15 if 75 yrs or older, 9 if 65–74 yrs, 5 if 55–64 yrs<br>Weight: 9 if <60 kg, 3 if 60.0–69.9 kg<br>Estrogen use: 2 if not currently taking estrogen |
| Age, Body Size, No Estrogen (ABONE) | Score ≥2 | Points are given for:<br>Age: 1 if >65 yrs<br>Weight: 1 if <63.5 kg<br>Estrogen use: 1 if never used oral contraceptives or estrogen therapy for at least 6 mos |
| Body weight criterion | | Weight <70 kg |

[a]ORAI is also applicable for use in premenopausal women aged 45 years or older.

[b]For the purpose of the area under receiver operating characteristic (AUROC) curve analysis, each factor was given 1 point. All those with at least 1 "NOF point" were identified for testing.

[c]NOF guidelines stipulate maternal/paternal theory of hip, wrist, or spine fracture when the parent was 50 years or older. These specific data were not collected in CaMos.

[d]Forearm/wrist were included as a history of wrist fracture.

*Source:* Reproduced with permission from Ravnikar V. Identifying women at risk for osteoporosis. Supplement to *Cont OB/GYN.* 2004:11. *Cont OB/GYN* is a copyrighted publication of Advanstar Communications Inc. All rights reserved.

460

## Recommended Regimens for the Prevention and Treatment of Postmenopausal Osteoporosis[a]

| Organization | Whom to Treat | Nonpharmacologic Intervention | Pharmacologic Intervention |
|---|---|---|---|
| National Osteoporosis Foundation | T score below −2.0 with no risk factors | 1200 mg calcium daily | Antiresorptive agents or anabolic agents |
| | T score below −1.5 with one or more risk factors | 400–800 IU vitamin D daily | |
| | Any spine or hip fracture | Regular weight-bearing exercise | |
| American Association of Clinical Endocrinology | T score below −2.5 | 1200 mg calcium daily | Antiresorptive or anabolic agents |
| | T score below −1.5 with fractures | 400–800 IU vitamin D daily | |
| | | Weight-bearing physical activity | |
| U.S. Surgeon General's Pyramid Approach[b] | No recommendations | 1200 mg calcium daily | Antiresorptive agents or anabolic agents |
| | | 600–800 IU vitamin D daily | |
| | | Regular weight-bearing activity (30 mins daily) | |
| | | Strength and balance training | |

[a]Data in this table are from the National Osteoporosis Foundation. Physician's guide to prevention and treatment of osteoporosis. 1999, updated January 2003; Hodgson SF, et al. American association of clinical endocrinologist medical guidelines for the prevention and treatment of postmenopausal osteoporosis: 2001 edition, with selected updates for 2003. *Endocr Pract.* 2003;9:544–564, and the Office of the Surgeon General. Bone health and osteoporosis: a report of the Surgeon General. Rockville, MD: Department of Health and Human Services, 2004:436. T scores are the number of standard deviations the bone mineral density measurement is above or below the young-normal mean bone mineral density.

[b]The pyramid approach consists, in ascending order, of lifestyle changes, the identification of a secondary cause of osteoporosis, and pharmacotherapy.

*Source:* Reproduced with permission from Rosen CJ. Postmenopausal osteoporosis. *N Engl J Med.* 2005;353(6):595–603. Copyright © 2005 Massachusetts Medical Society. All rights reserved.

# MENOPAUSE

## Current FDA-Approved Treatment Options for the Prevention and Treatment of Osteoporosis

| Drug | Year Approved | Prevention of Postmeno-pausal Osteoporosis | Treatment of Postmeno-pausal Osteoporosis | Reduction of Hip Fracture | Reduction of Non-vertebral Fractures | Reduction of Vertebral Fractures |
|---|---|---|---|---|---|---|
| Prempro™ (conjugated estrogens) | 1995 | √a | | | | |
| Fosamax® (alen-dronate) | 1997 | √ | √ | √ | | √ |
| Actonel® (risedronate) | 1998 | √ | √ | | √ | √ |
| Evista® (ralox-ifene) | 1998 | √ | √ | | | √ |
| Forteo® (teri-paratide) | 2001 | | √b | | √ | √ |
| Miacalcin® (calcitonin) | 2002 | | √c | | | |
| Boniva® (iban-dronate) | 2003 | √ | √ | | | √ |
| Fosamax Plus D™ (alen-dronate + vitamin D) | 2005 | | √ | √ | | √ |

aConsider alternatives if used solely for osteoporosis prevention.
bFor use in patients at high risk for fracture.
cFor use >5 yrs after menopause if hormone therapy is not tolerated.
*Source*: Derman RG, Kagan R, Simon JA. Practical steps to improve patient outcomes in the management of osteoporosis. Sponsored by the Postgraduate Institute for Medicine. August, 2005.

**Calcium and Vitamin D Supplementation for Postmenopausal Women**[a]

| Supplement | Preparation | Recommended Daily Total | Frequency of Doses | Comment |
|---|---|---|---|---|
| Calcium | | 1200–1500 mg | Two or three times daily | Side effects: nausea, constipation |
| Calcium carbonate | | 200–600 mg | Two or three times daily | Food enhances absorption |
| | Caltrate | 600 mg | Twice daily | With or without vitamin D, at a dose of 200 IU; food enhances absorption[b] |
| | OsCal | 250–600 mg | Two or four times daily | Fasting enhances absorption; with or without vitamin D |
| | Tums | 200–500 mg | Two or three times daily | Available as chewable antacid tablets and pills |
| | Viactiv | 500 mg | Twice daily | Available as flavored "chews"; with vitamin D[b] |
| Calcium lactate | | 42–84 mg | Five or six times daily | Requires taking many tablets very often |
| Calcium citrate | Citracal | 200–500 mg | Two or four times daily | With or without vitamin D, at a dose of 200 IU; food enhances absorption[b] |
| Calcium phosphate | Posture | 600 mg | Twice daily | Posture is the only calcium phosphate preparation available |
| Vitamin D | | 600–800 IU (15–20 mcg) daily | Daily | Taken any time of the day |
| | Multivitamin | 400 IU per pill | Daily or twice daily | Good absorption; may contain vitamin D2 or D3 |
| | Vitamin D | 400 IU per pill | Daily or twice daily | Good absorption |

*(continued)*

## Calcium and Vitamin D Supplementation for Postmenopausal Women[a] *(continued)*

| Supplement | Preparation | Recommended Daily Total | Frequency of Doses | Comment |
|---|---|---|---|---|
| | Calcium with vitamin D[b] | 125–400 IU per pill | Daily or twice daily | The dose of vitamin D varies in different supplements |
| | Ergocalciferol (vitamin D2) | 50,000 IU per capsule | Once weekly | For vitamin D deficiency, vitamin D3 is preferred |
| | Cholecalciferol (vitamin D3)[c] | 50,000 IU per capsule | Once weekly | For vitamin D deficiency |

[a]Adequate intake of vitamin D for older postmenopausal women, as established by the Institute of Medicine in 1997, is 600 IU daily; persons living in northern latitudes often have lower serum vitamin D levels and are thought to require 800 IU daily. The recommended daily totals are for elemental calcium and elemental vitamin D.

[b]Often calcium supplements contain vitamin D, but the dose and type of vitamin D vary (e.g., 125 IU to 400 IU per tablet). Similarly, vitamin D supplements often include calcium at various doses (e.g., 125 mg to 500 mg per tablet). Supplements need to be examined carefully by both the patient and the provider, so that proper doses are administered.

[c]Vitamin D3 is preferred for replacement in persons with vitamin D deficiency, because it can be measured more accurately than D2 and is absorbed better. However, high doses (e.g., 50,000 IU) can be difficult to obtain. Vitamin D2 is derived from plant sources. It can be obtained from most formularies and pharmacies. Regardless of the type of vitamin D, treatment with high doses should not continue beyond three months and should be followed by a repeated measurement of the serum 25 (OH) vitamin D level. If supplementation is successful in raising the serum level, a dose of 800 IU per day is used for maintenance. If supplementation is unsuccessful and the assay is valid, then consideration should be given to malabsorption, particularly gluten enteropathy.

*Source:* Reproduced with permission from Rosen CJ. Postmenopausal osteoporosis. *N Engl J Med.* 2005;353(6):595–603. Copyright © 2005 Massachusetts Medical Society. All rights reserved.

## Medications Approved by the Food and Drug Administration for the Treatment or Prevention of Postmenopausal Osteoporosis[a]

| Drug | Method of Administration and Dose | Reduction in Risk of Fracture | Side Effect | FDA Approval |
|---|---|---|---|---|
| Bisphosphonates | Oral | | Esophagitis, myalgias | For treatment and prevention[b] |
| Alendronate | 35–70 mg weekly, 5–10 mg daily | Vertebral, nonvertebral, and hip fracture | | |
| Risedronate | 30–35 mg weekly, 5 mg daily | Vertebral, nonvertebral, and hip fracture | | |
| Ibandronate | 150 mg monthly, 2.5 mg daily | Vertebral fracture | First dose[c] | |
| SERM | Oral | | | For treatment and prevention |
| Raloxifene | 60 mg daily | Vertebral fracture only | Hot flashes, nausea, DVT, leg cramps | |
| Anabolic agents | Subcutaneous, daily | | | |
| PTH (1–34) (teriparatide) | 20 mcg | Vertebral and nonvertebral fracture | Hypercalcemia, nausea, leg cramps | Approved for treatment only; generally used for severe osteoporosis |
| Calcitonin[d] | Subcutaneous or nasal, 100–200 IU | Vertebral fracture only | Nasal stuffiness, nausea | Approved for treatment only |
| Estrogens | Oral or transdermal | | Risk of DVT, risk of cardiovascular disease, breast cancer | Approved for prevention only |

*(continued)*

# MENOPAUSE

## Medications Approved by the Food and Drug Administration for the Treatment or Prevention of Postmenopausal Osteoporosis[a] (continued)

| Conjugated equine estrogens | Oral, 0.30–1.25 mg daily | Vertebral, non-vertebral, and hip fracture (at dose of 0.625 mg daily) | |
|---|---|---|---|
| 17β-Estradiol[e] | Oral, 0.025–0.10 mg, or transdermal twice weekly | No data from randomized, controlled trials | |
| | Ultra-low-dose (0.014 mg/day, given weekly) | No data available | For prevention only |

[a]All agents approved for treatment have demonstrated efficacy in reducing fractures, as determined in randomized, placebo-controlled trials with fracture as the primary end point. DVT denotes deep-vein thrombosis, SERM selective estrogen-receptor modulator, and PTH parathyroid hormone.

[b]There has been limited post-marketing experience with ibandronate for prevention.

[c]There may be a response to the first dose at 150 mg consisting of myalgias, joint aches, and low-grade fever, which is similar to a response to the first intravenous administration of bisphosphonates containing nitrogen.

[d]The use of calcitonin is not generally recommended.

[e]A reduction in the risk of hip fracture has not been established for 17β-estradiol in a randomized, controlled trial.

Source: Reproduced with permission from Rosen CJ. Postmenopausal osteoporosis. N Engl J Med. 2005;353(6):595–603. Copyright © 2005 Massachusetts Medical Society. All rights reserved.

## HORMONE REPLACEMENT THERAPY (1950s–1990s) → HORMONE THERAPY (2002 TO PRESENT)

- Although the Women's Health Initiative (WHI) estradiol ($E_2$)/progestin and estrogen-only studies (see Hormone Therapy Risks and Benefits section) are not perfect, the indications and duration of hormone therapy (HT) have been revised. Many areas are still controversial; the following are general recommendations:
  - Risks and benefits of these interventions for perimenopausal and naturally and surgically postmenopausal women are now more clearly defined.
  - Unopposed estrogen therapy does not ↑ breast cancer incidence (see WHI data below); the role of progestins in combined $E_2$/progestin HT is still controversial.
  - Data on prevention and treatment of osteoporosis with fracture outcomes (not just BMD) are more complete for estrogen therapy than for any other treatment option.
  - Role of HT in primary prevention of coronary heart disease (CHD) is controversial; current data suggest that neither primary nor secondary prevention of CHD is a valid indication for starting or continuing therapy.
  - Major indications for HT with estrogen ± progestin are relief of menopausal symptoms and prevention/treatment of osteoporosis.
  - For symptom relief, use the lowest effective dose for the shortest time.
  - Surgical menopause (MP) (bilateral salpingo-oophorectomy ± hysterectomy) and prevention/treatment of osteoporosis may be indications for longer-term treatment (>2–3 years). Use the lowest effective dose; review treatment every few years; and discuss risks, benefits, and alternative treatment options with the patient.
  - Women currently on long-term HT who are doing well should not automatically stop treatment but should be reevaluated and individually counseled. Stopping HT causes rapid loss of hip fracture protection (within 5 years) (Yates et al., 2004), so women who choose to stop HT need alternative therapy (selective estrogen receptor modulators, bisphosphonates) and/or BMD follow-up.

### Hormone Therapy in the Perimenopause

- Standard HT is not an adequate contraceptive.
  - Can use low-dose oral contraceptives (20 mcg ethinyl $E_2$) as HT for nonsmokers
  - Change to standard HT (oral, transdermal, and so forth) with lower estrogen doses 1–2 years after expected time of MP (mean, 51 years old).

# MENOPAUSE

## Classic Approach to Hormone Therapy (Based on Observational Studies Only)

1. Estrogen is good for you.
2. Start taking it now.
3. Take it for the rest of your life.

## Post–Women's Health Initiative Approach

- Individualize estimates of the benefit to risk ratio for HT.
  - Alleviating menopausal symptoms (no other treatment is as effective, but symptoms were not included in WHI main outcome measures).
  - Bone preserving (annual loss in bone mass after MP: 3–5%).
  - Risk of breast cancer: No ↑ risk found with $E_2$ alone in WHI study; questionable progestin (Provera) effect.
  - Cardioprotective: Observational data (e.g., Nurses' Health Study [NHS]) may well have overstated CHD reduction, *but* younger, healthier patients starting HT closer to MP may still reap benefit vs. older population, smokers, obese patients, and those farther from MP in WHI studies.
  - Memory preservation: weak data; ↓ **cognitive function in WHI studies.**

## Large Observational Studies

### Nurses' Health Study

- NHS: 48,470 postmenopausal women, 10-year prospective cohort study:

| Nurses' Health Study: $E_2$ Users vs. Nonusers | Relative Risk |
|---|---|
| ↑ Breast cancer in current hormone therapy users | 1.33 (1.12–1.57) |
| No significant effect on stroke | 0.97 (0.65–1.45) |
| ↓ Rate of CHD events in current $E_2$ users | 0.56 (0.40–0.80)[a] |
| ↓ CHD events in low-CHD-risk women[b] | 0.53 (0.31–0.91)[a] |
| ↓ CHD mortality in current/past $E_2$ users | 0.72 (0.55–0.95)[a] |

CHD, coronary heart disease; $E_2$, estradiol.
[a]Not supported by large randomized controlled trials (Women's Health Initiative).
[b]Low CHD risk: excludes smoking, diabetes mellitus, hypertension, ↑ cholesterol, or body mass index >90th percentile.
*Source:* Adapted from Stampfer MJ, Colditz GA, Willett WC, et al. Postmenopausal estrogen therapy and cardiovascular disease. Ten-year follow-up from the nurses' health study. *N Engl J Med.* 1991;325(11):756; and Colditz GA, Stampfer MJ, Willett WC et al. Type of postmenopausal hormone use and risk of breast cancer: 12-year follow-up from the Nurses' Health Study. *Cancer Causes Control.* 1992;3(5):433.

- NHS CHD data were based on 10 years follow-up (337,854 woman-years) and provided a rationale for the widespread use of HT for **primary prevention of CHD** in postmenopausal women.

- The finding of ↑ breast cancer risk in HT users was based on 12 years follow-up (480,665 woman-years) and was assessed for subgroups as follows:

| Nurses' Health Study: Breast Cancer Risks | Relative Risk |
|---|---|
| ↑ Breast cancer in unopposed $E_2$ users | 1.42 (1.19–1.70)[a] |
| Breast cancer in $E_2$ + progestin users | 1.54 (0.99–2.39) |
| Breast cancer in progestin-only users | 2.52 (0.66–9.63) |

$E_2$, estradiol.

[a]Not supported by large randomized controlled trials (Women's Health Initiative).

*Source:* Adapted from Stampfer MJ, Colditz GA, Willett WC, et al. Postmenopausal estrogen therapy and cardiovascular disease. Ten-year follow-up from the Nurses' Health Study. *N Engl J Med.* 1991;325(11):756; and Colditz GA, Stampfer MJ, Willett WC et al. Type of postmenopausal hormone use and risk of breast cancer: 12-year follow-up from the Nurses' Health Study. *Cancer Causes Control.* 1992;3(5):433.

- Neither the strong benefit for primary prevention of CHD nor the ↑ breast cancer risk with unopposed $E_2$ has been supported by later randomized controlled trials (Heart and Estrogen/Progestin Replacement Study [HERS] and the two WHI studies, see below).

## Randomized Controlled Trials

### Heart and Estrogen/Progestin Replacement Study

- HERS: 2321 women with CHD and a uterus:

| HERS: Estradiol + Progestins vs. Placebo | Hazard Ratio (Confidence Interval) |
|---|---|
| ↑ Venous thromboembolism | 2.08 (1.28–3.40) |
| ↑ Biliary tract surgery | 1.48 (1.12–1.95) |
| No significant effect on cancers | 1.19 (0.95–1.50) |
| No significant effect on hip, wrist, other fractures | ? Need ≥10-yr estrogen therapy |
| Similar rate of coronary heart disease events | 0.96 (0.77–1.19) |

*Source:* Adapted from Grady D, Herrington D, Bittner V et al. Cardiovascular disease outcomes during 6.8 years of hormone therapy: heart and estrogen/progestin replacement study follow-up (HERS II). *JAMA.* 2002;288(1):49; and Hulley S, Furberg C, Barrett-Connor E et al. Noncardiovascular disease outcomes during 6.8 years of hormone therapy: heart and estrogen/progestin replacement study follow-up (HERS II). *JAMA.* 2002;288(1):58.

### Raloxifene Use for the Heart

- Raloxifene use for the heart (RUTH): 10,101 postmenopausal women with CHD or multiple risk factors for CHD: RCT comparing raloxifene, 60 mg daily, vs. placebo; 5.6 year medial follow-up.
- Coronary events outcome defined as death from coronary causes, nonfatal MI or hospitalization for an acute coronary syndrome.

# MENOPAUSE

| Parameter | Hazard Ratio (Confidence Interval) | Absolute Risk[a] |
|---|---|---|
| ↑ Venous thromboembolism | 1.44 (1.06–1.95) | 1.2 |
| ↑ Fatal stroke | 1.49 (1.00–2.24) | 0.7 |
| Coronary events | 0.95 (0.84–1.07) | No difference |
| ↓ Invasive breast cancer | 0.56 (0.38–0.83) | 1.2 |
| ↓ Clinical vertebral fractures[b] | 0.65 (0.47–0.89) | 1.3 |

[a]Absolute risk: number of excess events per 10,000 women per year of treatment.
[b]No difference in non-vertebral fractures.
Source: Adapted from Barrett-Connor E, Mosca L, Collins P, et al. Effects of raloxifene on cardiovascular events and breast cancer in postmenopausal women. *New Engl J Med.* 2006;335(2):125.

## Women's Health Initiative

- **WHI E$_2$ + progestin:** 16,608 postmenopausal women without CHD: effect of E$_2$ + progestin in women *without* CHD; results at 5.2 years.

| Parameter | Hazard Ratio (Confidence Interval) | Absolute Risk[a] |
|---|---|---|
| ↑ Invasive breast cancer | 1.26 (1.00–1.59) | +8 |
| ↑ Coronary heart disease events | 1.29 (1.02–1.63) | +7 |
| ↑ Stroke | 1.41 (1.07–1.85) | +8 |
| ↑ Pulmonary embolism | 2.13 (1.39–3.25) | +8 |
| Endometrial cancer | 0.83 (0.47–1.47) | No difference |
| ↓ Colorectal cancer | 0.63 (0.43–0.92) | −6 |
| ↓ Hip fracture | 0.66 (0.45–0.98) | −5 |
| ↓ Vertebral fracture[b] | 0.66 (0.44–0.98) | −6 |
| ↓ Other osteoporotic fracture[b] | 0.77 (0.69–0.86) | −39 |

[a]Absolute risk: number of excess events per 10,000 woman-yrs of treatment.
[b]Not included in global index of main outcomes.
Source: Adapted from Rossouw JE, Anderson GL, Prentice RL et al. Risks and benefits of estrogen plus progestin in healthy postmenopausal women: principal results from the Women's Health Initiative randomized controlled trial. *JAMA.* 2002;288(3):321.

- **WHI E$_2$ alone:** 10,739 postmenopausal women without CHD; halted in February, 2004. Results from 6.8 years mean follow-up.

| Parameter | Hazard Ratio (Confidence Interval) | Absolute Risk[a] |
|---|---|---|
| ↑ Stroke | 1.39 (1.10–1.77) | +12 |
| Invasive breast cancer | 0.77 (0.59–1.01) | No difference |
| Coronary heart disease | 0.91 (0.75–1.12) | No difference |
| Pulmonary embolism | 1.34 (0.87–2.06) | No difference |
| Colorectal cancer | 1.08 (0.75–1.55) | No difference |
| ↓ Hip fracture | 0.61 (0.41–0.91) | −6 |

[a]Absolute risk: number of excess events per 10,000 woman-yrs of treatment.
Source: Adapted from Anderson GL, Limacher M, Assaf AR, et al.; Women's Health Initiative Steering Committee. Effects of conjugated equine estrogen in postmenopausal women with hysterectomy: the Women's Health Initiative randomized controlled trial. *JAMA.* 2004;291(14):1701.

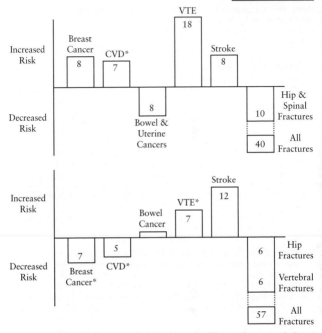

Annual risks and benefits after 5 years of combined (upper) and 7 years of estrogen-only (lower) HRT. *Not statistically significant. Numbers in bars are increased or decreased risk per 10,000 women. *Source:* Reproduced with permission from Hickey M, Davis SR, Sturdee DW. Treatment of menopausal symptoms: what shall we do now? *Lancet.* 2005;366(9483):409-421.

- **Women's Health Initiative Memory Study (WHIMS)** found adverse effects of conjugated equine estrogen (CEE) on cognitive function and ↑ dementia and ↑ mild cognitive impairment in both $E_2$/medroxyprogesterone acetate (MPA) and $E_2$-alone studies (Shumaker et al., 2004; Espeland et al., 2004), but these findings are based on a subset of WHI patients, as cognitive performance was not one of the primary outcome measures of the WHI study.

# MENOPAUSE

## Why the Discrepancy between Observational and Randomized Controlled Trials?

- Why did large observational studies (NHS) show ↓ CHD and ↑ breast cancer incidence in HT users, but these findings were not substantiated in recent large randomized controlled trials (HERS, two WHI studies)?

### In Favor of Hormone Therapy

- Primary vs. secondary prevention.
- Differences exist between the NHS population and the WHI subjects (e.g., mean age in NHS, 57 years old vs. WHI $E_2$/progestin study, 63 years old). WHI subjects thus started HT at an average of 12 years post-MP, in contrast with women in the NHS, who commenced hormones in the perimenopausal or early postmenopausal periods consistent with both primary prevention goals and with typical clinical practice.
- WHI studies combine a smaller (<20% of the study) primary prevention group of patients in their early 50s at the start of the study with a much larger secondary prevention group of patients in their late 50s to late 70s. In the $E_2$/MPA WHI study, only 33% of subjects and control subjects were 50–59 years old, and only 16–17% were within 5 years of the MP at enrollment (Naftolin et al., 2004).
- Despite their large overall size, the WHI trials are **severely underpowered** to detect a CHD reduction resulting from HT started in 50- to 54-year-olds soon after the MP (Naftolin et al., 2004).

### In Favor of the Women's Health Initiative Conclusions

- Observational studies like NHS suffer from the *healthy user effect*, in which nurses using HT were more likely to have confounding positive lifestyle factors, such as being less likely to smoke, leading to apparently ↓ CHD in HT users without a direct causative effect. Also, ↑ breast examinations/↑ mammography use may have ↑ breast cancer diagnosis in HT users for the NHS participants.
- NHS excluded silent myocardial infarction, whereas these were included in WHI data (Col and Pauker, 2003). Biases in the classification of deaths by unblinded investigators may have occurred in the NHS study.
- RCT data are less subject to confounding and bias such as the effects listed above.
- Estrogen and Thromboembolism Risk (ESTHER) multicenter case control study among 881 women found that women who took hormone pills were four times as likely to suffer a serious clot. Women who used hormone patches or gels were at no higher risk for blood clots than women who didn't take hormones at all (Canonico, 2007).

## Hormone Replacement Therapy Choices

| Active Ingredients | Drug Name | Company | Typical Daily Dosage Choices |
|---|---|---|---|
| **Estrogens** | | | |
| Conjugated equine estrogens (C | Premarin | Wyeth-Ayerst | 0.3, 0.625, 0.9, 125, 25 mg/continuous daily dosing or cyclic dosing |
| 17β-Estradiol (oral) | Estrace | Warner Chilcot | 0.5, 1, 2 mg/continuous daily dosing |
| 17β-Estradiol (transdermal) | Climera | Berlex | 0.025, 0.05, 0.075, 0.1 mg weekly patch |
| | Alora | Watson | 0.05, 0.075, 0.1 mg/change patch 2×/wk |
| | Esclim | Women First | 0.025, 0.0375, 0.05, 0.075, 0.1 mg/change patch 2×/wk |
| | Estraderm | Novartis | 0.05, 0.1 mg/change patch 2×/wk |
| | Vivelle dot | Novartis | 0.0375, 0.05, 0.075, 0.1 mg/change patch 2×/wk |
| Estropipate | Ogen | Pharmacia | 0.625, 1.25, 2.5 mg/continuous daily dosing or cyclic dosing |
| | Ortho-EST | Women First | 0.625, 1.25 mg/continuous daily dosing or cyclic dosing |
| Esterified estrogens | Estratab | Solvay | 0.3, 0.625, 2.5 mg/continuous daily dosing |
| | Menest | Monarch | 0.3, 0.625, 125, 25 mg/cyclic dosing (3 wk on therapy, 1 wk off) |
| Synthetic conjugated estrogens | Cenestin | Duramed/Solva | 0.625, 0.9, 1.25 mg/continuous daily dosing |
| **Oral Estrogen-Progestin Combination Therapy** | | | |
| Conjugated equine estrogens and medroxyprogesterone acetate (M | PremPro | Wyeth-Ayerst | 0.625 mg CEE plus 25 mg MPA, 0.625 mg CEE plus 5 mg MPA |
| | PremPhase | Wyeth-Ayerst | 0.625 mg CEE days 1–14, 0.625 mg CEE plus 5 mg MPA days 15–28 |
| ethinyl estradiol (EE), and norethindrone acetate (NE) | Fern HRT | Parke-Davis | 5 mcg EE plus 1 mg NE; continuous daily dosing |
| Micronized estradiol and norgestimate | Ortho-Prefest | Ortho-McNeil | 1 mg 17β-estradiol (continuous) and 0.09 mg norgestimate (pulsed in 3-day cycles) |
| Micronized estradiol and norethindrone acetate (NE) | Activella | Pharmacia | 1 mg 17β-estradiol and 0.5 mg NE; continuous daily dosing |

*(continued)*

**473**

# MENOPAUSE

## Hormone Replacement Therapy Choices *(continued)*

| Active Ingredients | Drug Name | Company | Typical Daily Dosage Choices |
|---|---|---|---|
| **Combination Oral Estrogen and Testosterone** | | | |
| Conjugated equine estrogens an methyltestosterone (MT) | Estratest | Solvay | 125 mg CEE plus 25 mg MT; cyclic dosing (3 wk on therapy, 1 wk off) |
| | Estratest-HS | | 0.625 mg CEE plus 1.25 mg MT; cyclic dosing (3 wk on therapy, 1 wk off) |
| **Transdermal Combination Therapy** | | | |
| 17β-Estradiol and norethindrone acetate (NE) | CombiPatch | Aventis | 0.05 mg 17β-estradiol and 0.14 mg NE or 0.05 mg 17β-estradiol and 0.25 mg NE; change patch 2×/wk |
| **Vaginal Estrogen Therapy** | | | |
| Conjugated equine estrogens | Premarin | Wyeth-Ayerst | 0.625 mg/gram; daily |
| 17β-Estradiol | Estrace | Warner-Chilcot | 0.1 mg/gram; daily then 1–3×/wk |
| Estropipate | Ogen | Pharmacia | 1.5 mg/gram; daily |
| Dienestrol | Ortho Dienestrol | Ortho-McNeil | 0.1 mg/gram; daily then 1–3×/wk |
| Estradiol | Vagifem | Pharmacia | 25 mcg tablets daily for 2 wks then 2×/wk |
| **Vaginal Estrogen Ring** | | | |
| Estradiol | Estring | Pharmacia | 2 mg reservoir; replace every 90 days |

## Common HRT Problems

| Solutions for Common HRT Problems | Additional Options |
|---|---|
| **PMS Symptoms** | |
| Increase exercise. Vitamin B6 50–100 mg daily. Decrease salt/sugar intake. | Change to low-dose oral contraceptive. Change to low-dose patch (e.g., Climara 0.025 mg) weekly during the progestin phase and extend into the menstrual week. Withdrawal bleeding will still occur. Consider using oral micronized progesterone 100–200 mg qhs during progestin phase (has sedative and anxiolytic properties). Consider Maxzide 25 mg qd for mild diuresis. |
| **Breast Tenderness** | |
| Restart HRT at lower estrogen dose and increase slowly. | Change HRT to a patch for steadier levels. Change progestin to norethindrone or oral micronized progesterone. Add methyltestosterone (e.g., HS Estratest). |
| **Hot Flashes** | |
| Double estrogen dosage for 3–6 mos then taper or change estrogen to a patch for steadier levels or add testosterone. | |
| **Insomnia** | |
| Recommend patient take estrogen in A.M. (stimulant) and to change the progestin to oral micronized progesterone at bedtime (sedative). Vaginal dryness Apply $^1/_2$ applicator of estrogen cream PV 2–3× weekly at bedtime or use the Estring vaginal ring (3 mos). | |
| **Breakthrough Bleeding** | |
| Consider endometrial biopsy if >35 yrs Change to cyclical combined or continuous sequential (see diagram). | Consider a progesterone IUD. Perform hysteroscopy and D&C. |
| **Breast Cancer Anxiety** | |
| Provide appropriate counseling. Consider using a lower dose of estrogen (e.g., 0.3 mg CEE or 0.5 mg estradiol) or use raloxifene. | |

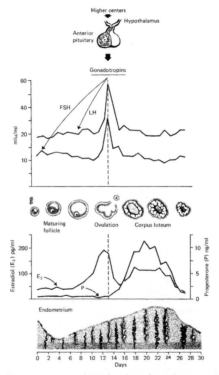

*Source:* Couchman GM, Hammond CB. Physiology of reproduction. In: Scott JR, DiSaia PD, Hammond CB, Spellacy WN, ed. *Danforth's Obstetrics and Gynecology.* 7th ed. Philadelphia: Lippincott, 1994. Reproduced with the permission of the publisher.

## PUBERTY

### Definition

- Puberty is the process of biologic and physical development through which sexual reproduction first becomes possible.
- Progression:
  - thelarche → adrenarche → peak growth spurt → menarche → ovulation

### Factors Affecting Time of Onset

- Genetics (average interval between menarche in monozygotic twins is 2.2 months compared with 8.2 months in dizygotic twins) (McDonough, 1998).
- Race (African-American girls enter puberty 1.0–1.5 years before white girls) (Herman-Giddens et al., 1997).
- Nutritional state (earlier with moderate obesity; delayed with malnutrition)
- General health.
- Geographic location (urban, closer to the equator, lower altitudes earlier than rural, farther from the equator, higher altitudes).
- Exposure to light (blind earlier than sighted).
- Psychological state.
- Several pathologic states influence the timing of puberty either directly or indirectly, contributing to a gaussian distribution.

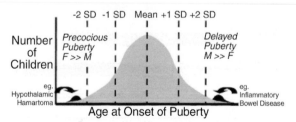

F, female; M, male; SD, standard deviation.
*Source:* Reproduced with permission from Palmert MR, Boepple PA. Variation in the timing of puberty: clinical spectrum and genetic investigation. *J Clin Endocrinol Metab.* 2001;86:2364.

# ENDOCRINOLOGY

## Physical Changes during Puberty

- Thelarche to menarche requires approximately 2–3 years.
  - Accelerated growth
  - Breast budding (thelarche)
  - Pubic and axillary hair growth (pubarche and adrenarche)
  - Peak growth velocity
  - Menarche
  - Ovulation (half the cycles are ovulatory approximately 1–3 years after menarche) (McDonough, 1998)
- Adrenarche can precede thelarche.
  - Prevalent in girls of African descent (McDonough, 1998)
- Average age of appearance of pubertal events:

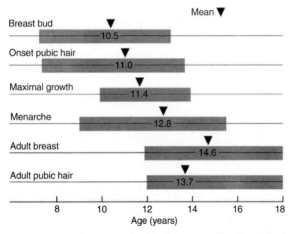

*Source:* Reproduced with permission from Gordon JD, Speroff L. Abnormal puberty and growth problems. In *Handbook for Clinical Gynecologic Endocrinology & Infertility.* 6th ed. Philadelphia: Lippincott–Raven, 2002:199.

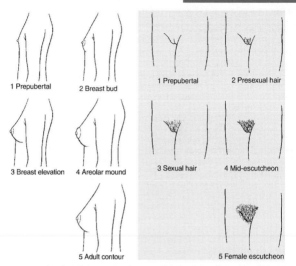

1 Prepubertal   2 Breast bud

1 Prepubertal   2 Presexual hair

3 Breast elevation   4 Areolar mound

3 Sexual hair   4 Mid-escutcheon

5 Adult contour

5 Female escutcheon

*Source*: Reproduced with permission from Gordon JD, Speroff L. Abnormal puberty and growth problems. In *Handbook for Clinical Gynecologic Endocrinology & Infertility*. 6th ed. Philadelphia: Lippincott–Raven, 2002:205.

| Pubertal Intervals | Mean ± Standard Deviation (Yrs) |
|---|---|
| B2 to peak height velocity | 1.0 ± 0.8 |
| B2 to menarche | 2.3 ± 1.0 |
| B2–PH5 | 3.1 ± 1.0 |
| B2–B5 (average duration of puberty) | 4.5 ± 2.0 |

B, breast; PH, pubic hair.

- Tanner staging (Marshall and Tanner, 1969)
  - Developed in 1969

# ENDOCRINOLOGY

■ Based on cohort of 192 British children of low socioeconomic status

| Classification | Description |
| --- | --- |
| Breast growth | |
| B1 | Prepubertal: elevation of papilla only. |
| B2 | Breast budding. |
| B3 | ↑ Breast with glandular tissue, without separation of breast contours. |
| B4 | 2nd mound formed by areola. |
| B5 | Single contour of breast and areola. |
| Pubic hair growth | |
| PH1 | Prepubertal: no pubic hair. |
| PH2 | Labial hair present. |
| PH3 | Labial hair spreads over mons pubis. |
| PH3 | Slight lateral spread. |
| PH4 | Further lateral spread to form inverse triangle and reach medial thighs. |

B, breast; PH, pubic hair.

## ABERRATIONS OF PUBERTAL DEVELOPMENT

### Delayed or Interrupted Puberty

- Difficult to define due to wide variation in normal development (most girls should enter puberty by 13 years; mean age of menarche is 16 years).

**Eugonadal** Well-estrogenized (26%)

- Müllerian agenesis or Mayer-Rokitansky-Kuster-Hauser syndrome (14%)
  - Second most common cause of primary amenorrhea after gonadal dysgenesis
  - Amenorrhea aside, pubertal development is normal (ovaries present).
  - 11–50% have skeletal abnormalities (scoliosis, phocomelia, lobster claw).
  - Up to 30% have unilateral renal agenesis or a single pelvic kidney.
  - Diagnosis: normal pubic hair (to differentiate from androgen insensitivity syndrome), ultrasound reveals absence of uterus and presence of ovaries.
  - Treatment: counseling, creation of a neovagina (through dilators or surgery), possible assisted reproductive technology with use of a surrogate.
  - Karyotype 46,XX.
- Vaginal septum (3%)
- Imperforate hymen (0.5%)
- Androgen insensitivity syndrome (1%)
  - Etiology: receptor absence, receptor defect, postreceptor defect
  - Complete: testes, female external genitalia, blind vaginal pouch, no Müllerian derivatives
  - Incomplete: above features as well as clitoral enlargement, labioscrotal fusion
  - Diagnosis: absent or significantly reduced pubic hair, male testosterone levels (to differentiate from Müllerian agenesis), karyotype
  - Treatment: gonadectomy after breast development, estrogen replacement therapy
  - Karyotype 46,XY
- Inappropriate positive feedback (7%): constitutional delay

**Hypogonadal** Hypoestrogenic (74%)

- Hypergonadotropic hypogonadism (follicle-stimulating hormone [FSH] >30 mIU/mL) (43%)
  - Turner syndrome (45,X or mosaic)
    ⇨ Lymphedema at birth, short stature, webbed neck, nevi and heart/kidney/skeletal/great vessel problems, streak ovaries secondary to oocyte depletion.
    ⇨ Check karyotype, complete physical exam, thyroid function tests, glucose, liver function tests, and intravenous pyelogram or renal ultrasound.
    ⇨ Treatment: growth hormone (GH) for height, then estrogen (gradually increase to 2× postmenopausal dose); later, progestins; counseling.

# ENDOCRINOLOGY

- Pure gonadal dysgenesis
  - ⇨ 46,XX
    - ❖ Idiopathic
    - ❖ FSH and luteinizing hormone (LH) receptor mutations
    - ❖ Steroidogenic acute regulatory protein, CYP17 (congenital adrenal hyperplasia [CAH]), and CYP19 mutations
  - ⇨ 46,XY
    - ❖ Swyer syndrome: point mutations in *sex-related Y* (SRY) or deletion of SRY
  - ⇨ No secondary sexual development, normal (or above average) height, normal but infantile female genitalia
    - ❖ Wilms' tumor suppressor gene mutations.
    - ❖ Hypogonadism, nephropathy, and Wilms' tumor.
    - ❖ Camptomelic dysplasia (SOX9 gene), SF-1, DAX1, Leydig cell hypoplasia.
    - ❖ Treatment: estrogen, gonadectomy if XY (20–30% risk of developing a gonadal tumor).
    - ❖ Must differentiate Swyer syndrome (–SRY) from LH-R mutation, as the latter involves a more technically challenging surgery because of the lack of landmarks.
- Hypogonadotropic hypogonadism (LH and FSH <5 mIU/mL) (31%)
  - Physiologic or constitutional delay is most common, but it is important to exclude other causes.
  - Sustained malnutrition: gastrointestinal malabsorption, anorexia nervosa, excessive exercise.
  - Endocrine disorders: hypothyroidism, Cushing disease or syndrome, CAH, hyperprolactinemia.
  - Hypothalamic-pituitary etiologies:
    - ⇨ Kallmann syndrome (anosmia, hypogonadism)
      - ❖ Absence of gonadotropin-releasing hormone (GnRH) neurons in hypothalamus
      - ❖ Treatment: hormonal therapy (oral contraceptives)
      - ❖ Fertility treatment: gonadotropins or pulsatile GnRH
    - ⇨ Pituitary insufficiency
    - ⇨ Pituitary tumors
      - ❖ Craniopharyngioma
    - ⇨ Signs: headache, visual changes, growth failure, delayed puberty
    - ⇨ Treatment: surgical, radiation treatment

## DISORDERS OF PUBERTY
### Relative Frequency of Delayed Pubertal Abnormalities

| Classification | | | |
|---|---|---|---|
| Hypergonadotropic hypogonadism | 43% | | |
| Ovarian failure, abnormal karyotype | | 26% | |
| Ovarian failure, normal karyotype | | 17% | |
| 46,XX | | | 15% |
| 46,XY | | | 2% |
| Hypogonadotropic hypogonadism | 31% | | |
| Reversible | | 18% | |
| Physiologic delay | | | 10% |
| Weight loss/anorexia | | | 3% |
| Primary hypothyroidism | | | 1% |
| Congenital adrenal hyperplasia | | | 1% |
| Cushing syndrome | | | 0.5% |
| Prolactinomas | | | 1.5% |
| Irreversible | | 13% | |
| GnRH deficiency | | | 7% |
| Hypopituitarism | | | 2% |
| Congenital CNS defects | | | 0.5% |
| Other pituitary adenomas | | | 0.5% |
| Craniopharyngioma | | | 1% |
| Malignant pituitary tumor | | | 0.5% |
| Eugonadism | 26% | | |
| Müllerian agenesis | | 14% | |
| Vaginal septum | | 3% | |
| Imperforate hymen | | 0.5% | |
| Androgen insensitivity syndrome | | 1% | |
| Inappropriate positive feedback | | 7% | |

GnRH, gonadotropin-releasing hormone.
*Source:* Speroff L, Glass RH, Kase NG. Abnormal puberty and growth problems. In: *Clinical Gynecologic Endocrinology and Infertility.* 6th ed. Philadelphia: Lippincott Williams & Wilkins, 1999. Reproduced with the permission of the publisher.

# ENDOCRINOLOGY

## Precocious Puberty

- Distribution of diagnoses in 80 girls referred for precocious puberty:

| Diagnosis | % |
|---|---|
| Premature adrenarche | 46 |
| Premature thelarche | 11 |
| True precocious puberty | 11 |
| Early breast development | 11 |
| Pubic hair of infancy | 6 |
| Premature menses | 6 |
| No puberty | 6 |

*Source:* Adapted from Kaplowitz P. Clinical characteristics of 104 children referred for evaluation of precocious puberty. *J Clin Endocrinol Metab.* 2004;89(8):3644.

- Most patients with Tanner stage 2 breast or pubic hair can be evaluated with only a history, physical exam, and review of the growth chart, without the need for hormonal studies and an estimate of bone age, provided that growth is normal (Kaplowitz, 2004).

### Definitions

- Traditional: thelarche before 8 years, pubarche before 9 years
- New (Kaplowitz and Oberfield, 1999)
  - Pubarche or thelarche before 7 years (white girls) or 6 years (African-American girls)
  - After ages 7 (white) or 6 (African-American) in conjunction with
    ⇨ Rapid progression of puberty
    ⇨ Central nervous system (CNS) findings: headache, neurologic symptoms, seizures
    ⇨ Pubertal progression that affects the emotional health of the family or girl

### Central or True Precocious Puberty

- Premature stimulation by GnRH (GnRH-dependent).
- Idiopathic is the most common.
- CNS tumors, infection, congenital abnormality, trauma, juvenile primary hypothyroidism, Russell-Silver syndrome.

### Peripheral Precocious Puberty

- GnRH independent.
- Peripheral precocious puberty may result in GnRH-dependent precocious puberty if left untreated.

### Isosexual Precocious Puberty

- Ovarian cysts
  - McCune-Albright syndrome
    ⇨ Gene mutation of the G protein α-subunit (leads to hormone receptor activation in absence of the hormone); toxic multinodular goiter, pituitary gigantism, Cushing syndrome, polyostotic fibrous dysplasia, café-au-lait spots
    ⇨ Treat with testolactone (aromatase inhibitor)
- Neoplasms (adrenal or gonadal); 11% of girls with precocious puberty have an ovarian tumor.
- Exogenous hormones (drugs, food)

### Heterosexual Precocious Puberty

- Prepubertal production of androgens with pubarche, adrenarche, and skeletal maturation
- CAH:
  - 21-Hydroxylase deficiency (virilizing, salt-wasting, nonclassic)
  - 3β-Hydroxysteroid dehydrogenase (classic, nonclassic)
- Exogenous androgen ingestion
- Androgen secreting tumor (i.e., adrenal masculinizing tumor)

### Pseudoprecocious Puberty

- Premature thelarche
  - Early isolated breast development
  - Normal bone age
  - Close follow-up to rule out true precocious puberty
- Premature adrenarche
  - Early isolated appearance of pubic or axillary hair (polycystic ovary syndrome [PCOS] precursor?)
  - Commonly seen in African-American girls
  - May be associated with excess androgen secretion secondary to deficiencies in other enzymes

### Evaluation

- Check bone age (increase in growth or bone age is more dramatic in girls with central precocious puberty or ovarian disease).
- High basal and GnRH-stimulated serum LH concentration = gonadotropin-dependent precocious puberty.

# ENDOCRINOLOGY

## Treatment

- Incomplete precocity
  - Premature thelarche or adrenarche → reexamine regularly
- GnRH- and gonadotropin-independent precocious puberty
  - Tumors of adrenal or ovary → surgery
  - McCune-Albright syndrome → testolactone (aromatase inhibitor)
- Central precocious puberty:
  - GnRH-agonist–induced pituitary-gonadal suppression ± GH when growth is slowed too much:
  - Regression of secondary sexual characteristics
  - Cessation of menstrual bleeding
  - Slowing of bone growth

| Classification | Female | Male |
|---|---|---|
| GnRH independent (true precocity) | | |
| Idiopathic | 74% | 41% |
| CNS problem | 7% | 26% |
| GnRH independent (precocious pseudopuberty) | | |
| Ovarian (cyst or tumor) | 11% | — |
| Testicular | — | 10% |
| McCune-Albright syndrome | 5% | 1% |
| Adrenal feminizing | 1% | 0% |
| Adrenal masculinizing | 1% | 22% |
| Ectopic gonadotropin production | 0.5% | 0.5% |

GnRH, gonadotropin-releasing hormone.
*Source:* Speroff L, Glass RH, Kase NG. Abnormal puberty and growth problems. In: *Clinical Gynecologic Endocrinology and Infertility.* 6th ed. Philadelphia: Lippincott Williams & Wilkins, 1999. Reproduced with the permission of the publisher.

## AMENORRHEA

### Definition
- No menses by age 14 in absence of 2° sexual characteristics (primary)
- No menses by age 16 despite 2° sexual characteristics (primary)
- No menses in 6 months (secondary)

### Etiology

#### Primary
43% Gonadal failure
14% Congenital absence of the vagina
10% Constitutional delay

#### Secondary
39% Chronic anovulation
20% Hypothyroidism/hyperprolactinemia
16% Weight loss/anorexia

### Vaginal Agenesis vs. Androgen Insensitivity Syndrome

|  | Mayer-Rokitansky-Kuster-Hauser Syndrome | Complete Androgen Insensitivity Syndrome |
|---|---|---|
| Vagina | Absent | Absent |
| Pubic hair | Present | Absent |
| Breasts | Present | Present |
| Gonads | Ovaries | Testes |
| Uterus | Absent | Absent |
| Karyotype | 46,XX | 46,XY |
| Other anomalies (renal, cardiac) | Increased | Not increased |

# ENDOCRINOLOGY

## Evaluation of Amenorrhea

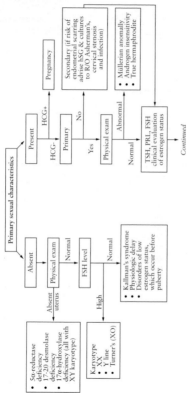

*Continued*

*Source*: Reproduced with permission from Berek JS, ed. *Novak's Gynecology*. 13th ed. New York: Lippincott Williams & Wilkins; 2002. pg. 810–811.

## Evaluation of Amenorrhea

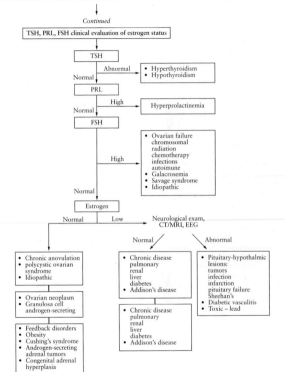

*Continued*

TSH, PRL, FSH clinical evaluation of estrogen status

**TSH**

Abnormal → • Hyperthyroidism
• Hypothyroidism

Normal

**PRL**

High → Hyperprolactinemia

Normal

**FSH**

High → • Ovarian failure
chromosomal
radiation
chemotherapy
infections
autoimmune
• Galacrosemia
• Savage syndrome
• Idiopathic

Normal

**Estrogen**

Normal | Low → Neurological exam, CT/MRI, EEG

Normal | Abnormal

• Chronic anovulation
• polycystic ovarian syndrome
• Idiopathic

• Ovarian neoplasm
• Granulosa cell androgen-secreting

• Feedback disorders
• Obesity
• Cushing's syndrome
• Androgen-secreting adrenal tumors
• Congenital adrenal hyperplasia

• Chronic disease
pulmonary
renal
liver
diabetes
• Addison's disease

• Chronic disease
pulmonary
renal
liver
diabetes
• Addison's disease

• Pituitary-hypothalmic lesions:
tumors
infection
infarction
pituitary failure
Sheehan's
• Diabetic vasculitis
• Toxic – lead

# ENDOCRINOLOGY

## STEROID BIOSYNTHESIS

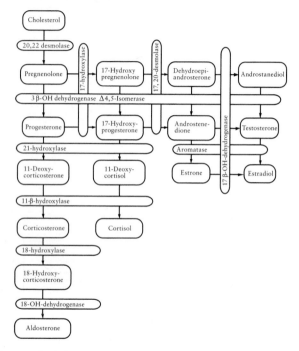

## Enzymatic Defects

### 20–22 Desmolase Deficiency (adrenal and ovary)

- Lethal
- Internal/external female βgenitalia
- Adrenal enlarged with cholesterol esters

## 17 α-Hydroxylase Deficiency (adrenal and ovary)

- Hypertension, hypokalemia
- Infantile female external genitalia
- Primary amenorrhea with elevated FSH and LH
- Genital ambiguity in male infants only

## 3 β-Hydroxysteroid Dehydrogenase Deficiency (adrenal and ovary)

- Infants severely ill at birth
- Rarely survive
- Females slightly virilized, males incompletely masculinized
- Milder non-classic cases may be common

## 21-Hydroxylase Deficiency (adrenal only)

- Most common form of congenital adrenal hyperplasia (>90%)
- Most frequent cause of sexual ambiguity
- Most frequent endocrine cause of neonatal death
  - Salt-wasting
  - Hypertension
- 3 clinical forms
  - Salt-wasting (cortisol and aldosterone)
  - Simple virilizing (cortisol production only)
  - Non-classic or late-onset
- Inherited as monogenic autosomal recessive
  - Close linkage to human leukocyte antigen complex on short arm of chromosome 6
- Diagnosis by increased 17-alpha-hydroxyprogesterone (OHP) (baseline or with ACTH stimulation test)

## 11 β-Hydroxylase Deficiency (adrenal only)

- 11-deoxycortisol not converted to cortisol
- Desoxycorticosterone not converted to corticosterone
- Variable affect on aldosterone levels
- Hypertension, hypokalemic acidosis (usually mild after several years of life)
- Diagnosis by high levels of deoxycorticosterone and compound S (11-deoxycortisol)

*Source:* Speroff L, Glass RH, Kase, NG. Normal and abnormal sexual development. In: *Clinical Gynecologic Endocrinology and Infertility.* 6th ed. Philadelphia: Lippincott Williams & Wilkins, 1999. Reproduced with the permission of the publisher.

# ENDOCRINOLOGY

## POLYCYSTIC OVARY SYNDROME
- ~8% of reproductive-aged women have PCOS
- Genetics

| Affected 1st-Degree Relative | Risk of Polycystic Ovary Syndrome (%) |
|---|---|
| Mother | 35 |
| Sister | 40 |

*Source:* Adapted from Kahsar-Miller MD, Nixon C, Boots LR et al. Prevalence of polycystic ovary syndrome (PCOS) in first-degree relatives of patients with PCOS. *Fertil Steril.* 2001;75(1):53.

- Mothers of women with PCOS have elevated low-density lipoprotein/androgen levels as well as markers of insulin resistance (IR) consistent with a heritable trait. (Sam S et al. *DNAS.* 2006;103(18):7030–7035.)
- PCOS patients frequently develop regular menstrual cycles when aging (Elting et al., 2000), due to ↓ size of the follicle cohort? Or due to ↓ inhibin?
- Theory of etiology: *enhanced serine phosphorylation unification theory* → ↑ CYP17 activity in the ovary (hyperandrogenism) and ↓ insulin receptor activity peripherally (IR) (Dunaif et al., 1995) lead to the endocrine dysfunction of PCOS.

## Clinical Signs and Symptoms
### Menstrual Dysfunction
- Onset at menarche: oligo/amenorrhea

### Infertility
- Ovulatory dysfunction

### Obesity
- Obesity occurs in 35–65% of women with PCOS (>80% are obese before puberty).
- Androgens converted to E1 in peripheral fat and can contribute to endometrial hyperplasia.
- Fat contributes to insulin insensitivity.

### Hirsutism
- Gradual onset over months to years; onset usually with puberty.
- Dark, coarse hairs in androgen-dependent locations.
- Associated with hyperandrogenemia (classic PCOS) and idiopathic increased end organ sensitivity.
- *Ferriman-Gallway* scores are used to quantify degree of hirsutism and grade responses to treatments (Ferriman and Gallway, 1961); on a day-to-day clinical basis, most endocrinologists rely on patient perceptions and frequency of waxing or electrolysis.

### Variable Other Signs and Symptoms
- **Acne:** no known correlation between the severity of acne and plasma-free T (Slayden and Azziz, 1997).

- **Acanthosis nigricans:** usually seen with significant insulin resistance; called the *hyperandrogenism, insulin resistance–acanthosis nigricans* (**HAIR-AN**) syndrome:
    - Dermal hyperkeratosis and papillomatosis presenting as a brown or gray, velvety, occasionally verrucous, hyperpigmented area over the vulva (most common), axillae, groin, umbilicus, and submammary areas
- IR (~30%) or overt non–insulin-dependent diabetes mellitus (NIDDM) (~8%) (Dunaif, 1997).
- Skin tags.
- **Polycystic-appearing ovaries** not necessarily a prerequisite for diagnosis (see criteria below); present in 30% of population:

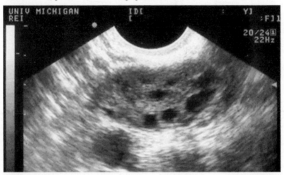

## Clinical Evaluation

- Dr. Andrea Dunaif (*personal communication*): "PCOS is like pornography: It's hard to define, but when you see it, you recognize it."
- Revised 2003 Rotterdam European Society for Human Reproduction and Embryology (ESHRE)/American Society for Reproductive Medicine (ASRM)–sponsored PCOS consensus on diagnostic criteria for PCOS (two out of three) (Rotterdam ESHRE/ASRM-Sponsored PCOS Consensus Workshop Group, 2004):

# ENDOCRINOLOGY

1. Oligo- and/or anovulation
2. Clinical and/or biochemical (total T >70 ng/dL; A⁴ >245 ng/dL; DHEA-S >248 mcg/dL) signs of hyperandrogenism
3. Polycystic ovaries (≥12 follicles [2–9 mm diameter] in each ovary)

   Exclusion of other etiologies (e.g., nonclassic congenital adrenal hyperplasia [NCAH], hyperprolactinemia, Cushing syndrome, and androgen-secreting tumors)

## Diagnostic Algorithm for the Polycystic Ovary Syndrome

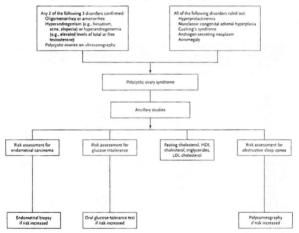

Source: Reprinted with permission from Ehrmann DA. Polycystic ovary syndrome. N Engl J Med. 2005;352:1223–1236. Copyright © 2005 Massachusetts Medical Society. All rights reserved.

## DIFFERENTIAL DIAGNOSIS OF POLYCYSTIC OVARY SYNDROME

### Virilizing Ovarian or Adrenal Tumor

- *Rapid* onset and *progressive* course of virilizing symptoms
- *Severe* hirsutism: male pattern balding, clitoromegaly, weight gain
- Total T >200 ng/dL or DHEA-S >700 mcg/dL
  - Positive predictive value of a repeat total T >250 ng/dL → 9%; negative predictive value of 100% (Waggoner et al., 1999)

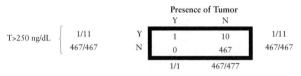

|  |  | Presence of Tumor | |  |
|---|---|---|---|---|
|  |  | Y | N |  |
| T>250 ng/dL | Y | 1 | 10 | 1/11 |
|  | 1/11 467/467 | | | 467/467 |
|  | N | 0 | 467 |  |
|  |  | 1/1 | 467/477 |  |

- Computed tomography (CT) of pelvis and adrenals with contrast if tumor suspected (may require selective venous catheterization of ovarian/adrenal veins)
  - Most common virilizing ovarian tumor: *arrhenoblastoma*
  - **Adrenal tumor:** suspect if DHEA-S >700 mcg/dL
  - Diagnosis: Dexamethasone, 0.5 mg PO q6hrs × 2 days
  - DHEA-S and 17-OHP, before and after
  - If no decrease to normal → virilizing adrenal tumor (Cushing syndrome), although some tumors may suppress DHEA-S
  - If levels decrease → NCAH vs. PCOS; need to check 17-OHP

### Cushing Syndrome

- If patient is hypertensive, assess 24-hour free urinary cortisol; >50 mcg consistent with Cushing syndrome
- Idiopathic hirsutism
- Clinical hyperandrogenism with normal androgen levels and regular ovulatory cycles
  - Women with PCOS have greater 5α-reductase activity than healthy women (Fassnacht et al., 2003). Only the 5α-reductase, type 1 isoform is associated with the severity of hirsutism (Goodarzi et al., 2006).
  - The enzyme responsible for the degradation of dihydrotestosterone (DHT) (3α-hydroxysteroid dehydrogenase, type III) may be deficient in some hirsute women (Steiner et al., 2004).

### Nonclassic Congenital Adrenal Hyperplasia

- Measure 17-OHP and $P_4$ to discriminate between PCOS and NCAH:
  - A.M. follicular phase, due to circadian variability

# ENDOCRINOLOGY

- The presenting signs of NCAH in children include premature pubarche, cystic acne, accelerated growth and advanced bone age. Patients are tall children but short adults (New, 2006).
  - 50% of those with NCAH have elevated DHEA-S.

| 17-Hydroxyprogesterone (17-OHP) (ng/mL) | Diagnosis |
|---|---|
| <2 | Polycystic ovary syndrome |
| 2–4 | Cortrosyn stimulation test[a] |
| >4 | Nonclassic congenital adrenal hyperplasia |

[a]Cortrosyn stimulation test: Measure 17-OHP at t = 60 after 0.25 mg IV adrenocorticotropic hormone administration (see list below).

t = 60 17-Hydroxyprogesterone (ng/mL):

>10 = Likely NCAH
>15 = NCAH

- **21-Hydroxylase deficiency** (gene: **CYP21A2**) (20–50% enzyme activity) is an autosomal-recessive trait with variable genotype-phenotype patterns. More than 40 CYP21A2 mutations have been found in association with NCAH due to 21-hydroxylase deficiency.
  - Incidence: 1/1000.
  - Treatment: 5.0–7.5 mg prednisone in two divided doses.
  - May restore ovulation but relatively ineffective for existing hirsutism; monitor for iatrogenic Cushing syndrome (rapid weight gain, hypertension, pigmented striae, and osteopenia).
  - Treatment efficacy is considered a target 17-OHP between 1 and 10 ng/mL measured at the nadir of steroid blood levels.
  - Treatment during pregnancy:
  - Pregnant women with NCAH should have A[4], T, and 17-OHP measured q2wks, and the glucocorticoid dose (avoid dexamethasone since it is transferred across the placenta and can suppress the fetal adrenal gland; hydrocortisone or prednisone preferred) should be increased, if necessary, to maintain the concentrations within the high–normal range for each trimester (TM) of pregnancy and ameliorate genital ambiguity* in affected female fetuses (Lo et al., 1999). Begin at the time of a positive pregnancy test and continue **only if** chorionic villus sampling shows a female with affected

*At <12 weeks of gestation, high fetal androgen levels lead to a varying degree of labioscrotal fusion and clitoral enlargement in the female fetus; exposure to androgen at >12 weeks induces clitoromegaly alone.

CYP21 genotype (Speiser and White, 2003). Even if androgen production cannot be suppressed to normal, placental aromatase activity protects the fetal genitalia and, presumably, the brain from masculinization (Lo et al., 1999).

- Diagnosis with ACTH stimulation test (0 and 60 min) (Lutfallah et al., 2002):

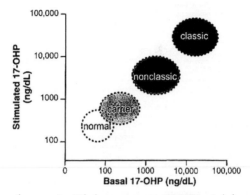

Nomogram for comparing 17-hydroxyprogesterone (17-OHP) ratio before and after administration of 0.25-mg IV cosyntropin (carriers = heterozygotes).
*Source:* Reproduced with permission from White PC, Speiser PW. Congenital adrenal hyperplasia due to 21-hydroxylase deficiency. *Endocr Rev.* 2000;21[3]:2454.

- **3β-Hydroxysteroid dehydrogenase deficiency** (gene: HSDB2) (less common and no consensus on this diagnosis)

# ENDOCRINOLOGY

## Pathophysiology of Polycystic Ovary Syndrome

### Endocrine Dysfunction

#### Hypersecretion/Elevation of Luteinizing Hormone

- ↑ Pulse amplitude and frequency, ↑ LH bioactivity (abnormal LH secretion is secondary to ovarian dysfunction)
  - Lack of negative feedback (↓ progesterone [$P_4$])?
  - Programming of the hypothalamic-pituitary axis by androgens?
  - ↓ Sex hormone–binding globulin (SHBG) from hyperinsulinemia and hyperandrogenemia leads to ↑ free estradiol levels, lowering FSH relative to LH.
  - Insulin is the most potent inhibitor of SHBG (Nestler et al., 1991).

#### Hyperinsulinemia

- Hyperinsulinemia leads to ↓ SHBG, ↓ IGF-binding protein-I, and ↑ free androgens.
- Total serum IGF-I levels are normal in PCOS, but ↓ IGF-binding protein-I concentrations can lead to ↑ free IGF-I.
- IGF-I and -II → ↑ LH stimulation of androgens in theca cells.
- Insulin may also ↑ androgen production directly or may ↑ LH secretion from the pituitary (Dorn et al., 2004).
- Waist-hip ratio >0.85 (central obesity) is significantly related to insulin sensitivity, but body mass index is not.

#### Androgen Excess

- Ovarian production: ↑ LH results in theca hyperplasia (theca cell dysfunction), resulting in ↑ testosterone (T), androstenedione ($A^4$), dehydroepiandrosterone (DHEA), 17-hydroxyprogesterone, and estrone ($E_1$). Ovarian estradiol ($E_2$) production is unchanged.
- Adrenal is a secondary source of elevated serum androgens. Nonclassic adrenal hyperplasia (NCAH)—a genetic defect in either the 21-hydroxylase or the 3β-hydroxysteroid dehydrogenase genes, results in elevated levels of primarily adrenal androgens (i.e., DHEA-sulfate [DHEA-S]).
- ↓ SHBG leads to ↑ free androgen and estrogen (↓ SHBG from elevated insulin, hyperandrogenemia, hyperprolactinemia).
- 30% of patients with PCOS show mild hyperprolactinemia (Isik et al., 1997).

## Prevalence of Different Androgen Excess Disorders in 950 Women Referred Because of Clinical Hyperandrogenism

|  | Number of Patients | % of Total Number of Patients |
|---|---|---|
| Classic PCOS | 538 | 56.6 |
| Ovulatory PCOS | 147 | 15.5 |
| Idiopathic hyperandrogenism | 150 | 15.8 |
| Idiopathic hirsutism | 72 | 7.6 |
| NCAH | 41 | 4.3 |
| Androgen-secreting tumors | 2 | 0.2 |

*Source:* Reproduced with permission from Carmina E, Rosato F, Janni A et al. Extensive clinical experience: relative prevalence of different androgen excess disorders in 950 women referred because of clinical hyperandrogenism. *JCEM.* 2006;91(1):2–6.

## Potential Long-Term Consequences of Polycystic Ovary Syndrome

| Definite or Very Likely Consequences of Polycystic Ovary Syndrome | Possible Consequences of Polycystic Ovary Syndrome |
|---|---|
| Insulin resistance; type II diabetes mellitus (greater than weight-matched controls) | Hypertension |
| | Coronary heart disease |
| Endometrial hyperplasia/atypia | Dyslipidemia |
| Gestational diabetes | Ovarian cancer (conflicting data) |
| Sleep apnea (even when controlled for body mass index) | Spontaneous abortion (may not be greater than for subfertility population) |

Hyperlipidemia (Mahabeer et al., 1990; Orio et al., 2004) reported to elevate plasminogen activator inhibitor (PAI; major inhibitor of fibrinolysis); PAI is an independent risk factor for atherosclerosis.

↑ Left ventricular mass index among asymptomatic women with PCOS compared with controls (Orio et al., 2004).

Studies showing no clear association between PCOS and cardiovascular events may be biased due to PCOS study patients having had wedge resection (Pierpoint et al., 1998; Wild et al., 2000).

Type II diabetes mellitus (DM): $3–7 \times$ ↑ incidence in PCOS patients.

# ENDOCRINOLOGY

## Treatment of Polycystic Ovary Syndrome

### Goals
- Prevent endometrial hyperplasia/cancer
- Restore normal menstruation; resolution of anovulation/infertility
- Improve hirsutism and acne

### Weight Reduction
- As little as 5–7% of body weight reduction can reduce hyperandrogenism, improve insulin sensitivity, and restore spontaneous ovulation and fertility in 75% of women with PCOS (Kiddy et al., 1992).
  - Low-calorie diet (1000–1500 kcal/day).
  - Waist-hip ratio >0.85 at greater risk for morbidity.
  - Metformin may stimulate weight loss.

### Oral Contraceptives
- 1st line of drug treatment (i.e., **Yasmin** [ethinyl estradiol, 30 mcg; drospirenone, 3 mg]; avoid norgestrel and levonorgestrel).
- Method of action: ↑ SHBG, suppression of LH, inhibition of 5α-reductase and androgen receptor binding.
- Greatest efficacy against acne (hirsutism usually requires the addition of antiandrogens).
- Avoid levonorgestrel-containing oral contraceptives (OCs), due to the androgenic properties of the progestin (e.g., Alesse, Levlen, Nordette, Triphasil).
- OCs ↓ LH but not to normal levels (Polson et al., 1988).
- GnRH-agonist plus add-back no better than OCs alone (Carr et al., 1995).

### Progestins
- Give progestins q month or q2–3mos to prevent endometrial hyperplasia.

### Antiandrogens
- Antiandrogens are effective in the treatment of hirsutism after 6–9 months; however, cessation of antiandrogen therapy is followed by recurrence (Yucelten et al., 1999).
  - **Spironolactone** (Aldactone, 100–200 mg/day) plus OCs (Lobo et al., 1985; Young et al., 1987). *Contraception is mandatory* with the use of spironolactone, as incomplete virilization of a male fetus may occur. Should wait ≥2 months after discontinuance of spironolactone to begin attempts at conception.
    ⇨ Aldosterone antagonist, K+-sparing diuretic:
    ❖ Inhibits steroidogenic enzymes and binds the DHT receptor at the hair follicle.
    ❖ Can cause irregular uterine bleeding.
    ❖ 25-mg tablets are generic and inexpensive.

- **Finasteride** (Proscar, 5 mg/day), type II 5α-reductase inhibitor; shows signs of being an excellent and safe antiandrogen.
  - ⇨ ↓ Circulating DHT levels; not effective topically (Price et al., 2000); not approved by the U.S. Food and Drug Administration (FDA) for this purpose
  - ⇨ Low dose (2.5 mg) every 3 days is as effective as continuous administration in ↓ hirsutism (Tartagni et al., 2004).
  - ⇨ *Contraception is mandatory* (Ciotta et al., 1995; Wong et al., 1995; Fruzzetti et al., 1999) because its use during the late first TM may ↑ risk of hypospadias and other genital abnormalities in male fetuses.
- **Cyproterone acetate** (Androcur), not approved in the United States (used extensively in Europe [Diane 35] and Israel for hirsutism).
  - ⇨ Androgen receptor antagonist, decreases 5α-reductase activity, impairs androgen synthesis.
  - ⇨ Reports of liver tumors in beagles have kept this effective drug from the U.S. market.
- **Eflornithine** (Vaniqa, 13.9% topical cream bid).
  - ⇨ Irreversibly inhibits ornithine decarboxylase to inhibit follicle polyamine synthesis necessary for hair growth.
  - ⇨ Effect seen over 4–8 weeks; *reversible* if medicine stopped.
  - ⇨ <1% systemic absorption, skin irritation may occur.
  - ⇨ Category C drug.

## Insulin Sensitizing Drugs

### Metformin (Glucophage)

- Biguanide oral hypoglycemic agent.
- ↓ Hepatic gluconeogenesis; ↓ intestinal glucose absorption; ↑ peripheral glucose uptake and utilization; no change in insulin secretion but ↓ fasting insulin levels; ↑ SHBG; ↓ LH, free T, and PAI-I.
  - 50% have improved menstrual function.
- May be used *whether or not* there is hyperandrogenism.
- If glucose to insulin ratio is <4.5, patient needs further testing to rule out diabetes, 1st check a 2-hour GTT to rule out overt diabetes.
  - >50% of women with PCOS have IR and this is independent of obesity (Dunaif et al., 1989).
- Avoid metformin if creatinine >1.2 mg/dL or liver function tests (LFTs) are elevated → ↑ risk of lactic acidosis.
  - Metformin may cause dizziness and/or gastrointestinal discomfort and should not be taken with IV contrast dye (e.g., hysterosalpingogram [HSG]); it is recommended to stop the drug 1 day before a contrast study.

# ENDOCRINOLOGY

- Metformin XR regimen (no consensus regarding optimal dose [Nestler, 2001]):

500 mg $\xrightarrow[\text{1 week}]{}$ 1000 mg $\xrightarrow[\text{1 week}]{}$ 1500 mg metformin XR QHS

- Stop at the end of the 1st TM, although preliminary studies suggest no teratogenicity (Gilbert et al., 2006).
- Significant weight loss is to be expected with protracted metformin (Harborne, 2005).

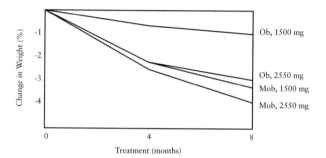

- Effectiveness of metformin alone for ovulation induction vs. placebo—Cochrane database: overall odds ratio = 3.91 (2.20, 6.95) (Lord et al., 2003).
- Single randomized, placebo-controlled study showing that lean women with PCOS and no IR respond favorably to metformin (Baillargeon et al., 2004).
- Insulin resistance and higher LH to FSH ratios (>2.5) may predict greater success with metformin (Kriplani and Agarwal, 2004; Eisenhardt et al., 2006).
- How long to give metformin before concluding that there is no effect? Unknown but effects on insulin and SHBG seen within 2–4 weeks (Khowann, 2006; Eisenhardt et al., 2006).
- Velazquez et al. (1997) found that:
  - Metformin therapy (500 mg PO t.i.d.) restored menstrual cyclicity in 21 of 22 (96%).
  - Most studies on *ovulatory rate*, not pregnancy rate.
- CMRMN Study (Legro, 2007).
  - 6-month randomized trial comparing clomiphene, metformin, or both for PCOS.

- Live-birth rate was 22.5% in clomiphene group, 7.2% in metformin group, and 26.8% in the combination group (*p* <0.001 for metformin vs. either other group).
- Rate of multiple pregnancy was 6% (clomiphene), 0% (metformin), and 3.1% (combination-therapy group).
- No significant difference in first TM loss although metformin was discontinued with a positive pregnancy test (not adequately powered).
- No placebo-only group.
- Can metformin ↓ early pregnancy loss (early pregnancy loss; 1st TM)? All prospective/historical studies, some with suspect methodology.

|  |  | Spontaneous Abortion Rate (%) | |
| --- | --- | --- | --- |
| Reference | Pregnancies (No.) | Historical Controls | Metformin-Treated |
| Glueck et al., 2002 | 46 | 62 | 26 |
| Jakubowicz et al., 2002 | 65 | 42 | 9 |
| Heard et al., 2002 | 20 | Not available | 35 |
| Thatcher et al., 2006 | 124 | 67 | 36 |

- Metformin and the incidence of preeclampsia and perinatal mortality—single study with unsubstantiated results (Hellmuth et al., 2000).
  - Metformin vs. insulin-treated: 32% vs. 10% incidence of preeclampsia (*p* <.001)
  - Metformin vs. insulin- or sulfonylurea-treated: 11.6% vs. 1.3% incidence of perinatal mortality (*p* <.02)
- In a randomized, controlled trial, metformin reduced the incidence of diabetes in persons at high risk (↓ 31%/3 years; number needed to treat = 14) (Jakubowicz et al., 2002).

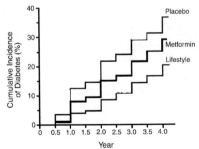

# ENDOCRINOLOGY

## Ovulation Induction

• See pg. 525 for ovulation induction protocols for PCOS.

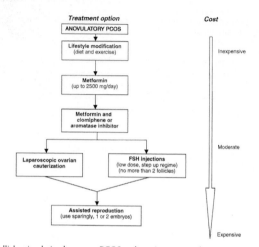

FSH, follicle-stimulating hormone; PCOS, polycystic ovary syndrome.

*Source:* Adapted from Norman RJ. Metformin—comparison with other therapies in ovulation induction in polycystic ovary syndrome. *J Clin Endocrinol Metab.* 2004;89 [10]:4797.

## Drug Treatments[a]

| Agent | Mechanism of Action | Advantages or Disadvantages | Examples | Uses | | | |
|---|---|---|---|---|---|---|---|
| | | | | Hirsutism, Acne | Oligomenorrhea or Amenorrhea | Ovulation Induction | Insulin Lowering |
| Combinations of estrogen and progestin | Increase SHBG, suppress LH and FSH, suppress ovarian androgen production; progestin can act as an antiandrogen | Cyclic exposure of endometrium to estrogen and progestin; effective for hirsutism and acne; may increase risk of thrombosis and metabolic abnormalities; beneficial antiandrogenic effects of drospirenone | Ethinyl estradiol and norgestimate (Ortho Cyclen); ethinyl estradiol and desogestrel (Orthocept); ethinyl estradiol and drospirenone (Yasmin) | X | X | | |
| Antiandrogens | Inhibit androgens from binding to the androgen receptor | Effective for hirsutism and acne; risk of hyperkalemia (spironolactone) or hepatitis (flutamide) | Cyproterone acetate, spironolactone, flutamide | X | | | |
| Glucocorticoids | Suppress corticotropin and thus adrenal androgen production | Attenuate adrenal component of androgen excess; long-term risks of glucose intolerance, insulin resistance, osteopenia, weight gain | Prednisone, dexamethasone | X | X | X | |
| 5α-Reductase inhibitors | Inhibit 5α-reductase | Do not specifically target the isoenzyme of 5α-reductase in the pilosebaceous unit | Finasteride (Propecia) | X | | | |
| Ornithine decarboxylase inhibitors | Inhibit ornithine decarboxylase | Minimal documented efficacy; used topically | Eflornithine hydrochloride (Vaniqa) | X | | | |

*(continued)*

# ENDOCRINOLOGY

**Drug Treatments[a]** (*continued*)

| Agent | Mechanism of Action | Advantages or Disadvantages | Examples | Uses | | | |
|---|---|---|---|---|---|---|---|
| | | | | Hirsutism, Acne | Oligomen-orrhea or Amenorrhea | Ovulation Induction | Insulin Lowering |
| Thiazolidinediones | Enhance insulin action at target-tissue level (adipocyte, muscle); may have direct effects on ovarian steroidogenesis | Extremely effective at lowering levels of insulin and androgens, modest effects on hirsutism; associated with weight gain | Pioglitazone (Actos), rosiglitazone (Avandia) | X | X | X | X |

[a]SHBG, sex hormone–binding globulin; LH, luteinizing hormone; FSH, follicle-stimulating hormone.
*Source:* Reproduced with permission from Ehrmann DA. Polycystic ovary syndrome. *N Engl J Med.* 2005;352(12):1223–1236.
Copyright © 2005 Massachusetts Medical Society. All rights reserved.

## HIRSUTISM

### Fast Facts

- Definition: male type body hair distribution (sexual hair areas).
  - Face—mustache, beard, sideburns
  - Body—chest, circumareolar, linea alba, abdominal trigone, inner thighs
- $1/3$ of women age 14–45 have excessive upper lip hair.
- 6–9% have unwanted chin/sideburn hair.
- Cushing disease.
  - Most common referral diagnosis, one of the least common final diagnoses
- Hair follicles laid down at 8 weeks gestation.
- Cyclic hair growth.
  - Anagen: growing phase
  - Catagen: rapid involution phase
  - Telogen: resting phase

### Differential Diagnosis

### Hypertrichosis

a. Drugs: phenytoin, streptomycin, steroids, penicillamine, diazoxide, minoxidil
b. Pathologic states: hypothyroidism, anorexia, dermatomyositis, porphyria
c. Normal states: older age, ethnic background, pregnancy

### Hirsutism (increase in sexual hair)

#### Endogenous Androgen Overproduction

**Tumors**

Adrenal: adrenocortical tumors, adenomas, carcinomas
Ovarian: arrhenoblastomas, hilar cell, Krukenberg
Pituitary: adenomas

**Non-tumors**

Adrenal: congenital adrenal hyperplasia

- 21-hydroxylase deficiency
- 11-hydroxylase deficiency

### Ovary: Androgenized Ovary Syndrome

- Polycystic ovaries
- Hyperthecosis

### Initial Laboratory Studies

- Testosterone (>200 ng/dL possible adrenal tumor)
- DHAS (>700 mg/dL adrenal hyperplasia or tumor)
- 17-OH progesterone (<300 ng/dL or suppressible rules out adrenal hyperplasia)
- Prolactin
- Thyroid-stimulating hormone (TSH)
- Endometrial biopsy (individualize)

# ENDOCRINOLOGY

## Sources of Androgen Production

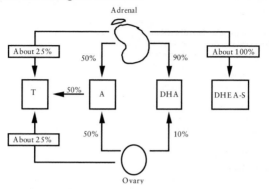

*Source:* Speroff L, Fritz MA. Hirsutism. In: *Clinical Gynecologic Endocrinology and Infertility.* 7th ed. Philadelphia:Lippincott Williams & Wilkins, 2004. Reproduced with the permission of the publisher.

# ENDOCRINOLOGY

## HYPERPROLACTINEMIA

### Definition
- Consistently elevated fasting serum prolactin (PRL) (>20 ng/mL) in the absence of pregnancy or postpartum lactation; nonpuerperal lactation

### Prolactin
- Little PRL = polypeptide hormone of 198 amino acids, but there are several different circulating forms.
- Circulating big PRL can be converted to little PRL by disulfide bond reduction.
- In the vast majority of cases, big-big PRL consists of a complex of PRL and an anti-PRL IgG autoantibody and is referred to as macroprolactin. Less commonly, big-big PRL is composed of either covalent or noncovalent polymers of monomeric PRL. This may account for 10% of hyperprolactinemia. A significant proportion of patients with macroprolactinemia appear to suffer from symptoms commonly associated with hyperprolactinemia and dopaminergic therapy may be beneficial. (Gibney I. *JCEM* 2005;90[7]:3927–3932.)

| Name | Molecular Weight | Biologically Active | Immunologically Active |
|------|------------------|---------------------|------------------------|
| Little PRL | 22 kd | Yes | Yes |
| Glycosylated little PRL | 25 kd | Yes, but decreased | No |
| Big PRL | 50 kd | No | Yes |
| Big-big PRL | >100 kd | No | Yes |

PRL, prolactin.

- Synthesized and stored in the pituitary gland in lactotrophs (also synthesized in decidua and endometrium, although not under dopaminergic control)
- Mean levels of 8 ng/dL in adult women; $t^1/_2$ = 20 minutes
- Cleared by the liver and kidney (hence ↑ PRL with renal failure)
- Functions:
  - Mammogenic → stimulates growth of the mammary tissue
  - Lactogenic → stimulates mammary tissue to produce and secrete milk

### Physiology
- Synthesis and release controlled by CNS neurotransmitters (usually inhibitory).
- Dopamine (DA; PRL-inhibiting factor) and cannabinoids inhibit secretion through $D_2$ DA receptors (DA-Rs) on lactotrophs (Pagotto et al., 2001).
- PRL-releasing peptide (PrRP), thyrotropin-releasing factor, and estrogen stimulate release (Rubinek et al., 2001).
- FSH may be suppressed by ↑ PRL through GnRH suppression.
- Episodic secretion varying throughout the day and cycle (↑ PRL at time of LH surge) (Djahanbakhch et al., 1984).

# ENDOCRINOLOGY

- No clinically relevant changes over the menstrual cycle, although there is a significant albeit subtle midcycle peak in PRL (Fujimoto et al., 1990).
- Hypertrophy and hyperplasia of lactotrophs in pregnancy in response to ↑ estrogen.
- PRL:
  - Steadily ↑ during pregnancy, reaching 200 ng/mL in the 3rd TM
  - Return to normal in nonlactating women 2–3 weeks postpartum
  - Return to normal in lactating women 6 months postpartum
  - ↑ With breast stimulation, exercise, sleep, stress

## Prevalence of Increased Prolactin with the Following Signs and Symptoms

| Sign/Symptom | ↑ Prolactin (%) |
| --- | --- |
| Anovulation | 15 |
| Amenorrhea | 15 |
| Galactorrhea | 30 |
| Amenorrhea + galactorrhea | 75 |
| Infertility | 34 |

*Source:* Adapted from Molitch ME, Reichlin S. Hyperprolactinemic disorders. *Dis Mon.* 1982;28(9):1.

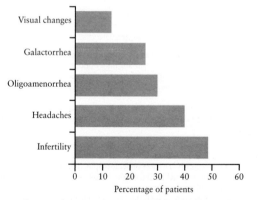

Most commonly reported symptoms in patients with hyperprolactinemia.
*Source:* Reproduced with permission from Bayrak A, Saadat P, Mor E et al. Pituitary imaging is indicated for the evaluation of hyperprolactinemia. *Fertil Steril.* 2005;84(1):181–185.

- ↑ PRL induces a dose-dependent ↑ DA secretion, which in turn inhibits GnRH pulsatile release through the $D_1$ receptor on GnRH neurons and by the activation of the β-endorphin neuronal system that further inhibits GnRH release (Seki et al., 1986).
- Autopsy: pituitary adenomas in 27% of women (Burrow et al., 1981) (PRL-secreting incidence in autopsies: 11%).

## Potential Causes of Hyperprolactinemia

| Cause | Example | Mechanism |
|---|---|---|
| Physiological | Pregnancy | Increasing estrogen levels |
| | Breast stimulation | Inhibition of dopamine via the autonomic nervous system |
| | Breastfeeding | Reduced dopamine stimulation |
| | Stress | |
| | Exercise | |
| | Sleep | |
| Pituitary disorders | Pituitary tumors: micro- or macroprolactinoma, adenoma, hypothalamic stalk interruption, hypophysitis (inflammation) | Disruption of dopamine delivery from the hypothalamus and/or secretion of growth hormone and prolactin |
| | Acromegaly | Prolactin secretion from a growth hormone adenoma |
| | Cushing syndrome | Prolactin secretion from a corticotroph adenoma |
| | Empty sella syndrome | Damage to/regression of the pituitary |
| | Rathke cysts | Compresses pituitary |
| | Infiltrative diseases (tuberculosis, sarcoidosis) | Infiltration of pituitary |
| Hypothalamic disorders | Primary hypothyroidism | Increased hypothalamic thyrotrophin-releasing hormone and decreased metabolism |
| | Adrenal insufficiency | |
| Medications | Anti-psychotics (phenothiazines, haloperidol, butyrophenones, risperidone, monoamine oxidase inhibitors, fluoxetine, sulpiride) | Inhibition of dopamine release |
| | Anti-emetics (metoclopramide, domperidone) | |
| | Antihypertensives (methyldopa, calcium channel blockers, reserpine) | |
| | Tricyclic antidepressants | |
| | Opiates | Stimulation of hypothalamic opioid receptors |
| | Estrogens | |

*(continued)*

| Cause | Example | Mechanism |
|-------|---------|-----------|
| Medications *(cont.)* | Verapamil | Positive action on lactotrophs |
| | Protease inhibitors | Unknown |
| Neurogenic | Chest wall injury | Peripheral triggers of autonomic control that interrupt central neurogenic pathways that attenuate dopamine release into the hypophyseal portal circulation; may act via the same nerves affected by nipple stimulation |
| | Spinal cord lesions | |
| Increased prolactin production | Polycystic ovarian syndrome | Usually transient |
| | Oophorectomy | |
| Reduced prolactin elimination | Renal failure | Less rapid clearance of prolactin from the systemic circulation plus central stimulation of prolactin |
| | Hepatic insufficiency | |
| Abnormal molecules | Macroprolactinemia | Polymeric form of prolactin formed following binding of prolactin to immunoglobulin G antibodies that cannot bind to the prolactin receptor |
| Idiopathic | Unknown | Unknown |

*Source:* Reproduced with permission from Crosignani PG. Current treatment issues in female hyperprolactinemia. *European Journal of Obstetrics & Gynecology and Reproductive Biology.* 2006;125:152–164.

- Islands of pituitary lactotrophs may be released from the normal tonic inhibitory effect of DA through spontaneous or estradiol ($E_2$)-dependent generation of arteriolar shunts (Elias and Weiner, 1984).
- Found in 10% of general population (most asymptomatic).
- **Found in 50% of women with hyperprolactinemia.**
- Incidence increases with (a) increasing PRL levels and (b) severity of symptoms.
- A genetic predisposition to hyperprolactinemia is suggested by an excess homozygosity for polymorphism 1 in exon 7 of the DRD2 gene (Hansen, 2005).
- Microadenoma <1 cm.
  - Prevalence of up to 27% in autopsy series (Burrow et al., 1981).
  - Enlargement uncommon (≤5%) (Schlechte et al., 1989).
  - Most regress spontaneously.
- Macroadenoma >1 cm and usually PRL >200 ng/mL.

## Prolactinoma (Most Common)

- Even with normal values or only mildly elevated PRL, patient may have a large tumor.
- Arise most commonly from the lateral wings of the anterior pituitary

**Correlation between the Pituitary Size and Serum PRL Level (ng/mL)**

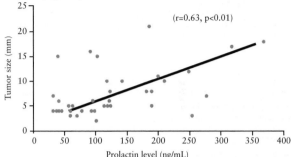

$(r=0.63, p<0.01)$

*Source:* Reproduced with permission from Bayrak A, Saadat P, Mor E et al. Pituitary imaging is indicated for the evaluation of hyperprolactinemia. *Fertil Steril.* 2005;84(1):181–185.

- Prevalence unknown
- The risk of diminished secretion of other pituitary hormones due to the presence of a prolactinoma is based on their proximity to the prolactinoma mass and their overall cell number: mnemonic for the adenohypophyseal hormones with the greatest to least propensity to be affected → **GnTAG** (% relates to the number of cells):
  - Gonadotropins (5%, close to lactotrophs), TSH (5%), ACTH (20%), GH (50%), antidiuretic hormone (rare, posterior pituitary)

## Acromegaly

- GH-secreting pituitary adenoma.
- Associated symptoms: macrognathia, spread teeth, sweaty palms, carpal tunnel syndrome.
- Affected patients experience symptoms of the disease ~7 years before diagnosis.
- GH can bind to PRL receptors (but PRL does not bind to GH receptors).
- ~20% of GH-secreting pituitary adenomas have concomitant hypersecretion of PRL.
- Check serum IGF-I (need age-adjusted and sex-adjusted IGF-I levels) as GH-secreting pituitary adenomas may not be visible on magnetic resonance imaging (MRI); IGF-I is produced primarily by the liver in response to GH.
- Diagnosis: elevated basal fasting GH and IGF-I; 1-hour glucose (100 mg) challenge test does not lead to GH levels <2 ng/mL in patients with acromegaly.
- Currently, surgery is the 1st choice for acromegaly.

# ENDOCRINOLOGY

## Cushing Disease

- Diagnosis: elevated 24-hour urinary free cortisol excretion and abnormal cortisol suppressibility to low-dose dexamethasone.
- Adenoma secretes ACTH. ↑ Supraclavicular/posterior dorsal fat.
- Patients present with hirsutism, coarse facial features, arthritis, and ↑ supraclavicular/posterior dorsal fat.
- 10% secrete PRL.

## Other Pituitary Tumors

- Clinically nonfunctioning pituitary tumor (most are classified as gonadotropic tumors; PRL usually ↓ with DA-agonist treatment), lymphocytic hypophysitis, craniopharyngioma, Rathke's cleft cyst, TSH-pituitary adenoma (rarest)

## Lactotroph Hyperplasia

- 8% of pituitary glands at autopsy.
- Can only be distinguished from microadenoma by surgery.
- Follistatin is a specific marker.

## Empty Sella Syndrome

- Congenital or acquired defect in the sella diaphragm.
- Intrasellar extension of the subarachnoid space results in compression of the pituitary gland and an enlarged sella turcica.
- 5–10% have hyperprolactinemia (usually <100 ng/mL).
- Diagnose with MRI.
- Benign course, although headaches (mostly localized anteriorly) are a frequent symptom (Catarci et al., 1994).

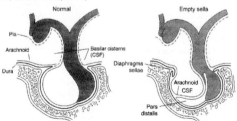

CSF, cerebrospinal fluid.
*Source:* Reproduced with permission from Jordan RM, Kendall JW, Kerber CW. The primary empty sella syndrome: analysis of the clinical characteristics, radiographic features, pituitary function and cerebrospinal fluid adenohypophysial hormone concentrations. *Am J Med.* 1977;62[4]:569.

## Hypothalamic Disease
- Alters normal portal circulation of DA
- Craniopharyngioma (most common)
- Infiltration of hypothalamus by sarcoidosis, histiocytosis, leukemia, carcinoma

## Pharmacologic Agents
- Interfere with DA production, action, uptake, or receptor binding.
- PRL levels range from 25–100 ng/mL.
- Return to normal level within days after the cessation of the offending drug (Rivera et al., 1976).
- Examples:
  - Neuroleptics (phenothiazines, haloperidol)
  - Antidepressants (selective serotonin reuptake inhibitors, not tricyclics)
  - Opiates
  - Antihypertensives ($\alpha$-methyldopa, reserpine, verapamil)
  - Metoclopramide (a DA-R blocker)
- H-2 blockers (intravenous cimetidine).

## Hypothyroidism
- Found in 3–5% of patients with hyperprolactinemia; 20–30% of patients with primary hypothyroidism have ↑ PRL.
- Galactorrhea secondary to ↑ thyroid-releasing hormone (TRH) → ↑ PRL.
- Primary hypothyroidism: ↓ thyroxine ($T_4$) → ↑ TRH → pituitary → ↑ TSH and ↑ PRL.
- Secondary hypothyroidism (from a pituitary tumor): normal TSH! Therefore, need to check $T_4$.

## Chronic Renal Disease
- ↓ PRL clearance and ↑ production rate

## Chronic Breast Nerve Stimulation
- Status post–thoracic surgery, herpes zoster, chest trauma

## Idiopathic Hyperprolactinemia
- PRL levels later return to normal in $^1/_3$.
- Unchanged PRL levels in nearly $^1/_2$.
- 10% have radiographic evidence of a pituitary tumor during a 6-year follow-up (Sluijmer and Lappohn, 1992).

# ENDOCRINOLOGY

## Evaluation of Elerated Prolactin

### Magnetic Resonance Imaging with Gadolinium Enhancement
- Preferred technique with resolution to 1 mm
- Accurate soft-tissue imagery without radiation exposure

### Laboratory Studies

| |
|---|
| Fasting a.m. laboratory tests: PRL, IGF-I, T4, TSH. |
| IGF-I obtained because 25% of acromegalics secrete ↑ PRL. |
| T4 obtained to rule out other pituitary tumor leading to low-normal TSH and low T4. |
| Cortisol, LH, FSH, α-subunit, if hyperprolactinemia and no response to medication, especially in cases with hypertension. |
| Routine breast examination does not acutely alter serum PRL levels in normal women (Hammond et al., 1996). |
| If PRL values are <200 ng/mL, and a macroadenoma (>10 mm) is seen on MRI, it is most likely not a prolactinoma (probably gonadotrope tumor or nonsecretory). |

### Three Caveats on the PRL Assay
1. The upper limit of PRL detection is usually between 180 and 200 ng/mL, so if the sample is not diluted, the value may be misleadingly reported as "200 ng/mL" when, in reality, with adequate dilution, the actual value is 2000 ng/mL or higher.
2. When present in very high concentrations, prolactin saturates both the capture and signal antibodies, blocks formation of the capture antibody-prolactin-signal antibody "sandwich," and results in falsely decreased prolactin results (referred to as the high-dose hook effect). Dilution of the sample eliminates the analytic artifact in these cases.
3. Macroprolactin due to immunoglobulins can be screened for with polyethylene glycol serum precipitation.

### Management
- Microadenoma or functional hyperprolactinemia: risk of progression for PRL-secreting tumors to macroadenomas is <7% (Gillam, 2005).
  - Most patients with microadenomas verified by MRI may be monitored by serial PRL as it is very rare for a prolactinoma to grow significantly without an increase in PRL (Hofle, 1998).
- Macroadenomas should be treated no matter the severity of symptoms.
- Without treatment of microadenomas, there is a 24% chance of PRL normalization within 5 years, and 95% do not grow (Schlechte et al., 1989).

## Goals of Treatment

| Low $E_2$ (<40 pg/mL) |
| --- |
| Estrogen treatment or oral contraceptives (OCs) (no ↑ size of microadenoma or ↑ [serum PRL]) to prevent osteopenia/osteoporosis |
| Yearly PRL levels |
| **Normal $E_2$** |
| Normal cycles |
| Yearly PRL levels |
| Oligomenorrhea or amenorrhea and $E_2$ >40 pg/mL |
| Progestin withdrawal or OCs |
| Yearly PRL levels |

## Treatment Endpoints (Effects of Medical Therapy)

- Bromocriptine (Parlodel) or cabergoline is used to achieve desired fertility (80% restored), relieve intolerable galactorrhea (60% eradicated), and reduce mass effect (reduced tumor size in 80–90%).

# ENDOCRINOLOGY

## Dopamine Agonists Commonly Used in the Treatment of Hyperprolactinemia

| | Bromocriptine | Cabergoline (Dostinex®) | Quinagolide (Norprolac®)[a] |
|---|---|---|---|
| Dopamine receptor target sites | $D_1$ and $D_2$ | $D_1$ (low affinity) and $D_2$ (high affinity) | $D_2$ |
| Duration of action | 8–12 hrs | 7–14 days | 24 hrs |
| Half-life (hours) | 3.3 | 65 | 22 |
| Available doses | 1.0 and 2.5 mg scored tablets; 5 and 10 mg capsules | 0.5 mg scored tablets | 25, 50, 75, and 150 mcg tablets |
| Typical dose | 2.5 mg/day in divided doses | 0.5 mg/week or twice weekly | 75 mcg/day |
| Dosing regimens, starter packs, dosage | Start on 1.25–2.5 mg/day at bedtime. Gradually increase to a median of 5.0–7.5 mg/day and a maximum of 15–20 mg/day | Start at 0.25–0.5 mg twice weekly. Adjust by 0.25 mg twice weekly up to 1 mg twice weekly every 2–4 mos according to serum prolactin levels | Start at 25 mcg/day. Increase over 1 week up to 75 mcg/day. Starter pack (3× 25 mcg tablets + 3× 50 mcg tablets) allows quick and convenient titration |
| Advantages | Long history of use; does not appear to be teratogenic; inexpensive | Good efficacy; low frequency of adverse events; may be useful in bromocriptine-resistant patients; weekly or twice-weekly dose | Good efficacy and tolerability; once-daily dosing; simple titration; pituitary selective; use to the time of confirmed pregnancy |
| Disadvantages | Tolerance; recurrence; resistance; multiple daily dosing | Not yet indicated for use during pregnancy | Not currently available in the United States or Japan |
| Common side effects | Nausea, headache, dizziness, abdominal pain, syncope, orthostatic hypotension, fatigue | Milder and less frequent compared with bromocriptine | Milder and less frequent compared with bromocriptine |

[a]Quinagolide is not registered for treatment of hyperprolactinemia in the United States or Japan.

*Source:* Reproduced with permission from Crosignani PG. Current treatment issues in femal hyperprolactinemia. *European Journal of Obstetrics & Gynecology and Reproductive Biology.* 2006;125:152–164.

## THYROID DISEASE

See also pg. 199 in Obstetrics chapter.

### Fast Facts

- Thyroid dysfunction is very common with 13 million Americans with some sort of thyroid disorder.
- Hypothyroidism occurs in 2% of adults and subclinical hypothyroidism in 5–17%.
- Early treatment of subclinical hypothyroidism may improve pregnancy outcome.

### Common Symptoms

### Hyperthyroidism

Anxiousness
Tremulousness
Rapid heartbeat
Feeling of warmth
Difficulty concentrating
Muscle weakness
Weight loss

### Hypothyroidism

Fatigue
Weakness
Weight gain
Constipation
Memory impairment
Cold intolerance
Muscle cramps
Infertility

# ENDOCRINOLOGY

## THYROID DISEASE
### Evaluation

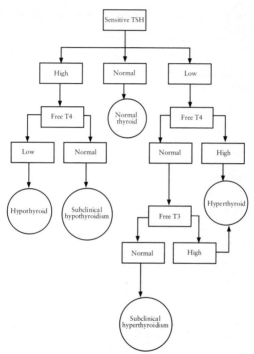

*Source:* Speroff L, Glass RH, Kase NG. Reproduction and the thyroid. In: *Clinical Gynecologic Endocrinology and Infertility.* 6th ed. Philadelphia: Lippincott Williams & Wilkins, 1999. Reproduced with the permission of the publisher.

## THYROID DISEASE
### Etiologies

| Primary Hypothyroidism | Central Hypothyroidism |
| --- | --- |
| Autoimmune thyroiditis (Hashimoto's) | Hypothalamic/pituitary disease |
| Postthyroidectomy | Tumors |
| Postradioactive iodine ablation | Infiltrative diseases |
| **Abnormal thyroid hormone biosynthesis** | Radiation therapy |
| Iodine deficiency | Postpartum pituitary necrosis |
| Inherited enzyme defects | Lymphocytic hypophysitis |
| Antithyroid drugs | Head trauma |
| **Thyroiditis (transient)** | |
| Silent thyroiditis | |
| Subacute thyroiditis | |
| Postpartum thyroiditis | |
| **Infiltrative thyroid diseases** | |
| Sarcoid | |
| Amyloidosis | |
| Hemochromatosis | |

| Primary Hyperthyroidism | Central Hyperthyroidism |
| --- | --- |
| **High radionuclide uptake** | **High radionuclide uptake** |
| Graves' disease | TSH-secreting pituitary adenoma |
| Toxic nodular goiter[a] | Thyroid hormone resistance |
| Toxic nodule[a] | |
| HCG-induced hyperthyroidism | |
| **Low radionuclide uptake** | |
| **Thyroiditis (transient)** | |
| Silent thyroiditis | |
| Subacute thyroiditis | |
| Postpartum thyroiditis | |
| **Excessive thyroid hormone** | |
| Ectopic thyroid tissue (struma ovarii) | |

[a]Radionuclide uptake may be within normal range.
*Source:* Reproduced with permission from Mulder JE. Thyroid disease in women. *Med Clin North Am.* 1998;82(1):103–125.

# INFERTILITY

## BASIC INFERTILITY

### Fast Facts

- 12% of all couples are childless.
  - Monthly pregnancy rate (PR) in couples with unexplained subfertility after 18 months duration → 1.5–3.0%.
  - Cumulative PRs for couples with unexplained subfertility 1 year and 3 years after the first visit are 13% and 40%, respectively.
- Approximately 50% of healthy women become clinically pregnant during the first two cycles, and between 80% and 90% during the first 6 months (Gnoth et al., 2003; Wang et al., 2003).

### Definitions

- **Subfertility:** failure to conceive after 6 months of unprotected intercourse (Gnoth, 2005)
- **Fecundability:** conception rate, usually *per month*
  - Normal → 20%
  - 38-year-old with 3-year history of infertility → 2%
- **Fecundity:** birth rate per 1 month

### Etiology

| Cause of Infertility | % |
|---|---|
| Tubal factor | 11 |
| Endometriosis | 6 |
| Ovulatory dysfunction | 6 |
| Diminished ovarian reserve | 7.9 |
| Uterine factor | 1.3 |
| Male factor | 18.5 |
| Other cause(s)[a] | 7 |
| Unexplained cause[b] | 12 |
| Multiple factors (female only) | 11.7 |
| Multiple factors (female + male) | 18.4 |

[a]Includes immunologic problems, chromosomal abnormalities, cancer chemotherapy, and serious illness.
[b]No cause of infertility found in either partner.
*Source:* Adapted from the Centers for Disease Control and Prevention. 2004 Assisted Reproductive Technology Success Rates, December 2006.

## Maternal Age

• Fertility decreases with maternal age.

| Age | Subfertile (%) |
| --- | --- |
| ≤30 yrs old | 25 |
| 30–35 yrs old | 33 |
| 35–40 yrs old | 50 |
| >40 yrs old | >90 |

**Effect of Age on the Cumulative Pregnancy Rate in a Donor Insemination Program**

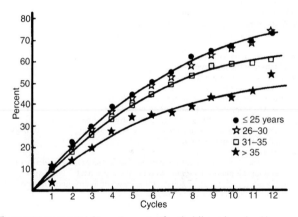

The younger age groups (<31 years) were significantly different from the older groups. *Source:* Reproduced with permission from Schwartz D, Mayaux MJ. Female fecundity as a function of age: results of artificial insemination in 2193 nulliparous women with azoospermic husbands. Federation CECOS. *N Engl J Med.* 1982;306:404. Copyright © 1982 Massachusetts Medical Society. All rights reserved.

# INFERTILITY

## Diagnostic Evaluation of the Infertile Couple

- History
  - Family history of endometriosis, early menopause
  - Previous surgeries
  - Menstrual irregularity
  - Dysmenorrhea, dyspareunia
  - Sexual dysfunction
- Physical exam/transvaginal ultrasound
  - Uterine appearance
  - Ovarian morphology and antral follicle count
  - Presence of ovarian cysts
- Laboratory testing
  - Prolactin/TSH
  - Assessment of ovarian reserve (see page 525)
    - ⇨ D3 FSH and estradiol
    - ⇨ CCCT
  - Semen analysis (see page 527)
- Evaluation of tubal patency
  - Hysterosalpingogram (HSG)
    - ⇨ Perform CD 6–12.
    - ⇨ Consider prophylactic antibiotics in high-risk patients.
      - ❖ Azithromycin 1 g PO qhs night before HSG
      - ❖ Doxycycline 100 mg PO bid night before and day of HSG
    - ⇨ Treat with extended antibiotics (doxycycline 100 mg bid × 7–10 days) if HSG reveals hydrosalpinx.
  - Laparoscopy
    - ⇨ Consider early in evaluation in patient with sonographic evidence of endometrioma or in patients who do not desire ART
    - ⇨ Useful in patients undergoing ART in cases of hydrosalpinx as removal will increase IVF success rates (see page 535)

## DIMINISHED OVARIAN RESERVE

### Definition
- *Diminished ovarian reserve* (DOR) refers to the condition of having a low number of normal oocytes or having poor quality oocytes (Scott et al., 1995).

### Background
- ↑ Age is associated with ↓ fecundity (ability to get pregnant), ↓ live birth rate, ↑ early follicular phase FSH levels, ↑ miscarriage rates, and ↑ IVF cancellation rates due to poor stimulation (Pearlstone et al., 1992; Pellestor et al., 2003; Stein, 1985).
- Despite age, some young, normally cycling women do not become pregnant with repetitive cycles of IVF, experience frequent miscarriage, or do not respond well to exogenous gonadotropins.
- From 1969 to 1994, the number of women older than 30 years having their first child ↑ from 4.1% to 21.2% (Heck et al., 1997).

### Implications
- Women with low ovarian reserve have ↓ fecundity with IVF cycles and natural cycles.
- Some of these women should be offered donor eggs and counseled about adoption.
- This **does not mean** that they do not ovulate, that they will not respond to gonadotropins or oral ovulation induction, or that there are **no** good eggs remaining within the ovary.
- It **does mean**, however, that **there are no means by which to selectively stimulate the good eggs to ovulate.**
- Before embarking on aggressive surgery or infertility treatment to enhance fertility, it is a good idea for some patients to undergo ovarian reserve testing.
- ↑ Incidence of Down syndrome in women with ↑ FSH, regardless of age (van Montfrans et al., 1999).

### Hormonal Tests

#### Caveats
- Different assays may report varying hormone levels from the same serum samples; it is important to calibrate the assay to that in the original studies (Sharara et al., 1998).
  - Dr. Toner's rule of thumb (Toner, 2003):

| Age = egg quality, whereas CD 3 FSH = egg quantity |
| --- |

# INFERTILITY

Ovarian reserve testing determines the number and quality of eggs present before infertility treatment:

| | |
|---|---|
| Day 3 FSH, E$_2$ | FSH on day 3 of <10 is normal. Levels between 10 and 14 are a gray zone with decreasing fertility as levels rise. FSH >14 results in a <1% chance of a live birth per cycle (Levi et al., 2001). E$_2$ should be <60 on day 3. Higher levels suggest early follicular recruitment, which results in a poor prognosis. |
| Clomiphene citrate challenge test | A more extensive test of ovarian reserve. Indicated for women ≥35 yrs old, smokers, those with one ovary or unexplained infertility, and patients in whom decreased ovarian reserve is suspected. Involves standard day 3 laboratory tests, as described above, along with the administration of clomiphene citrate, 100 mg days 5–9, and a repeat FSH on day 10. Day 10 FSH thresholds should be the same as those on day 3. |

E$_2$, estradiol; FSH, follicle-stimulating hormone.

- Understanding how the clomiphene citrate challenge test (CCCT) works:
  - Clomid blocks the effects of E$_2$ at the hypothalamus and pituitary, mimicking a hypoestrogenic state; the hypothalamic-pituitary axis responds by releasing a flood of FSH.
    ⇨ A woman with a normal, healthy cohort of follicles will produce enough E$_2$ and inhibin B to dislodge the Clomid and suppress FSH.
    ⇨ A woman with a poor cohort and aging follicles cannot generate enough E$_2$ or inhibin B to clear the Clomid or suppress FSH, respectively; therefore, FSH stays high.
    ⇨ A meta-analysis of CCCT studies concluded that there was too little difference between basal FSH(D3) and CCCT prediction to justify the additional cost and drug exposure (Jain et al., 2004).

## EVALUATION OF MALE FACTOR INFERTILITY

### Semen Analysis

- Collect × 2 if 1st one is abnormal; one test is not enough. Patient must be abstinent for 2–3 days before collection of semen.
- Collected by masturbation or by intercourse using special semen collection condoms that do not contain substances detrimental to sperm.
- Collected at home or in the laboratory; should be kept at room temperature during transport and examined within 1 hour of collection.
- Parameters can vary widely over time, even among fertile men, and exhibit seasonal variation.

| Parameter | Reference Value | Possible Pathologies |
|---|---|---|
| Volume | 1.5–5.0 mL (pH, 7.2) | Low: ejaculatory dysfunction, hypogonadism, poor collection technique |
| | | Acidic semen: ejaculatory duct obstruction, congenital absence of the vasa deferentia |
| Concentration | >20 million/mL | Azoospermia or oligospermia: varicocele, genetic, cryptorchidism, endocrinopathy, drugs, infections, toxins or radiation, obstruction, idiopathic |
| Total motile count | ≥10 million | — |
| Motility | >50% | Asthenospermia: prolonged abstinence, anti-sperm antibodies, partial obstruction, infection, sperm structural defects, idiopathic |
| Normal morphology | >30% normal (World Health Organization, 1999) | Teratospermia: varicocele, genetic, cryptorchidism, drugs, infections, toxins or radiation, idiopathic |
| | >14% normal (Kruger and Coetzee, 1999) | |
| Indirect immuno-bead assay (sperm antibodies) | ≥20% | Ductal obstruction, prior genital infection, testicular trauma, and prior vasovasostomy or vasoepididymostomy (50–70% incidence) |

Source: Adapted from World Health Organization. *WHO Laboratory Manual for the Examination of Human Semen and Semen-Cervical Mucus Interaction.* New York: Cambridge University Press, 1999.

### Total Motile Count

- Total motile count (TMC) *before processing* (million = volume × concentration × % motility):
- 10–20 million: IUI helpful

# INFERTILITY

- 5–10 million: IVF
- <5 million: intracytoplasmic sperm injection (ICSI)

## Morphology

| Morphology | Other | Recommendation |
|---|---|---|
| >4% | Irrespective | IUI |
| ≤4% | IMC >1 million<br>Motility >50%<br>≥2 follicles | 4 IUI cycles |
| ≤4% | IMC <1 million<br>Motility <50% | Intracytoplasmic sperm injection/*in vitro* fertilization |

IMC, inseminating motile count; IUI, intrauterine insemination.
*Source:* Adapted from Van Waart J, Kruger TF, Lombard CJ, et al. Predictive value of normal sperm morphology in intrauterine insemination (IUI): a structured literature review. *Hum Reprod Update* 7. 2001;(5):495.

## Antisperm Antibodies

- SperMAR ≥20% necessitates obtaining immunobead testing wherein head-binding antibodies are worse than tail, and >50% head-binding antibodies are worrisome (Clarke et al., 1985).
- Pregnancy rates are lower when >50% of sperm are antibody-bound (Ayvaliotis et al., 1985).
- ICSI can circumvent adverse effects of antisperm antibodies (ASAs).
- **Screen for ASA** when there is isolated asthenospermia with normal sperm concentration, sperm agglutination, or an abnormal postcoital test.
- ASAs found on the surface of sperm by direct testing are more significant than ASAs found in the serum or seminal plasma by indirect testing.
- ASA testing is not needed if sperm are to be used for ICSI.

## Round Cells

- Leukocytes and immature germ cells appear similar and are properly termed *round cells.*
- When >5 million/mL or >10/ high power fields (high power fields = 40× magnification), must differentiate using cytologic staining and immunohistochemical techniques.
- Mild prostatitis, epididymitis? (Treatment: ciprofloxacin [Cipro]).

## Hormones

- Evaluation of the pituitary-gonadal axis (1.7% incidence of abnormalities); evaluate if <10 million/mL sperm concentration, impaired sexual function, or other clinical findings suggestive of a specific endocrinopathy.

- Testosterone: ↓ if prolactinoma or hypogonadotropism.
- If low, obtain a repeat measurement of total and free testosterone.
- FSH: ↑ in germ cell aplasia.
- Prolactin: ↓ libido/impotence.
- Thyroid-stimulating hormone: leads to hyperprolactinemia.

| Clinical Condition | Follicle-Stimulating Hormone | Luteinizing Hormone | Testosterone | Prolactin |
|---|---|---|---|---|
| Normal spermatogenesis | Normal | Normal | Normal | Normal |
| Hypogonadotropic hypogonadism | Low | Low | Low | Normal |
| Abnormal spermatogenesis[a] | High/normal | Normal | Normal | Normal |
| Complete testicular failure/hypergonadotropic hypogonadism | High | High | Normal/low | Normal |
| Prolactin-secreting pituitary tumor | Normal/low | Normal/low | Low | High |

[a]Many men with abnormal spermatogenesis have a normal serum follicle-stimulating hormone, but a marked elevation of serum follicle-stimulating hormone is clearly indicative of an abnormality in spermatogenesis.

## Cystic Fibrosis Gene Mutations (Autosomal Recessive)
- Strong association between congenital bilateral absence of vas deferens (CBAVD) and mutations of the cystic fibrosis (CF) transmembrane regulator gene on chromosome 7.
  - CBAVD is associated with mutations within the CF gene in 70–80% of men.
  - CBAVD in 1% of infertile males.
- Besides CF gene mutations, a second genetic etiology involves abnormal differentiation of the mesonephric ducts.
- One of the more common diagnoses in patients with obstructive azoospermia.
- Seminal volume low (<1 cc), pH <7.0.
- Important to test patient's partner before performing a treatment that uses his sperm, because of the risk that his partner may be a CF carrier.

## Chromosomal Abnormalities Resulting in Impaired Testicular Function
- Prevalence of karyotypic abnormalities in infertile men: 7%.
- Frequency is inversely proportional to sperm count.
- 10–15% in azoospermic men.
- 5% in oligospermic men.
- <1% in normospermic men.

# INFERTILITY

- Klinefelter's syndrome (47,XXY or 46,XY/47,XXY) accounts for $^2/_3$ of the chromosomal abnormalities observed in subfertile men.
- Structural abnormalities of the autosomal chromosomes, such as inversions and translocations, are also observed at a higher frequency in infertile men than in the general population.
- Couple is at increased risk for miscarriages and children with chromosomal and congenital defects when the male has gross karyotypic abnormalities.
- Karyotyping should be offered to men who have nonobstructive azoospermia (NOA) or severe oligospermia (<5 million/mL) before IVF with ICSI.
- Genetic counseling should be provided whenever a genetic abnormality is detected.

## Y-Chromosome Microdeletions Associated with Isolated Spermatogenic Impairment

- Y-chromosome analysis should be offered to men who have NOA or severe oligospermia (<1 million/mL) before ICSI.
- Found in approximately 10% of men with azoospermia or severe oligospermia
- Too small to be detected by standard karyotyping but can be found by using polymerase chain reaction.
- The intervening large segment of the Y chromosome, known as the *male specific Y*, contains many genes involved in spermatogenesis.
- Regions prone to microdeletion: *AZFa, AZFb,* and *AZFc.*

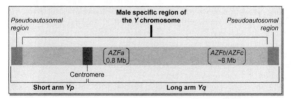

*Source:* Adapted from Oates RD. The genetics of male reproductive failure: what every clinician needs to know. *Sexuality, Reproduction and Menopause.* 2004;2(4):213.

- Microdeletion in *AZFc* region in 1 in 4000 men; most common molecular cause of NOA.
  - Approximately 70% of men with an *AZFc* microdeletion possess sperm.
  - 13% of men with NOA are *AZFc* microdeleted.
  - Approximately 6% of men with severe oligospermia, <5 million/mL, are *AZFc* microdeleted.

## Evaluation of Male Subfertility

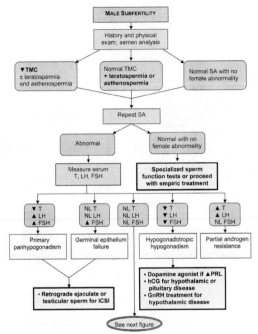

FSH, follicle-stimulating hormone; GnRH, gonadotropin-releasing hormone; hCG, human chorionic gonadotropin; ICSI, intracytoplasmic sperm injection; LH, luteinizing hormone; NL, normal; PRL, prolactin; SA, semen analysis; T, testosterone; TMC, total motile count. *Source:* Adapted from Swerdloff RS, Wang C. Evaluation of male infertility. UpToDate Patient Information Web site: http://www.utdol.com. Accessed February, 2005.

# INFERTILITY

## Evaluation of Male Subfertility

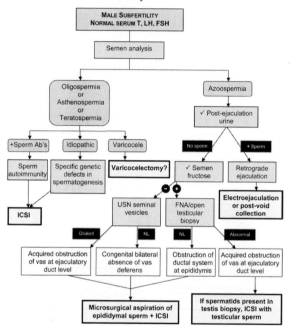

Abs, antibodies; FNA, fine-needle aspiration; FSH, follicle-stimulating hormone; ICSI, intracytoplasmic sperm injection; LH, luteinizing hormone; NL, normal; T, testosterone; USN, ultrasound.

*Source:* Adapted from Swerdloff RS, Wang C. Evaluation of male infertility. UpToDate Patient Information Web site: http://www.utdol.com. Accessed February, 2005.

## NON-ART TREATMENT OF INFERTILITY
### Ovulation Induction/Superovulation
### Clomiphene Citrate (Serephene, Clomid)
- Weak estrogen that functions as anti-estrogen.
- Requires intact hypothalamic-pituitary-ovarian axis.
  - Rule of 5s
    - ⇨ Oral progestin 10 mg q day × 5 days (after negative β-hCG).
    - ⇨ Begin clomiphene on day 5 of bleeding.
    - ⇨ 50 mg clomiphene q day × 5 days.
    - ⇨ Timed coitus 5 days later and for 5 days every other day.
  - Rule of 7s
    - ⇨ Check estradiol 7 days after last pill (CD#16) to assess recruitment.
    - ⇨ Check progesterone 7 days after estradiol to confirm ovulation.
    - ⇨ Check β-hCG 7 days after progesterone and perform pelvic exam/sonogram to assess prior to next clomiphene cycle.
- Increase clomiphene by 50 mg until ovulation obtained, 50% will ovulate on 50 mg.
- Follow follicular size with ultrasound.
- Consider IUI especially in couple with unexplained infertility.
  - Give 5000–10,000 mIU hCG when follicle 20–22 mm.
  - Ovulation will occur about 41 hours after hCG (Profasi).
- 15% of patients develop poor cervical mucus.
- Treatment usually limited to 4 ovulatory cycles as most pregnancies occur during 1st 4 cycles.

### Gonadotropins (FSH or FSH/Luteinizing Hormone (LH) Combinations) (see pg. 536)
- Candidates
  - Hypothalamic-pituitary failure
  - Hypothalamic-pituitary dysfunction
    - ⇨ PCOS or other anovulatory menstrual disorders
  - Unexplained infertility or minimal endometriosis
- Informed consent essential
  - Risk of multiple gestation (20%)
  - Risk of ovarian hyperstimulation depends on stimulation
- Administer hCG (Profasi) when estradiol 500–1500 pg/mL and lead follicle 20–22 mm
  - Timed intercourse that day and 2 days later or perform IUI

### Surgical Treatment of Tubal Factor Infertility
- Operative laparoscopy
- Hydrosalpinx: remove or clip hydrosalpinx
  - Meta-analysis: hydrosalpinx ↓ PR by 50% and ↑ spontaneous abortion × 2 (Camus et al., 1999)
  - Mechanism of adverse effect (Strandell and Lindhard, 2002)
    - ⇨ ↓ Nutrients in hydrosalpinx fluid
    - ⇨ Toxic effect of fluid on embryos (Sachdev et al., 1997) and/or sperm (Ng et al., 2000)
    - ⇨ ↓ Expression: $\alpha_v\beta_3$, leukemia inhibitory factor, HOXA10 (Meyer et al., 1997)
    - ⇨ Wash-out effect from fluid

⇨ ↑ Endometrial peristalsis due to hydrosalpinx fluid
⇨ ↓ Endometrial and subendometrial blood flow (Ng et al., 2006)
⇨ ↑ Endometrial inflammatory cells (Copperman, 2006)

- Ligation of the hydrosalpinx or salpingectomy restores normal PR (Johnson et al., 2002; Strandell et al., 2001a).
- Number needed to treat calculation: Seven to eight women would need to have a salpingectomy before *in vitro* fertilization (IVF) to gain one additional live birth (Johnson et al., 2002). A cost-effectiveness analysis of salpingectomy prior to IVF proved this to be a reasonable intervention (Strandell, 2005).
- Salpingectomy if hydrosalpinx seen on ultrasound:
  ⇨ No compromise of ovarian stimulation (Strandell et al., 2001b)
  ⇨ Randomized controlled trial (RCT) (192 patients; outcome = birth rate after first embryo transfer):

|  | Birth Rate (%)[a] |
|---|---|
| Salpingectomy | 28.6 |
| No intervention | 16.3 |

[a] $p < 0.05$.
*Source:* Adapted from Strandell A, Lindhard A, et al. Hydrosalpinx and IVF outcome: a prospective, randomized multicentre trial in Scandinavia on salpingectomy prior to IVF. *Hum Reprod.* 1999;14:2762–2769.

## Unexplained Infertility

- Intercourse, IUI, CC, CC/IUI, FSH, FSH/IUI, IVF
  - Retrospective analysis of 45 reports (Guzick et al., 1998)

| Method | Pregnancy Rate (%) |
|---|---|
| Intercourse | 4 |
| IUI | 4 |
| CC | 5.6 |
| CC + IUI[a] | 8 |
| FSH | 7.7 |
| FSH + IUI[a] | 17 |
| *In vitro* fertilization[a] | 21 |

CC, clomiphene citrate; FSH, follicle-stimulating hormone; IUI, intrauterine insemination.
*Note:* No randomized controlled trial: CC vs. CC/IUI; CC vs. FSH.
[a] Statistically significant difference.
*Source:* Adapted from Guzick DS, et al. Efficacy of treatment for unexplained infertility. *Fertil Steril* 70:207, 1998.

- IUI vs. FSH/IUI (randomized) (Guzick et al., 1999)

| Method | Pregnancy Rate (%) | LB/Couple (%) | LB/Cycle (%) |
|---|---|---|---|
| IUI | 18 | 13 | 4 |
| Follicle-stimulating hormone/IUI[a] | 33 | 22 | 8 |

IUI, intrauterine insemination; LB, live birth.
[a] Statistically significant difference.
*Source:* Adapted from Guzick DA, et al. Efficacy of superovulation and intrauterine insemination in the treatment of infertility. National Cooperative Reproductive Medicine Network. *N Engl J Med.* 1999;340:177.

## ASSISTED REPRODUCTIVE TECHNOLOGIES

### Fast Facts

- ART by definition are any fertility treatments in which **both egg and sperm** are handled. Accordingly, ART procedures involve the surgical removal of eggs, known as *egg retrieval.*
- IVF is the most common ART procedure; IVF has been used in the United States since 1981, and data are collected by the Centers for Disease Control and Prevention and published annually (http://www.cdc.gov/reproductivehealth/art.htm).
  - In 2004, 127,977 ART cycles were performed in over 400 fertility clinics.
  - 36,760 live births yielding 49,458 babies.

### Definitions

- IVF: ovulation induction, oocyte retrieval, and fertilization of the oocytes in the laboratory; embryos are then cultured for 3–5 days with subsequent transfer transcervically under abdominal ultrasound guidance into the uterine cavity.
- **Gamete intrafallopian transfer**: ovarian stimulation and egg retrieval along with laparoscopically guided transfer of a mixture of unfertilized eggs and sperm into the fallopian tubes.
- **Zygote intrafallopian transfer**: ovarian stimulation and egg retrieval followed by fertilization of the eggs in the laboratory and laparoscopic transfer of the day 1 fertilized eggs (*zygotes*) into the fallopian tubes.
- **Donor egg IVF**: used for patients with poor egg numbers or egg quality; involves stimulation of an egg donor with typical superovulation followed by standard egg retrieval; eggs are then fertilized by the sperm of the infertile woman's partner, and embryos are transferred to the infertile woman in a standard IVF-like process.
- ICSI: developed in the early 1990s to help couples with severe male factor infertility; one sperm is injected directly into each mature egg, typically resulting in a 50–70% fertilization rate.

# INFERTILITY

## Gonadotropin Preparations

| Trade Name, Manufacturer | Source |
|---|---|
| FSH/LH-containing preparations | |
| Pergonal, Serono[a] | Urine of menopausal women |
| Repronex, Ferring | Urine of menopausal women |
| Menopur, Ferring | Urine of menopausal women |
| Humegon, Organon[a] | Urine of menopausal women |
| FSH-containing preparations | |
| Bravelle, Ferring | Urine of menopausal women |
| Fertinex, Serono[a] | Urine of menopausal women |
| Gonal-F, Serono | Recombinant, Chinese hamster ovary cells |
| Follistim, Organon | Recombinant, Chinese hamster ovary cells |
| LH-only–containing preparation | |
| Luveris, Serono | Recombinant |

FSH, follicle-stimulating hormone; LH, luteinizing hormone.
[a]Drug has been discontinued.

## Human Chorionic Gonadotropin Preparations

| Trade Name, Manufacturer | Source | Formulations |
|---|---|---|
| Profasi, Serono[a] | Urine of pregnant females | 10,000 IU IM |
| Pregnyl, Organon | Urine of pregnant females | 10,000 IU IM |
| Novarel, Ferring | Urine of pregnant females | 10,000 IU IM |
| Chorex, Hyrex | Urine of pregnant females | 10,000 IU IM |
| Ovidrel, Serono | Recombinant, Chinese hamster ovary cells | 250 mcg SC |

[a]Drug has been discontinued.

## Gonadotropin-Releasing Hormone Agonist/Antagonist Preparations

| Trade Name, Manufacturer | Formulations |
|---|---|
| Lupron Depot, TAP (agonist) | 1 mg/0.2 mL = 20 U SC |
| Synarel, Searle (agonist) | 2 mg/mL intranasal |
| Zoladex, AstraZeneca (agonist) | 3.6 mg SC |
| Ganirelex, Organon (antagonist) | 250 mcg/0.5 mL SC |
| Cetrotide, Serono (antagonist) | 250 mcg/1 mL SC |

## Stimulation Protocols and Doses

- Estimating the patient's responsiveness to the fertility agents:
  - Age, body mass index, day 3 FSH/estradiol ($E_2$), ovarian volume, antral follicle count, response to prior ovarian stimulation

## Oral Contraceptive–Gonadotropin-Releasing Hormone Agonist Stimulation Protocol

- Oral contraceptives (OCs) can help with scheduling of IVF cycles and may help synchronize the ovary and result in a better cohort size. OCs typically increase the amount of medications required during stimulation and may decrease the number of eggs in older women.

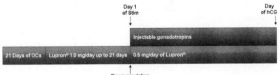

Oral contraceptive (OC)/gonadotropin-stimulating hormone agonist stimulation (Stim). hCG, human chorionic gonadotropin.

1. Start OCs between days 1 and 3 of menstrual cycle. Typically administer for 15–21 days.
2. Start GnRH-a 3–5 days before the completion of the OCs. This overlap of OCs and GnRH-a helps to prevent ovarian cyst formation.
3. Spontaneous menses expected 10–12 days after the 1st day of GnRH-a.
4. Start ovarian stimulation and continue GnRH-a. Stimulation is typically a step-down protocol, using a higher dose of medicine early in the stimulation and gradually decreasing the dose. Stimulation can be with FSH, human menopausal gonadotropin (HMG), or a combination of FSH and HMG.
5. Serial ultrasounds and $E_2$ levels monitor follicular development; $E_2$ should ↑ by 50% each day of stimulation.
6. Once follicle size reaches 18–22 mm, administer hCG, typically 5000–10,000 U SC or IM.
7. Oocyte retrieval 34–35 hrs after hCG.

# INFERTILITY

## Luteal Gonadotropin-Releasing Hormone Agonist Stimulation Protocol

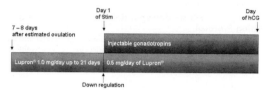

Gonadotropin-releasing hormone agonist stimulation (Stim). hCG, human chorionic gonadotropin.

1. Start GnRH-a on day 21 of menstrual cycle. The luteal start is typically confirmed by a serum progesterone level >4 ng/mL. The luteal start of GnRH-a helps to prevent ovarian cyst formation.
2. Spontaneous menses expected 10–12 days after the 1st day of GnRH-a.
3. Start ovarian stimulation and continue Lupron at lower dose. Stimulation is typically a step-down protocol, using a higher dose of medicine early in the stimulation and gradually decreasing the dose. Stimulation can be with FSH, HMG, or a combination of FSH and HMG.
4. Serial ultrasounds and $E_2$ levels monitor follicular development; $E_2$ should ↑ by 50% each day of stimulation.
5. Once follicular size reaches 18–22 mm, administer hCG, typically 5000–10,000 U SC or IM.
6. Oocyte retrieval 34–35 hours after hCG.

## Microdose Gonadotropin-Releasing Hormone Agonist Flare Stimulation Protocol

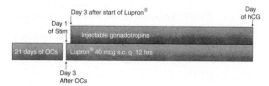

Microdose gonadotropin-releasing hormone agonist flare stimulation (Stim). hCG, human chorionic gonadotropin; OCs, oral contraceptives.

1. Start of OCs between days 1 and 3 of menstrual cycle and administer for 21 days. (Note: Many programs do not use OCs at all for this protocol.)
2. Start Lupron, 40 mcg SC q12hrs, 3 days after the end of the OC course (i.e., day 24).
3. Start ovarian stimulation with FSH, HMG, or a combination of FSH and HMG 3 days after the start of Lupron (i.e., day 27) and continue Lupron. (Note: Many programs start the gonadotropins on the same day as the microdose Lupron.)
4. Serial ultrasounds and $E_2$ levels monitor follicular development; $E_2$ should ↑ by 50% each day of stimulation.
5. Once follicular size reaches 18–22 mm, administer hCG, typically 5000–10,000 units SC or IM.
6. Oocyte retrieval 34–35 hours after hCG.

## Oral Contraceptive–Gonadotropin-Releasing Hormone Antagonist Stimulation Protocol

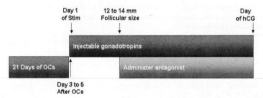

Gonadotropin-releasing hormone antagonist stimulation (Stim). hCG, human chorionic gonadotropin; OCs, oral contraceptives.

1. Start of OCs between days 1 and 3 of menstrual cycle. Typically, administer for 15–21 days.
2. Start ovarian stimulation 3–5 days after discontinuing OCs. Stimulation is typically a step-down protocol, using a higher dose of medicine early in the stimulation and gradually decreasing the dose. Stimulation can be with FSH, HMG, or a combination of FSH and HMG.
3. Serial ultrasounds and $E_2$ levels to monitor follicular development; $E_2$ should rise 50% per day.
4. Once a follicular size of 14 mm is reached, start GnRH antagonist. Administration of the GnRH antagonist can lower endogenous $E_2$ levels. Typically, no further decrease in gonadotropin dose is recommended. Rather, most clinicians add back FSH/LH drugs at time of antagonist start.
5. Once follicular size reaches 18–22 mm, administer hCG, typically 5000–10,000 U SC or IM.
6. Oocyte retrieval 34–35 hours after hCG.

# INFERTILITY

## Embryology Primer

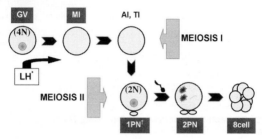

*Arrested at prophase I until luteinizing hormone (LH) surge. †Arrested at metaphase II until fertilization. AI, anaphase I; GV, germinal vesicle; MI, metaphase I; N, nuclei; PN, pronuclei; TI, telophase I.

- Retrieved eggs are identified in the follicular aspirate. Once they are identified, they are removed from the aspirate and placed in culture dishes.
- Standard IVF insemination is performed by culturing the identified eggs for approximately 16 hours with ≥50,000 sperm/mL. The next morning, the eggs are identified and evaluated for fertilization. The first sign of fertilization is two pronuclei within the cytoplasm.
- ICSI is performed in cases of severe male factor infertility, failed fertilization in a previous cycle, or severe antisperm antibody levels. After identification of the eggs in the follicular aspirate, the eggs are then placed into culture dishes. The cumulus cell complex surrounding the eggs is then removed in a process called *stripping*. Once the eggs are stripped, they are evaluated for maturity. Only metaphase 2 (MII) eggs can be fertilized. All MII eggs are then inseminated by taking one motile, morphologically normal-appearing sperm and injecting it into each mature egg.
- Fertilization rate with standard insemination is approximately 70%. With ICSI fertilization, rates range from 50–70%.
- Embryos are then cultured, typically for 3–5 days, in incubators maintained at body temperature and media specific for human embryo culture. Embryos are typically evaluated on day 3 for their cell number and overall morphology.
- It is most common for embryo transfer to be performed on day 3. In some centers, patients with a large number of embryos of high cell count and grade are placed into extended embryo culture for 2 additional days, referred to as the *blastocyst stage*.

- Extended embryo culture to the blastocyst stage may help to identify embryos with the highest prognosis for pregnancy. Cochrane Review concludes that there is little difference in the major pregnancy outcome parameters between day 2–3 embryo transfer and blastocyst culture (Blake et al., 2002).
- Blastocyst embryo transfer seems to increase the risk of monozygotic twins compared to day 2–3 embryo transfers (Behr et al., 2000).

## Postretrieval Hormonal Management

- Due to the use of GnRH-a and antagonists, there is concern about diminished progesterone secretion by the corpus luteum. Accordingly, the vast majority of ART cycles use supplemental progesterone via IM progesterone or vaginally administered progesterone. This is typically continued until 9–12 weeks of pregnancy.
- Some centers also replace $E_2$, which is also concomitantly secreted by the corpus luteum.

## Embryo Transfer

- On either day 3 or day 5, the embryos are typically transferred transcervically into the uterine cavity.
- The number of embryos transferred is ultimately based on the patient's age, prior IVF history, egg quality, embryo quality, and the IVF center's success rates.
- ASRM practice committee guidelines on number of embryos transferred:

## Recommended Limits on the Numbers of Embryos to Transfer

| | Cleavage Stage Embryos[a] | | | |
|---|---|---|---|---|
| Prognosis | Age <35 | Age 35–37 | Age 38–40 | Age >40 |
| Favorable[b] | 1–2 | 2 | 3 | 5 |
| All others | 2 | 3 | 4 | 5 |
| | Blastocysts[a] | | | |
| Favorable[b] | 1 | 2 | 2 | 3 |
| All others | 2 | 2 | 3 | 3 |

[a]See text for more complete explanations. Justification for transferring more than the recommended number of embryos should be clearly documented in the patient's medical record.
[b]Favorable = first cycle of *in vitro* fertilization, good embryo quality, excess embryos available for cryopreservation, or previous successful *in vitro* fertilization cycle.
*Source:* Adapted from Guidelines on the number of embryos transferred. The Practice Committee of the Society for Assisted Reproductive Technology and the American Society for Reproductive Medicine. *Fertil Steril.* 2006;86(4).

- Embryo transfer is typically performed under ultrasound guidance. A full bladder helps provide acoustic window and decreases the anterior bend of the cervix in patients with an anteverted uterus. This can ease embryo transfer.
- Patients are typically asked to rest for 12–24 hours after embryo transfer.

# INFERTILITY

## ASSISTED REPRODUCTIVE TECHNOLOGY SUCCESS RATES
### Pregnancy and Live Birth Rates by Age (non-donor eggs)

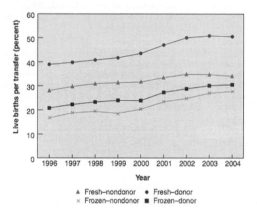

▲ Fresh–nondonor    ● Fresh–donor
× Frozen–nondonor    ■ Frozen–donor

Live births per transfer, by type of assisted reproductive technology cycle, 1996–2004. *Source:* Reproduced with permission from the Centers for Disease Control and Prevention (CDC). Section 5: Trends in ART. *2004 Assisted Reproductive Technology (ART) Report. 1996–2004.*

**Numbers of Assisted Reproductive Technology Cycles Performed, Live-Birth Deliveries, and Infants Born Using Assisted Reproductive Technology, 1996–2004**

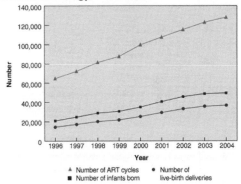

▲ Number of ART cycles    ● Number of
■ Number of infants born    live-birth deliveries

**Live Births Per Transfer for Assisted Reproductive Technology Cycles Using Fresh Embryos from Own and Donor Eggs, by Assisted Reproductive Technology Patient's Age, 2004**

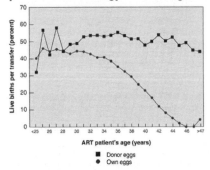

■ Donor eggs
● Own eggs

*Source:* Reproduced with permission from the Centers for Disease Control and Prevention (CDC). Section 5: Trends in ART. *2004 Assisted Reproductive Technology (ART) Report.* 1996–2004.

# INFERTILITY

## Comparison of the Cumulative Delivery Rates According to the Age and Number of Intracytoplasmic Sperm Injection Cycles

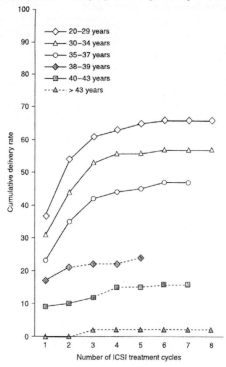

The plots illustrate the markedly reduced success rate of assisted reproductive technology in women aged >40 years. Increasing the number of intracytoplasmic sperm injection cycles improved the final success rate considerably in women aged 20–37 years but scarcely in older women.
*Source:* Reproduced with permission from Poppe K, Velkeniers B, Glinoer D. Thyroid disease and female reproduction. *Clin Endocrinol (Oxf).* 2007;66(3):309–321.

# OVARIAN HYPERSTIMULATION SYNDROME

## Incidence

- Iatrogenic complication of superovulation induction therapy (rarely clomiphene citrate) with a varied spectrum of clinical and laboratory manifestations
- Incidence in superovulation induction cycles:
  - Mild ovarian hyperstimulation syndrome (OHSS) → 33%
  - Moderate OHSS → 3–4%
  - Severe OHSS → 0.1–0.2%
- ↑ Incidence with:
  - Young age
  - More aggressive ARTs
  - Anovulatory women with PCOS
  - Large numbers of small/medium follicles at time of hCG administration

## Pathophysiology

- Ovarian enlargement with multiple cysts.
- Edema of stroma.
- ↑ Capillary permeability (marked arteriolar vasodilation) with acute fluid shift out of intravascular space.
  - ↑ Permeability secondary to a *factor* secreted by corpora lutea? *Factors:* Prostaglandins? Endothelin-I? Vascular endothelial growth factor? Angiotensin-II?
- Shift of fluid from intravascular space into the abdominal cavity → massive 3rd spacing
- Follicular aspirations may offer partial protection against OHSS.
- Early vs. late form (Papanikolaou et al., 2004):
  - **Early-onset OHSS** is related to exogenous hCG and is associated with a higher risk for preclinical miscarriage; presents 3–7 days after hCG administration.
  - **Late-onset OHSS** is more likely associated with pregnancy and tends to be more severe with a relatively low risk for miscarriage; presents 12–17 days after hCG administration.

## Hyperreactio Luteinalis

- Hyperreactio luteinalis (HL) can mimic OHSS (Foulk et al., 1997).
- HL is the benign hyperplastic luteinization of ovarian theca-interna cells, leading to multicystic ovaries (bilateral) and occasional hyperandrogenism.
- Both may be managed conservatively.
- Comparison features of OHSS and HL:

| Ovarian Hyperstimulation Syndrome | Hyperreactio Luteinalis |
| --- | --- |
| Ovulation induction | Absence of ovulation induction |
| 1st TM | Any time during pregnancy (54%, 3rd TM; 16%, 1st TM) |
| Associated with polycystic ovary syndrome, hypothyroidism | Associated with trophoblastic disease |

TM, trimester.

# INFERTILITY

## Management

- Conservative management leading to spontaneous resolution with time:
  - 7 days in nonpregnant women
  - 10–20 days in pregnant women
- Have patient drink ≥1 L fluid/day (Gatorade).
- ↓ Physical activity.
- Pelvic rest.
- Laboratory tests:
  - Electrolytes, creatinine
  - Complete blood count with platelets
  - Prothrombin time/partial thromboplastin time
- Management scheme:

| Classification | Clinical Characteristics/ Biochemical Parameters | Management |
|---|---|---|
| A: Mild | Abdominal distention Inconvenience | Accept as inevitable |
| B: Moderate | A plus: Ascites on sonogram Variable ovarian enlargement | Instruct patient carefully Self-monitoring of body weight Bed rest Abundant fluid intake Frequent follow-up (outpatient basis) |
| C: Severe | B plus: Massive ascites Hypovolemia | Hospitalization Consider paracentesis IV fluids (crystalloids/plasma expanders/ albumin) Monitoring fluid balance Low-dose heparin prophylaxis Diuretics only when hemodilution achieved Correction of electrolytes |
| D: Critical | C plus: Hematocrit >55% Impaired renal perfusion Thromboembolism Impending multiorgan failure | Intensive care unit Continuous monitoring of hemodynamics Perform paracentesis/transvaginal drainage IV heparin/SC heparin Consider termination of pregnancy |

*Source:* Adapted from Beerendonk CC, van Dop PA, Braat DD, et al. Ovarian hyperstimulation syndrome: facts and fallacies. *Obstet Gynecol Surv.* 1998;53:439.

## Treatment Algorithm for OHSS

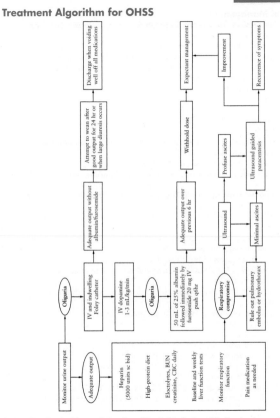

The algorithm contains the following elements:

- Monitor urine output
  - Oliguria → IV and indwelling Foley catheter → Adequate output without albumin/furosemide → Attempt to wean after good output for 24 hr or when large diuresis occurs → Discharge when voiding well off all medications
  - IV dopamine 1–3 mL/kg/min
  - Oliguria → 50 mL of 25% albumin followed immediately by IV push q6hr furosemide 20 mg IV push q6hr → Adequate output over previous 6 hr → Withhold dose
  - Adequate output → Heparin (5000 units sc bid)
- High-protein diet
- Electrolytes, BUN creatinine, CBC daily
- Baseline and weekly liver function tests
- Monitor respiratory function
  - Respiratory compromise → Rule out pulmonary embolus or hydrothorax
    - Ultrasound → Profuse ascites → Ultrasound guided paracentesis
    - Minimal ascites
- Pain medication as needed
- Expectant management
  - Improvement
  - Recurrence of symptoms

# INFERTILITY

## Hospital Management
### Admission Orders for Severe Ovarian Hyperstimulation Syndrome

1. Daily weight
2. Strict intake and output
3. Complete blood count, prothrombin time/partial thromboplastin time, electrolytes, liver function tests, and β-hCG on admission and p.r.n.
4. Chest x-ray and arterial blood gas if short of breath
5. Bed rest with bathroom privileges
6. Enoxaparin (Lovenox) if hemoconcentrated
   - Prophylaxis: 30 mg SC q12hours
   - Treatment: 1 mg/kg SC q12hours
7. Regular diet
8. IV fluid dextrose 5% in normal saline solution at 120 mL/hour without added potassium (see below)
9. Continue progesterone for luteal support
10. Acetaminophen with narcotics as needed; avoid nonsteroidal antiinflammatory drugs
11. Paracentesis/transvaginal aspiration for discomfort, shortness of breath, and/or persistent oliguria
12. If hypovolemic, oliguric (<30 cc/hour), see treatment algorithm on the previous page

- No pelvic/abdominal examinations secondary to fragility of ovaries (can precipitate ovarian rupture and hemorrhage)
- Chest x-ray if shortness of breath ensues
- White blood cell count >22,000 is an ominous sign of imminent thromboembolism (Kodama et al., 1995).
- K-exchange resins (i.e., Kayexalate) p.r.n.; no diuretics; electrocardiogram PRN for elevated K
- Anticoagulation in severely hemoconcentrated patients
- Transvaginal aspiration of ascites or of follicular structures
- Fluid replacement management (also see treatment algorithm above):
  - **Initial:** 1 L of normal saline × 1 hour (lactated ringer solution not recommended, as patients with severe OHSS are hyponatremic)
  - **Maintenance:** dextrose 5% in normal saline solution at 125–150 mL/hour; assess urinary output (UO) q4hours
  - **On diuresis:** Restrict oral fluids to 1 L/day and stop IV fluid
- A falling Hct + diuresis is an indication of resolution, not hemorrhage.

## Complications

### Tension Ascites

- Manifestation of capillary leakage.
- Pleural effusions may be associated with tension ascites.
- Treatment with paracentesis suggested by some.

### Thromboembolic Phenomena

- Coagulation abnormalities
- Hemoconcentration → arterial thromboemboli

### Liver Dysfunction

- Hepatocellular and cholestatic changes

### Renal Impairment

- Prenal failure secondary to ↓ perfusion from hypovolemia
- Sign of recovery from OHSS = ↑ urine output
- Renal-dose dopamine after restoration of plasma volume

### Acute Respiratory Distress Syndrome

- Due to ↑ capillary leakage
- Treat with positive end-expiratory pressure respiration

## Prevention

- Choice of stimulation protocol may help avoid this situation.
- Cancel cycle, withhold hCG.
- Give hCG, aspirate, then cryopreserve all embryos.
  - Aspiration of follicles has a protective effect (decreasing volume of granulosa cells and subsequent vascular endothelial growth factor production for late-onset OHSS but not necessarily for early-onset OHSS).
- Induce ovulation/oocyte maturation with:
  - Minimal effective dose of hCG: 5000 IU and avoid hCG in luteal phase

# INFERTILITY

## DIETHYLSTILBESTROL EXPOSURE

### Fast Facts
- 90% of those with clear cell carcinoma have adenosis of vagina.
- 20% have cervical hood, vaginal ridge, cockscomb cervix.
- 63% have uterus with T-shaped cavity and constrictions at cornu.
- 64% were fertile.

### Pregnancy Outcome (First Pregnancy)

| Result | Diethylstilbestrol Exposed (n = 150) | Unexposed (n = 181) |
|---|---|---|
| Term | 59 (52%) | 106 (83%) |
| Preterm (>26 weeks or <2500 g) | 23 (20%) | 8 (6%) |
| 2nd Trimester loss (14–26 weeks) | 5 (3%) | 2 (1%) |
| 1st Trimester loss (<13 weeks) | 19 (13%) | 12 (7%) |
| Ectopic | 8 (7%) | 0 |

*Source:* Herbst AL, Hubby MM, Azizi F, Makii MM. Reproductive and gynecologic surgical experience in diethylstilbestrol-exposed daughters. *Am J Obstet Gynecol.* 1981;141(8):1019-28.

### Exam

#### Diethylstilbestrol (DES) Exposed Female Offspring
- Start at 14 years or menarche or any age with symptoms.
1. Inspect the introitus and hymen to assess vaginal patency.
2. Palpate the vaginal membrane with the index finger. Note areas of induration or exophytic regions.
3. Perform speculum exam with the largest speculum that can be comfortably inserted. Adenosis will appear red and granular (strawberry surface).
4. Obtain cytologic specimens from the cervical os and the upper $^1/_3$ of the vagina.
5. Perform colposcopic exam on initial visit.
6. Biopsy indurated, exophytic lesions or colposcopically abnormal areas.
7. Perform bimanual exam.

### Follow-Up
- If no DES changes then yearly exam with Pap, colposcopy as indicated
- If has DES changes then q6mos exams with Paps and colposcopy q2yrs
- Male DES changes
  - Epididymal cysts, undescended testes, low sperm counts but NO malignancy

550

# RECURRENT PREGNANCY LOSS

## Incidence

- Fetal viability is only achieved in 30% of all human conceptions, 50% of which are lost before the first missed menses (Edmonds et al., 1982).
- **15–20%** of clinically diagnosed pregnancies are lost in the 1st or early 2nd trimester (TM) (Warburton and Fraser, 1964; Alberman, 1988).
- Risk of loss:
  - 12% after one successful pregnancy
  - 24% after two consecutive losses
  - 30% after three consecutive losses
  - 40% after four consecutive losses
- Risk of a 4th loss after three prior losses:
  - If no prior live birth → 40–45%
  - If ≥1 prior live birth → 30%
- ↑ Rate of pregnancy loss with advanced maternal age (most commonly, isolated nondisjunction) as well as advanced paternal age (Kleinhaus, 2006).
- 80% of spontaneous abortions (SABs) occur within first 12 weeks of pregnancy, and 60% of these are due to chromosome abnormalities.
- Recurrent pregnancy loss (RPL) is a risk factor for ectopic pregnancies (2.5%), complete molar gestations (5 in 2500), and neural tube defects (Adam, 1995).
- Prognostic value of transvaginal ultrasound observation of embryonic heart activity:

| Maternal Age (Yrs) | Risk of Loss (%) |
|---|---|
| ≤35 | <5 |
| 36–39 | 10 |
| ≥40 | 29 |
| History of recurrent pregnancy loss | 15–25 |

*Sources:* Adapted from van Leeuwen I, Branch DW, et al. First-trimester ultrasonography findings in women with a history of recurrent pregnancy loss. *Am J Obstet Gynecol.* 1993;168(1 Pt 1):111; Laufer MR, Ecker JL, et al. Pregnancy outcome following ultrasound-detected fetal cardiac activity in women with a history of multiple spontaneous abortions. *J Soc Gynecol Investig.* 1994;1(2):138; and Deaton JL, Honore GM, et al. Early transvaginal ultrasound following an accurately dated pregnancy: the importance of finding a yolk sac or fetal heart motion. *Hum Reprod.* 1997;12(12):2820.

## Definitions

- RPL (≥3 consecutive losses ≤20 weeks) occurs in approximately 1–4% (by chance the incidence would be 15% × 15% × 15% = 0.3%) (Salat-Baroux, 1988).
- Abortion: pregnancy loss before 20 weeks gestation or a fetal weight of <500 g.
- Primary RPL: refers to a woman who has never carried a pregnancy to viability.

# INFERTILITY

- **Secondary RPL:** refers to a history of ≥1 viable term pregnancy before a series of losses.
- **Early pregnancy loss:** refers to a loss <12 weeks estimated gestational age (EGA).
- **Late pregnancy loss:** refers to a loss between 12 and 20 weeks EGA.

## Etiology

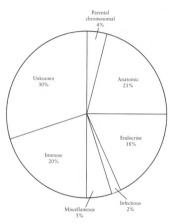

Etiologies of recurrent pregnancy loss.

- In approximately 30% of couples with RPL, there is no identifiable cause after sufficient workup (Boue et al., 1985).

### Genetic Factors
#### Parental Chromosome Abnormality
- Approximately 4% in couples with RPL (vs. 0.2% in normal population).
- The maternal to paternal ratio is 2 to 1.
- 4% probability that either parent is a carrier of a balanced translocation if there are ≥2 SABs or one SAB + a malformed fetus.
- Majority of abnormalities are balanced translocations (no DNA is lost and phenotype of the parent is normal), resulting in an unbalanced translocation in the fetus.

- Approximately 60% of balanced translocations are **reciprocal,** and 40% are **Robertsonian:**

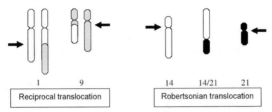

| 1 | 9 | | 14 | 14/21 | 21 |
|---|---|---|---|---|---|
| Reciprocal translocation | | | Robertsonian translocation | | |

*Source:* Reproduced with permission from PROLOG. *Reproductive Endocrinology and Infertility,* 4th ed. Washington, DC: American College of Obstetricians and Gynecologists, 2000:23.

- **Reciprocal translocation:** even exchange of chromatin between two nonhomologous chromosomes; *risk of a malformed, chromosomally abnormal liveborn varies depending on the size, specific translocation, and breakpoint: approximately 10–15%.*
- **Robertsonian translocation:** involves group D (13–15) and G (21 and 22) chromosomes (i.e., 14/21 translocation = long arms join up, but some short-arm material may be lost; breakage occurs close to the centromere; there are 45 chromosomes present (one normal 14 and 21, along with the balanced 14/21); *risk of an abnormal live birth ~10% if the mother is the carrier of a 21 translocation and 1% if the father carries the translocation.*

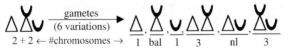

Robertsonian transfer. Robertsonian translocation: $^1/_3$ of gametes are normal (including balanced). Reciprocal translocation: $^1/_2$ of gametes are normal (including balanced). bal, balanced; nl, normal.

- ⇨ Robertsonian translocation of homologous chromosomes (incidence of 1 in 2500 with RPL) necessitates donor gametes for the affected partner.
- *De novo* translocations (Warburton, 1991):
  - ⇨ Reciprocal translocation: 1 in 2000
  - ⇨ Robertsonian translocation: 1 in 9000

# INFERTILITY

- Parental chromosomal testing may or may not demonstrate abnormality; there may be single gene defects that are not manifested by abnormalities; if an abnormal chromosome pattern is defined, there is nothing that can be done to lessen the chance for another loss (may offer controlled ovarian hyperstimulation with FSH); the parents should be referred to genetic counseling/prenatal diagnosis.
- Preimplantation genetic aneuploidy screening may improve the rate of live-births for unexplained RPL although, at this point, preimplantation genetic aneuploidy screening should not be performed on a routine basis.
- Turner mosaics are more susceptible to spontaneous miscarriages (Tarani et al., 1998):
  - Out of 160 pregnancies:
    ⇨ 29%: spontaneous loss
    ⇨ 20%: malformed babies (Turner syndrome [TS], trisomy 21, and so forth)
    ⇨ 7%: perinatal death

## Fetal Chromosomal Abnormality
- Approximately 60–75% of SABs (Fritz et al., 2001).
- Karyotyping of the conceptus may reveal need for parental karyotype testing.
- The karyotype of a 2nd successive spontaneous loss was abnormal in approximately 50–70% when aneuploidy was found in the 1st abortus, but in only 20% of cases in which the 1st abortus was chromosomally normal (Daniely et al., 1998; Hassold, 1980).
- It is generally held that fetal chromosomal abnormalities play a prominent role in affecting single pregnancy losses but not recurrent losses; in fact, as the number of losses increases, the chance of a fetal chromosomal aberration decreases (Ogasawara et al., 2000; Christiansen et al., 2002).
- According to one controlled clinical study, a significant proportion of unexplained RPL couples have microdeletions in the proximal portion of the AZFc region of the Y chromosome (Dewan, 2006).

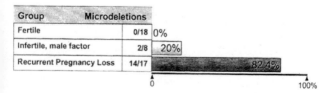

| Group | Microdeletions | |
|---|---|---|
| Fertile | 0/18 | 0% |
| Infertile, male factor | 2/8 | 20% |
| Recurrent Pregnancy Loss | 14/17 | 82.4% |

0                                                      100%

- A woman who loses a chromosomally abnormal fetus has a greater chance of a live birth than the woman losing a euploid embryo.

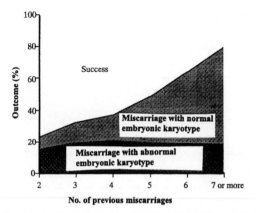

**No. of previous miscarriages**

*Source:* Reproduced with permission from Ogasawara M, Aoki K, et al. Embryonic karyotype of abortuses in relation to the number of previous miscarriages. *Fertil Steril.* 2000;73(2):300.

- As a group, the trisomies are the most common anomaly, and of these, trisomy 16 is the *most common trisomy* found in abortuses, although the *single most common aneuploidy* for 1st TM losses is 45,XO.

# INFERTILITY

## Anatomic Factors
### Congenital Uterine Anomalies

- Incidence of uterine malformations

| Defect | Fertile (n = 1289) (%) | RPL (n = 868) (%) |
|---|---|---|
| Arcuate | 1.6 | 1.0 |
| Septate | 1.5 | 2.0 |
| Bicornuate | 0.4* | 1.9 |
| Total | 3.8* | 6.3 |

| Defect | Controls (n = 1976) (%) | RPL (n = 509) (%) |
|---|---|---|
| Arcuate | 3.6* | 6.9 |
| Septate | 1.4* | 5.3 |
| Bicornuate | 0.2* | 1.2 |
| Total | 5.3* | 23.8 |

*p <0.05
Source: Adapted from Raga F, Bauset C et al. Reproductive impact of congenital Mullerian anomalies. Hum Reprod. 1977;12(10):2277 and Salim R, Regan L et al. A comparative study of the morphology of congenital uterine anomalies in women with and without a history of recurrent first trimester miscarriage. Hum Reprod. 2003;18(1):162. Note: Raga study classified RPL patients as having at least 2 consecutive losses; Salim study restricted to those with at least 3 consecutive losses although their controls had only a 54% live birth rate.

- Reproductive performance of different uterine malformations

| | Spontaneous Abortion (%) | Preterm Delivery (%) | Live Birth (%) |
|---|---|---|---|
| Didelphys | 20.0 | 53.3[b,c] | 40.0[f] |
| Unicornuate | 37.5[b] | 25.0[b] | 43.7[f] |
| Bicornuate | 25.0 | 25.0[b] | 62.5[e] |
| Septate | 25.5 | 14.5[b,d] | 62.0[e] |
| Arcuate | 12.7[a] | 4.5[a] | 82.7[e] |

Note: Statistical significance by column: a/b = p <0.05; c/d = p <0.01; e/f = p <0.001.
Source: Adapted from Raga F, Bauset C et al. Reproductive impact of congenital Mullerian anomalies. Hum Reprod. 1997;12(10):2277.

- A more recent study suggested that a bicornuate uterus is not generally associated with RPL (Proctor and Haney, 2003).
- Incomplete caudal to cephalad septum reabsorption, type V (**septate**) anomaly, is associated with a 60% rate of RPL (Buttram, 1983).
- *Note:* The vascular density in uterine septa removed at the time of metroplasty is similar to that of the normal uterine wall (Dabirashrafi et al., 1995).
- Pregnancy loss is more common among women with DES exposure (Kaufman et al., 2000).
- Benefit of metroplasty on pregnancy outcome has not been assessed by an RCT.

### Acquired Uterine Anomalies

- Intrauterine synechiae (also known as *Asherman syndrome*) from vigorous uterine curettage have been found to occur in 5% of women with RPL.
- Submucosal leiomyomas may cause an unfavorable implantation site by interfering with vascularization or by reducing the intrauterine cavity size; likewise, subserosal and myometrial fibroids may cause reproduction failure if they distort the uterine cavity. Submucosal leiomyomas lower *HOXA10* gene expression (important for implantation) (Cermik, 2002).
- Miscarriage rates are reduced after removal of large intramural fibroids (>5 cm) (Bajekal and Li, 2000).
- Uterine polyps may act like a foreign body and disrupt pregnancy; RCT of polypectomy vs. diagnostic hysteroscopy revealed greater pregnancy rate for definitive surgery (63% vs. 28%, *p* <0.001) (Perez-Medina, 2005).
- **Primary method of treatment in all cases is corrective surgery.** In the case of congenital anomalies, unification procedures such as the Strassman procedure are rarely undertaken. Septum resection is warranted. In the case of Asherman syndrome, hysteroscopy to lyse adhesions is advisable. Hysteroscopic myomectomy, when feasible, is recommended for submucosal fibroids.

## Endocrinologic Factors

### Luteal Phase Deficiency

- The insufficient level of progesterone, presumably from a deficient corpus luteum in the 2nd half of the menstrual cycle, is hypothesized to prevent implantation of conceptus or impair maintenance of pregnancy; luteal phase deficiency (LPD) is more clearly associated with RPL than subfertility; histologic differences between fertile and infertile women are not significant (Coutifaris et al., 2004); diagnose LPD if duration of luteal phase is <13 days (from positive LH kit to start of menses).
  - Normal women have endometrial histology suggestive of LPD in up to 50% of single menstrual cycles and 25% of sequential cycles (Davis et al., 1989).
  - Suggested treatment options include aromatase inhibitor, clomiphene citrate, recombinant human FSH, hCG, and progesterone supplementation (beginning 3 days after positive ovulation prediction kit until 10 weeks EGA).
  - Hyperprolactinemia has been shown to induce an LPD (possibly by ↓ progesterone from luteal cells); diagnose by prolactin level and treat with bromocriptine or cabergoline.

## Microbiologic Factors

- Several infectious agents have been implicated as etiologic factors in sporadic pregnancy loss, but no infectious agent has been clearly proven to cause RPL.
- Studies of women with RPL show an increased colonization with *Ureaplasma urealyticum* in the endometrium (Kundsin et al., 1981).

# INFERTILITY

- Other commonly linked infections include *Toxoplasma gondii*, rubella, herpes simplex virus, measles, cytomegalovirus, coxsackievirus, *Listeria monocytogenes*, and *Mycoplasma hominis*, although none has been convincingly associated with RPL.
- Bottom line: more cost effective and time efficient to empirically treat each partner with azithromycin (1 g × 1 **dose**) or doxycycline (100 mg bid × 10 days) than to pursue multiple and repeated cultures.
- Reasonable to omit infectious testing or treatment.

## Inherited Thrombophilia

- **Factor V Leiden (FVL)** thrombophilias and **prothrombin G20210A** mutation, found in approximately 9% (1% of these are homozygous for the FVL mutation) and 3%, respectively, of white women in the United States; these mutations are associated with approximately 25% of isolated thrombotic events and approximately 50% of familial thrombosis.
- Although all who carry the FVL mutation show phenotypic resistance to activated protein C (PC), approximately 15% of all cases of activated PC resistance are not due to being a carrier of the FVL mutation.
- RPL and maternal FVL or prothrombin G20210A.
  - Positive association with RPL prior to 10 weeks (Rey, 2003; Kovalevsky, 2004; Robertson, 2006)
  - No association with RPL prior to 10 weeks (Roque, 2004)
- There is a negative impact if ≥1 hereditary thrombophilia are found in EITHER partner, RR 1.9 (1.2, 2.8) (Jivraj, 2006).
- Only 2 small controlled studies (poor quality) assessed treatment efficacy; there was NO EFFECT (di Nisio, 2005).
- Bottom line—there is no evidence-based benefit of hereditary thrombophilia screening for early RPL.
- Other less common thrombophilias include autosomal-dominant deficiencies of the anticoagulants **PC, protein S (PS**; bad if <60%, then test antigenic levels of PS), **antithrombin III deficiency**, or **hyperhomocystinemia**.
- Methylene *tetrahydrofolate reductase* mutations and low vitamin B6 or B12 may lead to **hyperhomocystinemia:**
  - Mild: 16–24 mcmol/L
  - Moderate: 25–100 mcmol/L
  - Severe: >100 mcmol/L
  - Supplementation (see Treatment section for recommended doses) with vitamin B6, B12, and folate can often reduce homocysteine levels to normal, but this therapy has not yet been shown to result in a ↓ risk of thrombosis (Makris, 2000).
  - Compound heterozygotes for FVL and methylene tetrahydrofolate reductase alleles may experience worse outcomes.

- Risk of pregnancy loss (early + late pregnancy losses):

| Defect | Prevalence in Control Subjects (%) | Prevalence in Women with Pregnancy Loss[a] (%) | Risk of Pregnancy Loss (Odds Ratio) |
|---|---|---|---|
| Factor V Leiden | 9 | 8–32 | 2–5 |
| Prothrombin G20210A | 3 | 4–13 | 2–9 |
| Antithrombin III deficiency | 0–1.4 | 0–2 | 2–5 |
| Protein C deficiency | 0–2.5 | 6 | 2–3 |
| Protein S deficiency | 0–0.2 | 5–8 | 3–40 |
| Hyperhomocystinemia | 5–16 | 17–27 | 3–7 |

[a]Defined as first or recurrent early and/or late pregnancy loss.
*Source:* Adapted from Martinelli et al., 1998; Brenner et al., 1999; Ridker et al., 1998; Foka et al., 2000; Preston et al., 1996; Rai et al., 2001; Many et al., 2002; Sanson et al., 1996.

## Treatment

- Hereditary thrombophilia and history of RPL; there is no evidence of treatment efficacy although some treat women with thrombophilias and a history or RPL as follows:

| Defect | Treatment |
|---|---|
| Factor V Leiden, prothrombin G20210A, activated protein C resistance, protein S | ASA + LMWH/prophylactic heparin |
| Antithrombin III deficiency | ASA + full coagulation |
| ↑ Homocysteine | ASA + B6 (50 mg/day), B12 (1 mg/day), folate (0.8 mg/day) |

ASA, acetylsalicylic acid; LMWH, low-molecular-weight heparin.

## Immunologic Factors

### Autoimmunity (Self-Antigens) or Acquired Thrombophilia

- **Antiphospholipid-Ab syndrome** (APS or Hughes syndrome) believed to be a cause in approximately 5% of women with RPL; fetal loss more commonly occurs >10 wks of gestation (Simpson et al., 1998).
  - APS actually comprises two syndromes:
    - ⇨ Not associated with another illness (*primary APS*)
    - ⇨ Additional burden of systemic lupus erythematosus or other rheumatic disease (*secondary APS*)
  - $^1/_3$ of patients with lupus have antiphospholipid Abs.
  - Mechanism: uteroplacental thrombosis and vasoconstriction **secondary to** immunoglobulin binding to platelets and vascular endothelial membrane phospholipids; alternative mechanism is through activation of complement thereby increasing the inflammatory reaction at the placenta (Girardi, 2004).
    - ⇨ Note: True blood flow through placental vasculature does not occur until 9 to 10 weeks EGA (Jaffe et al., 1997).

# INFERTILITY

## Revised Classification Criteria for the Antiphospholipid Syndrome

Antiphospholipid antibody syndrome is present if at least one of the clinical criteria and one of the laboratory criteria that follow are met[a]

Clinical criteria

1. Vascular thrombosis[b]

One or more clinical episodes[c] of arterial, venous, or small vessel thrombosis,[d] in any tissue or organ. Thrombosis must be confirmed by objective validated criteria (i.e. unequivocal findings of appropriate imaging studies or histopathology). For histopathologic confirmation, thrombosis should be present without significant evidence of inflammation in the vessel wall.

2. Pregnancy morbidity

(a) One or more unexplained deaths of a morphologically normal fetus at or beyond the 10th wk of gestation, with normal fetal morphology documented by ultrasound or by direct examination of the fetus, or

(b) One or more premature births of a morphologically normal neonate before the 34th wk of gestation because of: (i) eclampsia or severe preeclampsia defined according to standard definitions, or (ii) recognized features of placental insufficiency,[e] or

(c) Three or more unexplained consecutive spontaneous abortions before the 10th wk of gestation, with maternal anatomic or hormonal abnormalities and paternal and maternal chromosomal causes excluded.

In studies of populations of patients who have more than one type of pregnancy morbidity, investigators are strongly encouraged to stratify groups of subjects according to a, b, or c above.

Laboratory criteria[f]

1. Lupus anticoagulant present in plasma, on two or more occasions at least 12 wks apart, detected according to the guidelines of the International Society on Thrombosis and Haemostasis (Scientific Subcommittee on LAs/phospholipid-dependent antibodies)

2. Anticardiolipin antibody of IgG and/or IgM isotype in serum or plasma, present in medium or high titer (i.e., >40 IgG phospholipid or IgM antiphospholipid, or > the 99th percentile), on two or more occasions, at least 12 wks apart, measured by a standardized enzyme-linked immunosorbent assay.

3. Anti-$\beta_2$ glycoprotein-I antibody of IgG and/or IgM isotype in serum or plasma (in titer > the 99th percentile), present on two or more occasions, at least 12 wks apart, measured by a standardized enzyme-linked immunosorbent assay, according to recommended procedures.

[a]Classification of antiphospholipid antibody syndrome should be avoided if less than 12 wks or more than 5 yrs separate the positive antiphospholipid test and the clinical manifestation.
[b]Coexisting inherited or acquired factors for thrombosis are not reasons for excluding patients from APS trials. However, two subgroups of APS patients should be recognized, according to: (a) the presence, and (b) the absence of additional risk factors for thrombosis. Indicative (but not exhaustive) such cases include: age (>55 in men, and >65 in women), and the presence of any of the established risk factors for cardiovascular disease (hypertension, diabetes mellitus, elevated LDL or low HDL cholesterol, cigarette smoking, family history of premature cardiovascular disease, body mass index ≥30 kg m$^{-2}$, microalbuminuria, estimated glomerular filtration rate <60 mL min$^{-1}$), inherited thrombophilias, oral contraceptives, nephrotic syndrome, malignancy, immobilization, and surgery. Thus, patients who fulfil criteria should be stratified according to contributing causes of thrombosis.
[c]A thrombotic episode in the past could be considered as a clinical criterion, provided that thrombosis is proved by appropriate diagnostic means and that no alternative diagnosis or cause of thrombosis is found.
[d]Superficial venous thrombosis is not included in the clinical criteria.
[e]Generally accepted features of placental insufficiency include: (i) abnormal or non-reassuring fetal surveillance test(s), e.g., a non-reactive non-stress test, suggestive of fetal hypoxemia, (ii) abnormal Doppler flow velocimetry waveform analysis suggestive of fetal hypoxemia, e.g., absent end-diastolic flow in the umbilical artery, (iii) oligohydramnios, e.g., an amniotic fluid index of 5 cm or less, or (iv) a postnatal birth weight less than the 10th percentile for the gestational age.
[f]Investigators are strongly advised to classify APS patients in studies into one of the following categories: I, more than one laboratory criteria present (any combination):IIa. LA present alone; IIb, aCL antibody present alone; IIc, anti-$\beta_2$ glycoprotein-I antibody present alone.

*Source:* Reproduced with permission from Miyakis S, Lockshin MD, Atsumi T et al. International consensus statement on an update of the classification criteria for definite antiphospholipid syndrome (APS). *J Thromb Haemost.* 2006;4:295–306.

## Treatment of APS

- **Low-molecular-weight heparin (LMWH) may be an effective alternative to unfractionated heparin** (Rai et al., 1997; Greer, 2002); initiate at positive pregnancy test, should stop at 36 weeks and potentially convert to unfractionated heparin to reduce risk of epidural hematoma.

> **Enoxaparin (Lovenox)**, 40 mg SC daily (Rai et al., 1997); adjust doses by weight (1 mg/kg/day) if obese (therapeutic dose: 1 mg/kg/day SC; full dose: q12hrs)
>
> Dalteparin (Fragmin), 5000 IU SC daily; adjust doses by weight (200 IU/kg/day) if obese (therapeutic dose: 100 IU/kg SC divided q12hrs)

- **Therapeutic unfractionated heparin levels** recommended if history of thrombosis (may use prophylactic unfractionated heparin, 5000 U bid, if no history of thrombosis).
- **Risk of thrombosis presumably highest first 6 weeks postpartum.**
- Initiating heparin before conception is potentially dangerous because of the risk of hemorrhage at the time of ovulation.
- Need close maternal and fetal surveillance secondary to high risk for complications (i.e., preeclampsia, fetal distress, intrauterine growth restriction, preterm labor, and so forth).
- Low-dose aspirin vs. placebo prospective study now under way.
- If surgery planned while on LMWH, stop 18–24 hours before procedure and restart 12 hours postprocedure. If emergent, can reverse with protamine sulfate; slow infusion, no need to reverse if >18 hours from last dose. For enoxaparin, use mg/mg, for dalteparin, 50 mg/5000 IU.

### Alloimmunity

- Controversy on how to diagnose and treat
- Refers to all causes of recurrent abortion related to an abnormal maternal immune response to antigens on placental or fetal tissues (i.e., T-helper [Th] 1 immunity)
- Th1 immunodystrophism: a dichotomous **Th1** (↑) and **Th2** (↓) cytokine profile directed toward trophoblasts (Hill et al., 1995); although an aberrant cytokine profile by peripheral blood mononuclear cells was not seen in RPL patients by one more recent report (Bates and Hill, 2002).
- Aberrant cytokine profile not detected in peripheral serum
- Treatment: immunosuppressive doses of progesterone vaginal suppositories (100 mg bid, beginning 3 days after ovulation)
- It has been proposed that maternal production of blocking factors may prevent maternal rejection of fetus, and RPL mothers do not make this blocking factor (Sargent et al., 1988):

# INFERTILITY

- Treatment: Immunotherapy to stimulate maternal immune tolerance of fetal material is **not effective** (Ober et al., 1999).
- Furthermore, agammaglobulinemic women are not at ↑ risk for fetal loss.
- APS: low-dose aspirin (81 mg/day) + LMWH with positive pregnancy test.

## Prognosis for Viable Birth (Derived from >1000 Cases at Brigham and Women's Hospital)

| Status | Intervention | Viable Births (%) |
|---|---|---|
| Genetic factors | Timed intercourse and supportive care | 20–90 |
| Anatomic factors | Surgery and supportive care | 60–90 |
| Endocrine factors | | |
|   Luteal phase deficiency | Progesterone ± ovulation induction and supportive care | 80–90 |
|   Hypothyroidism | Thyroid replacement and supportive care | 80–90 |
|   Hyperprolactinemia | Dopamine agonist | 80–90 |
| Infections | Antibiotics and supportive care | 70–90 |
| Antiphospholipid syndrome | Acetylsalicylic acid, heparin, and supportive care | 70–90 |
| Unknown factors | Timed intercourse and supportive care | 60–90 |

*Source:* Adapted from Hill JA. *Recurrent Pregnancy Loss: Male and Female Factor, Etiology and Treatment.* Frontiers in Reproductive Endocrinology. Washington, DC: Serono Symposia USA, Inc., 2001.

## ADVANCED CARDIAC LIFE SUPPORT (ACLS)

| Maneuver | Adult<br>Lay rescuer: ≥8 yrs<br>HCP: Adolescent and older | Child<br>Under 1 yr of age<br>HCP: 1 yr to adolescent | Infant |
|---|---|---|---|
| Airway | Head tilt-chin lift (HCP; suspected trauma, use jaw thrust) | | |
| **Breathing** (Initial) | 2 breaths at 1 sec/breath | 2 effective breaths at 1 sec/breath | |
| HCP: Rescue breathing without chest compressions | 10 to 12 breaths/min (approximate) | 12 to 20 breaths/min (approximate) | |
| HCP: Rescue breaths for CPR with advanced airway | 8 to 10 breaths/min (approximately) | | |
| Foreign body airway obstruction | Abdominal thrusts | | Back slaps and chest thrusts |
| **Circulation HCP:** Pulse check (≤10 sec) | Carotid | | Brachial or femoral |
| Compression landmarks | Lower half of sternum, between nipples | | Just below nipple line (lower half of sternum) |
| Compression method<br>Push hard and fast<br>Allow complete recoil | Heel of one hand, other hand on top | Heel of one hand as for adults | 2 or 3 fingers<br>HCP (2 rescuers): 2 thumb-encircling hands |
| Compression depth | 1¹/₂ to 2 in | Approximately one third to one half the depth of the chest | |
| Compression rate | Approximately 100/min | | |
| Compression-ventilation ratio | 30:2 (one or two rescuers) | 30:2 (single rescuer)<br>HCP: 15:2 (2 rescuers) | |
| **Defibrillation** AED | Use adult pads<br>Do not use child pads | Use AED after 5 cycles of CPR (out of hospital)<br><br>Use pediatric system for child 1 to 8 yrs if available<br><br>HCP: For sudden collapse (out of hospital) or in-hospital arrest use AED as soon as available | No recommendation for infants<br><br><1 yr of age |

AED, automated external defibrillator; CPR, cardiopulmonary resuscitation; HCP, maneuvers used by **only** healthcare providers.
*Source:* Reproduced with permission from the American Heart Association. *Circulation.* 2005;112 (24)suppl.

## ACLS

### Adult Basic Life Support Healthcare Provider Algorithm

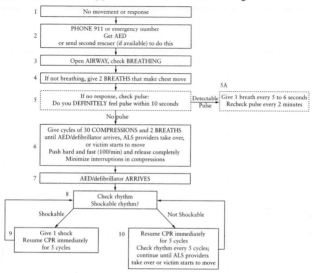

Boxes bordered with dotted lines indicate actions or steps performed by the healthcare provider but not the lay rescuer.

*Source:* Reproduced with permission from the American Heart Association. *Circulation.* 2005;112(24)suppl.

## Bradycardia Algorithm

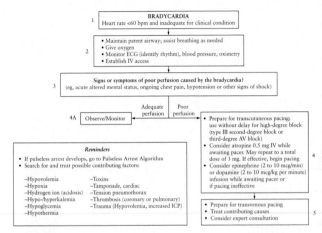

**1** BRADYCARDIA
Heart rate <60 bpm and inadequate for clinical condition

**2**
- Maintain patent airway; assist breathing as needed
- Give oxygen
- Monitor ECG (identify rhythm), blood pressure, oximetry
- Establish IV access

**3** Signs or symptoms of poor perfusion caused by the bradycardia?
(eg, acute altered mental status, ongoing chest pain, hypotension or other signs of shock)

Adequate perfusion → **4A** Observe/Monitor

Poor perfusion →

**4**
- Prepare for transcutaneous pacing; use without delay for high-degree block (type III second-degree block or third-degree AV block)
- Consider atropine 0.5 mg IV while awaiting pacer. May repeat to a total dose of 3 mg. If effective, begin pacing
- Consider epinephrine (2 to 10 mcg/min) or dopamine (2 to 10 mcg/kg per minute) infusion while awaiting pacer or if pacing ineffective

**5**
- Prepare for transvenous pacing
- Treat contributing causes
- Consider expert consultation

***Reminders***
- If pulseless arrest develops, go to Pulseless Arrest Algorithm
- Search for and treat possible contributing factors:

  –Hypovolemia         –Toxins
  –Hypoxia             –Tamponade, cardiac
  –Hydrogen ion (acidosis)  –Tension pneumothorax
  –Hypo-/hyperkalemia  –Thrombosis (coronary or pulmonary)
  –Hypoglycemia        –Trauma (Hypovolemia, increased ICP)
  –Hypothermia

*Source:* Reproduced with permission from the American Heart Association. *Circulation.* 2005;112(24)suppl.

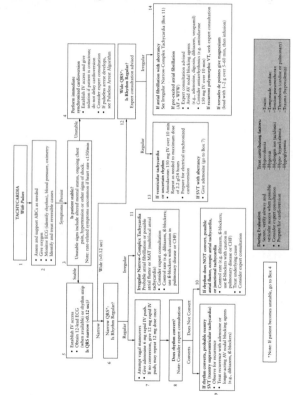

*Source:* Reproduced with permission from the American Heart Association. *Circulation.* 2005;112(24)suppl.

## ACLS Pulseless Arrest Algorithm

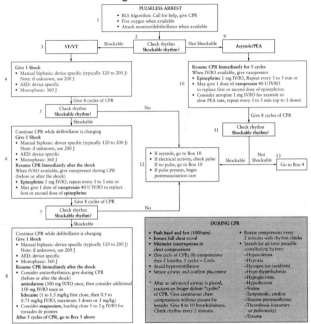

*Source:* Reproduced with permission from the American Heart Association. *Circulation.* 2005;112(24)suppl.

# ACLS

## Acute Coronary Syndromes Algorithm

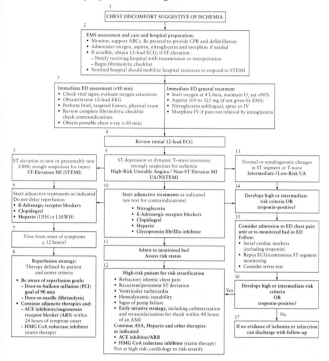

*Source:* Reproduced with permission from the American Heart Association. *Circulation.* 2005;112(24)suppl.

## Goals for Management of Patients with Suspected Stroke Algorithm

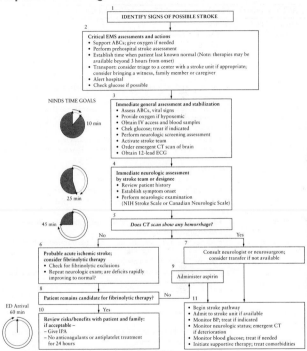

1
**IDENTIFY SIGNS OF POSSIBLE STROKE**

2
**Critical EMS assessments and actions**
- Support ABCs; give oxygen if needed
- Perform prehospital stroke assessment
- Establish time when patient last known normal (Note: therapies may be available beyond 3 hours from onset)
- Transport: consider triage to a center with a stroke unit if appropriate; consider bringing a witness, family member or caregiver
- Alert hospital
- Check glucose if possible

**NINDS TIME GOALS**

10 min

3
**Immediate general assessment and stabilization**
- Assess ABCs, vital signs
- Provide oxygen if hypoxemic
- Obtain IV access and blood samples
- Chek glucose; treat if indicated
- Perform neurologic screening assessment
- Activate stroke team
- Order emergent CT scan of brain
- Obtain 12-lead ECG

25 min

4
**Immediate neurologic assessment by stroke team or designee**
- Review patient history
- Establish symptom onset
- Perform neurologic examination (NIH Stroke Scale or Canadian Neurologic Scale)

45 min

5
**Does CT scan show any hemorrhage?**

No → 6
Yes → 7

6
**Probable acute ischemic stroke; consider fibrinolytic therapy**
- Check for fibrinolytic exclusions
- Repeat neurologic exam; are deficits rapidly improving to normal?

7
Consult neurologist or neurosurgeon; consider transfer if not available

9
Administer aspirin

8
**Patient remains candidate for fibrinolytic therapy?**

ED Arrival 60 min

No → 11

Yes → 10

10
**Review risks/benefits with patient and family: if acceptable –**
– Give IPA
– No anticoagulants or antiplatelet treatment for 24 hours

11
- Begin stroke pathway
- Admit to stroke unit if available
- Monitor BP; treat if indicated
- Monitor neurologic status; emergent CT if deterioration
- Monitor blood glucose; treat if needed
- Initiate supportive therapy; treat comorbidities

*Source:* Reproduced with permission from the American Heart Association. *Circulation.* 2005;112(24)suppl.

# ACLS

## Primary and Secondary ABCD Surveys: Modifications for Pregnant Women

| ACLS Approach | Modifications to BLS and ACLS Guidelines |
|---|---|
| Primary ABCD Survey | **Airway**<br>• No modifications.<br>**Breathing**<br>• No modifications.<br>**Circulation**<br>• Place the woman on her left side with her back angled 15° to 30° back from the left lateral position. Then start chest compressions.<br>   or<br>• Place a wedge under the woman's right side (so that she tilts toward her left side).<br>   or<br>• Have one rescuer kneel next to the woman's left side and pull the gravid uterus laterally. This maneuver will relieve pressure on the interior vena cava.<br>**Defibrillation**<br>• No modifications in dose or pad position.<br>• Defibrillation shocks transfer no significant current to the fetus.<br>• Remove any fetal or uterine monitors before shock delivery. |
| Secondary ABCD Survey | **Airway**<br>• Insert an advanced airway early in resuscitation to reduce the risk of regurgitation and aspiration.<br>• Airway edema and swelling may reduce the diameter of the trachea. Be prepared to use a tracheal tube that is slightly smaller than the one you would use for a nonpregnant woman of similar size.<br>• Monitor for excessive bleeding following insertion of any tube into the oropharynx or nasopharynx.<br>• No modifications to intubation techniques. A provider experienced in intubation should insert the tracheal tube.<br>• Effective preoxygenation is critical because hypoxia can develop quickly.<br>• Rapid sequence intubation with continuous cricoid pressure is the preferred technique.<br>• Agents for anesthesia or deep sedation should be selected to minimize hypotension.<br>**Breathing**<br>• No modifications of confirmation of tube placement. Note that the esophageal detector device may suggest esophageal placement despite correct tracheal tube placement. |

| ACLS Approach | Modifications to BLS and ACLS Guidelines |
|---|---|

- The gravid uterus elevates the diaphragm:
  - —Patients can develop hypoxemia if either oxygen demand or pulmonary function is compromised. They have less reserve because functional residual capacity and functional residual volume are decreased. Minute ventilation and tidal volume are increased.
  - —Tailor ventilatory support to produce effective oxygenation and ventilation.

Circulation

- Follow standard ACLS recommendations for administration of resuscitation medications.
- Do not use the femoral vein or other lower extremity sites for venous access. Drugs administered through these sites may not reach the maternal heart unless or until the fetus is delivered.

Differential Diagnosis and Decisions

- Decide whether to perform emergency hysterectomy.
- Identify and treat reversible causes of the arrest. Consider causes related to pregnancy and causes considered for all ACLS patients.

ACLS, advanced cardiac life support; BLS, basic life support.
*Source:* Reproduced with permission from the American Heart Association. *Circulation.* 2005;112 (24)suppl.

# ACLS

## Neonatal Resuscitation

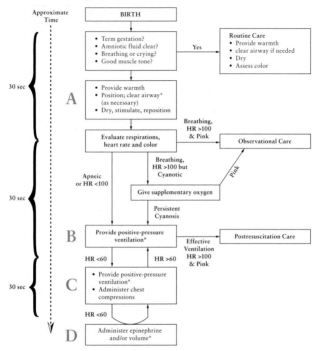

Approximate Time

**BIRTH**

- Term gestation?
- Amniotic fluid clear?
- Breathing or crying?
- Good muscle tone?

Yes →

**Routine Care**
- Provide warmth
- clear airway if needed
- Dry
- Assess color

30 sec

**A**

- Provide warmth
- Position; clear airway* (as necessary)
- Dry, stimulate, reposition

**Evaluate respirations, heart rate and color**

Breathing, HR >100 & Pink → **Observational Care**

Apneic or HR <100

Breathing, HR >100 but Cyanotic

Pink

**Give supplementary oxygen**

30 sec

Persistent Cyanosis

**B**

**Provide positive-pressure ventilation***

Effective Ventilation HR >100 & Pink → **Postresuscitation Care**

HR <60 | HR >60

30 sec

**C**

- Provide positive-pressure ventilation*
- Administer chest compressions

HR <60

**D**

**Administer epinephrine and/or volume***

*Endotracheal intubation may be considered at several steps

*Source:* Reproduced with permission from the American Heart Association. *Circulation.* 2005;112(24)suppl.

# LIFE-THREATENING ELECTROLYTE ABNORMALITIES

1) **Potassium (K⁺)**

   A) K⁺ gradient across cell membranes determines excitability of nerve and muscle cells (i.e., myocardium).

   B) Hyperkalemia.

      i) Defined as K⁺ >5 mEq/L; moderate (6–7 mEq/L) and severe (>7 mEq/L) are life-threatening.

      ii) Signs and symptoms: weakness, ascending paralysis, respiratory failure.

      iii) ECG findings: peaked T waves (tenting) → flattened P waves, prolonged PR interval (1st degree heart block), widened QRS complex, deepened S waves, and merging of S and T waves. If left untreated, a sine-wave pattern, idioventricular rhythms and asystolic cardiac arrest may develop.

---

**Common Causes of Hyperkalemia**

Endogenous Causes

   Chronic Renal Failure

   Metabolic acidosis (e.g., diabetic ketoacidosis)

   Pseudohypoaldosteronism type II (also known as Gordon's syndrome; familial hyperkalemia and hypertension)

   Chemotherapy causing tumor lysis

   Muscle breakdown (rhabdomyolysis)

   Renal tubular acidosis

   Hemolysis

   Hypoaldosteronism (Addison's disease, hyporeninemia)

   Hyperkalemic periodic paralysis

Exogenous Causes

   Medications: K⁺-sparing diuretics, ACE (angiotensin-converting enzyme) inhibitors, nonsteroidal anti-inflammatory drugs, potassium supplements, penicillin derivatives, succinylcholine, heparin therapy (especially in patients with other risk factors), β-blockers

   Blood administration (particularly in large transfusions of older "bank" blood)

   Diet (rarely the sole cause), salt substitutes

   Pseudohyperkalemia (due to blood sampling or hemolysis, high white blood cell count, high platelets, tumor lysis syndrome)

---

*Source:* Part 10.1: Life-threatening electrolyte abnormalities. *Circulation.* 2005;112:121–125.

      v) Treatment:

         (1) First

            (a) Stop sources of exogenous K⁺.

            (b) Evaluate drugs that can increase K⁺ (i.e., K⁺-sparing diuretics, angiotensin-converting enzyme inhibitors, nonsteroidal anti-inflammatory agents).

(2) For *mild* elevation (5–6 mEq/L), remove K$^+$ from body with
  (a) Diuretics: furosemide 40–80 mg IV
  (b) Resins: Kayexalate 15–30 g in 50–100 mL of 20% sorbitol PO or by retention enema
(3) For *moderate* elevation (6–7 mEq/L), shift K$^+$ intracellularly with
  (a) Glucose + insulin: mix 25 g (50 mL of D50) glucose and 10 U regular insulin and give IV over 15–30 minutes
  (b) Sodium bicarbonate: 50 mEq IV over 5 minutes
  (c) Nebulized albuterol: 10–20 mg nebulized over 15 minutes
(4) For *severe* elevation (>7 mEq/L with toxic ECG changes)
  (a) Shift K$^+$ into cells.
    (i) Calcium chloride (10%): 500–1000 mg (5–10 mL) IV over 2–5 minutes to reduce the effects of K$^+$ at the myocardial cell membrane (lowers risk of ventricular fibrillation)
    (ii) Sodium bicarbonate: 50 mEq IV over 5 minutes
    (iii) Glucose plus insulin: mix 25 g (50 mL of D50) glucose and 10 U regular insulin and give IV over 15–30 minutes
    (iv) Nebulized albuterol: 10–20 mg nebulized over 15 minutes
  (b) Promote K$^+$ excretion.
  (c) Diuresis: furosemide 40–80 mg IV.
  (d) Kayexalate 15–30 g in 50–100 mL of 20% sorbitol PO or per rectum.

C) Hypokalemia
  i) Defined as K$^+$ <3.5 mEq/L.
  ii) Signs and symptoms: weakness, fatigue, paralysis, respiratory difficulty, constipation, paralytic ileus, and leg cramps; more severe hypokalemia will alter cardiac tissue excitability and conduction.
  iii) Most common causes: GI loss (diarrhea, laxatives), renal loss, intracellular shift (alkalosis or a rise in pH), and malnutrition.
  iv) ECG findings: U waves, T-wave flattening, and arrhythmias (particularly ventricular arrhythmias); pulseless electrical activity or asystole may develop.
  v) Treatment
    (1) For K$^+$ <2.5 mEq/L or with arrhythmia
      (a) Gradual IV K$^+$ replacement with maximum amount of 10–20 mEq/hour with continuous ECG monitoring.
    (2) For rapid conversion if patient is clinically unstable
      (a) 10 mEq IV over 5 minutes, repeat once if needed.

       (b) Note in the chart that rapid infusion is intentional in response to life-threatening hypokalemia.

2) **Sodium (Na⁺)**

A) Na⁺ is the major intravascular ion that influences serum osmolality; acute changes in serum Na⁺ will produce free water shifts into and out of the vascular space.

    i) An acute fall → free water movement into the interstitial space and possible cerebral edema

    ii) An acute rise → shift of free water into the vascular space

    iii) Correct serum Na⁺ slowly over 48 hours avoiding overcorrection

B) Hypernatremia

    i) Defined as Na⁺ >145–150 mEq/L.

    ii) Causes include gains in Na⁺ (hyperaldosteronism, Cushing syndrome, excessive hypertonic saline or sodium bicarbonate administration) or loss of free water (GI losses or renal excretion).

    iii) Signs and symptoms: neurologic symptoms such as altered mental status, weakness, irritability, focal neurologic deficits and even coma or seizures.

    iv) Treatment

        (1) Reduce ongoing water loss and correct water deficit; for stable patients, replacement of fluid by mouth or NG tube is effective.

        (2) For hypovolemic patients: normal saline or a 5% dextrose in half-normal saline to prevent a rapid fall in serum Na⁺. Avoid D5W since this will reduce the Na⁺ too rapidly. Monitor serum Na⁺ closely.

        (3) Quantity of water needed:

           (a) Water deficit (in liters) =

$$\text{(i)} \quad \frac{\text{plasma Na}^{+}\text{concentration} - 140}{140} \times \begin{array}{c} \text{total body water} \\ (0.4 \times \text{weight in kg}) \end{array}$$

              (ii) Administer fluid to lower serum Na⁺ at a rate of 0.5–1 mEq/h with a decrease of no more than ~ 12 mEq/L in the first 24 hours and the remainder over the next 48–72 hours.

C) Hyponatremia

    i) Defined as Na⁺ <130–135 mEq/L.

    ii) Caused by reduced renal excretion of water with continued water intake or by loss of sodium in the urine (use of thiazide diuretics, renal failure, ECF depletion, syndrome of inappropriate antidiuretic hormone secretion, edematous states, hypothyroidism, adrenal insufficiency).

iii) Most cases are associated with low serum osmolality with the exception of uncontrolled diabetes when hyperglycemia leads to a hyperosmolar state despite a low $Na^+$.

iv) Signs and symptoms: usually asymptomatic unless it is acute or severe (<120 mEqL). An abrupt fall can lead to cerebral edema and resultant nausea, vomiting, headache, irritability, lethargy, seizures, coma or even death.

v) Treatment:

  (1) Administration of $Na^+$ and elimination of intravascular free water.

    (a) If SIADH → restrict fluid intake to 50–66% of estimated maintenance requirement.

  (2) Correction of asymptomatic hyponatremia should be gradual:

    (a) Increase the $Na^+$ by 0.5 mEq/L per hour to a maximum change of about 12 mEq/L in the first 24 hours.

    (b) If the patient develops neurologic compromise, administer 3% saline IV immediately to raise the serum $Na^+$ at a rate of 1 mEq/L per hour until neurologic symptoms are controlled. After neurologic symptoms are controlled, provide 3% saline IV to raise the serum $Na^+$ at a rate of 0.5 mEq/L per hour.

  (3) Quantity of sodium required to correct the deficit:

    (a) $Na^+$ deficit =

      (i) (desired $[Na^+]$ – current $[Na^+]$) × 0.5*× body wt (kg) (*Use 0.5 for women).

    (b) Once the deficit is estimated, divide the deficit by 513 mEq/L to determine the volume of 3% saline necessary to correct the deficit.

  (4) Plan to increase the $Na^+$ by 1 mEq/L per hour over 4 hours (or until neurologic symptoms resolve); then increase the $Na^+$ by 0.5 mEq/L per hour.

    To calculate the amount, use the amount you wish to correct the $Na^+$ in an hour (i.e., 0.5 mEq/L) and multiply by 0.5 (for women) and then multiply by the body weight (kg); that will calculate the amount of $Na^+$ to administer that hour.

  (5) Check serum $Na^+$ frequently and monitor neurologic status.

3) **Magnesium ($Mg^{++}$)**

  A) $Mg^{++}$ is necessary for the movement of $Na^+$, $K^+$, and $Ca^{++}$ into and out of cells; low $K^+$ in combination with low $Mg^{++}$ is a risk factor for severe arrhythmias.

B) Hypermagnesemia.
  i) Defined as $Mg^{++}$ >2.2 mEq/L.
  ii) Signs and symptoms: muscular weakness, paralysis, ataxia, drowsiness, and confusion; severe hypermagnesemia can lead to depressed level of consciousness, bradycardia, cardiac arrhythmias, hypoventilation, and cardiorespiratory arrest.
  iii) Most common cause is renal failure.
  iv) Treatment:
    (1) Cardiorespiratory support may be needed until $Mg^{++}$ levels are reduced.
    (2) 10% calcium chloride solution (5–10 mL [500–1000 mg] IV) will often correct lethal arrhythmias, may repeat if needed. The calcium removes $Mg^{++}$ from serum.
    (3) Dialysis is the treatment of choice for severe hypermagnesemia.
C) Hypomagnesemia
  i) Defined as $Mg^{++}$ <1.3 mEq/L; interferes with the effects of parathyroid hormone resulting in hypocalcemia.
  ii) Signs and symptoms: muscular tremors and fasciculations, ocular nystagmus, tetany, altered mental state, and cardiac arrhythmias such as torsades de pointes; other symptoms include ataxia, vertigo, seizures, and dysphagia.
  iii) Caused by decreased absorption or increased loss of $Mg^{++}$ (i.e., diarrhea); alterations in thyroid hormone function and certain medications (i.e. diuretics, alcohol).
  iv) Treatment:
    (1) For severe or symptomatic hypomagnesemia
        1–2 g IV $MgSO_4$ over 5–60 minutes.
    (2) For torsades de pointes with cardiac arrest
        1–2 g $MgSO_4$ IV push over 5–20 minutes.
    (3) If seizures are present
        2 g IV $MgSO_4$ over 10 minutes.
    (4) Patients with hypomagnesemia are also hypocalcemic.
4) **Calcium ($Ca^{++}$)**
  A) $Ca^{++}$ is the most abundant mineral in the body.
  B) Total serum $Ca^{++}$ is directly related to serum albumin:
      Total $Ca^{++}$ will increase 0.8 mg/dL for every 1 g/dL rise in serum albumin and will fall similarly.
  C) Ionized $Ca^{++}$ is inversely related to serum albumin:
      The lower the serum albumin, the higher the fraction of ionized $Ca^{++}$ so that in the presence of hypoalbuminemia, although total $Ca^{++}$ may be low, the ionized $Ca^{++}$ may be normal.

D) Hypercalcemia

   i) Defined as $Ca^{++}$ >10.5 mEq/L (or ionized $Ca^{++}$ >4.8 mg/dL).

   ii) Signs and symptoms when $Ca^{++}$ ≥12–15 mg/dL: depression, weakness, fatigue, and confusion at lower levels; at higher levels→ hallucinations, disorientation, hypotonicity, seizures, and coma; cardiovascular symptoms are variable but can lead to complete heart block when the total serum $Ca^{++}$ is >15–20 mg/dL; GI symptoms include dysphagia, constipation, peptic ulcers, and pancreatitis; kidney effects include diminished ability to concentrate urine with resultant loss of $Na^+$, $K^+$, $Mg^{++}$, and phosphate.

   iii) Primary hyperparathyroidism and malignancy account for >90% of reported cases.

   iv) Treatment:

      (1) Treat if symptomatic or $Ca^{++}$ >15 mg/dL.

         (a) Restore intravascular volume and promote $Ca^{++}$ excretion in the urine:

            (i) 0.9% saline at 300–500 mL/hour until fluid deficit is replaced and diuresis occurs (urine output ≥200–200 mL/hour).

            (ii) Once adequate rehydration has occurred, lower saline infusion to 100–200 mL/hour.

            (iii) Monitor $K^+$ and $Mg^{++}$ closely.

            (iv) If patient has heart failure→ hemodialysis; chelating agents may be used for extreme conditions.

            (v) Note: Use of furosemide may foster release of $Ca^{++}$ from bone, thus worsening hypercalcemia.

E) Hypocalcemia

   i) Defined as $Ca^{++}$ <8.5 mg/dL (or ionized Ca <4.2 mg/dL).

   ii) Signs and symptoms: paresthesias of the extremities and face, followed by muscle cramps, carpedal spasm, stridor, tetany, and seizures; hyperreflexia and positive Chvostek and Trousseau signs; cardiac effects include decreased myocardial contractility and heart failure.

   iii) Caused by toxic shock syndrome, abnormal serum $Mg^{++}$, thyroid surgery, fluoride poisoning, and tumor lysis syndrome.

   iv) Treatment:

      (1) Treat acute hypocalcemia with 10% calcium gluconate, 93–186 mg elemental $Ca^{++}$ (10–20 mL) IV over 10 minutes.

      (2) Follow this with an IV infusion of 540–720 mg of elemental $Ca^{++}$ (58–77 mL of 10% calcium gluconate) in 500–1000 mL D5W at 0.5–2 mg/kg per hour (10–15 mg/kg).

(3) Measure serum Ca$^{++}$ every 4–6 hours aiming for a total serum Ca$^{++}$ concentration of 7–9 mg/dL.

(4) Correct Mg$^{++}$, K$^+$, and pH abnormalities simultaneously. Note that untreated hypomagnesemia will often make hypocalcemia refractory to therapy.

# ANATOMY

## FETAL CIRCULATION

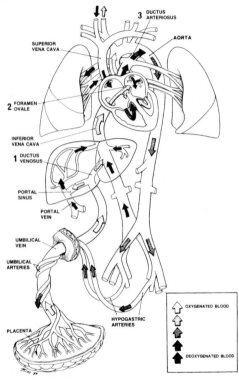

*Source:* Cunningham FG, MacDonald PC, Gant NF et al. The morphological and functional development of the fetus. In: *Williams Obstetrics.* 20th ed. Stamford, CT: Appleton & Lange, 1997. Reproduced with the permission of the publisher.

# PELVIC BLOOD SUPPLY

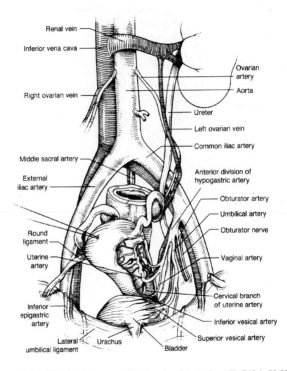

*Source:* DiSaia PJ. Clinical anatomy of the female pelvis. In: Scott JR, DiSaia PJ, Hammond CB, Spellacy WN, eds. *Danforth's Obstetrics and Gynecology.* 7th ed. Philadelphia: Lippincott, 1994. Reproduced with the permission of the publisher.

# ANATOMY

## LOCATION OF THE URETER

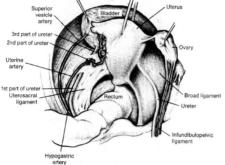

*Source:* DiSaia PJ, Creasman WT. Invasive cervical cancer. In: *Clinical Gynecologic Oncology.* 4th ed. St. Louis: Mosby Year Book, 1993. Reproduced with the permission of the publisher.

## BONY PELVIS

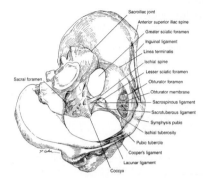

- Sacroiliac joint
- Anterior superior iliac spine
- Greater sciatic foramen
- Inguinal ligament
- Linea terminalis
- Ischial spine
- Lesser sciatic foramen
- Obturator foramen
- Obturator membrane
- Sacrospinous ligament
- Sacrotuberous ligament
- Symphysis pubis
- Ischial tuberosity
- Pubic tubercle
- Cooper's ligament
- Lacunar ligament
- Coccyx
- Sacral foramen

## LUMBAR/SACRAL NERVE PLEXUSES

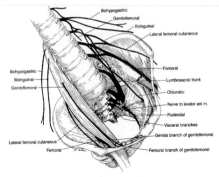

- Iliohypogastric
- Genitofemoral
- Ilioinguinal
- Lateral femoral cutaneous
- Iliohypogastric
- Ilioinguinal
- Genitofemoral
- Femoral
- Lumbosacral trunk
- Obturator
- Nerve to levator ani m.
- Pudendal
- Visceral branches
- Genital branch of genitofemoral
- Femoral branch of genitofemoral
- Lateral femoral cutaneous
- Femoral

*Source:* Burnett LS. Anatomy. In: Jones HW, Wentz AC, Burnett LS, eds. *Novak's Textbook of Gynecology.* 11th ed. Baltimore: Williams & Wilkins, 1988. Reproduced with the permission of the publisher.

# EPIDEMIOLOGY

## DEFINITION
• The study of health and health problems in populations

### Alternative Definitions
• Medical student: The worst taught class in medical school
• Resident: A very scary field in medicine filled with math
• David Grimes' mother: A dermatology subspecialty

### Epidemiologic Study Designs
• Descriptive Studies
• Analytic Studies
• Cohort Studies
• Case-Control Studies
• Experimental Studies
• Randomized Clinical Trials

### Basic Terms

*Prevalence*  $\dfrac{\text{\# of people who have a disease at one point in time}}{\text{\# of persons at risk at the point}}$

*Incidence*  $\dfrac{\text{\# of new cases of disease over a period of time}}{\text{\# of persons at risk during that period}}$

*Sensitivity*  The proportion of subjects with the disease who have a positive test (a/a+c)

*Specificity*  The proportion of subjects without the disease who have a negative test (d/b+d)

*Predictive value*
• Positive—likelihood a positive test indicates disease (a/a+b)
• Negative—likelihood a negative test indicates lack of disease (d/d+c)

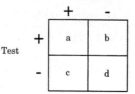

584

## DESCRIPTIVE STUDIES

### Advantages
- Data are relatively easy to obtain.
- Cost of obtaining data is relatively low.
- Ethical problems are minimal since the researcher does not decide which health services are to be received.

### Disadvantages
- No comparison group.
- Cause and effect relationships are suggested only.

### Study Design

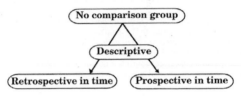

### Analysis
- Tables
- Histogram
- Line graphs
- Scatter diagrams
- Other graphic representation

## ANALYTIC STUDIES

### Essential Features

### There are at least 2 study groups:
- A group of subjects with the outcome or exposure of interest and a group of individuals without the health problem or exposure of interest.
- Association between exposure and outcome can be examined.
- Study subtypes named according to the determination of the study groups.

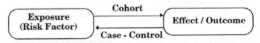

# EPIDEMIOLOGY

## COHORT STUDIES

### Advantages
- Avoids having to withhold treatment from those who wish to receive it
- Uses prospective data collection allowing standardization of eligibility criteria, the maneuver and outcome assessment
- Uses concurrent control group; co-intervention less likely to influence results since it should affect both groups
- Uses prospective data collection
- Can match for potential confounders during sample selection

### Disadvantages
- Impossible to ensure known confounding variables are equally distributed between groups
- Impossible to ensure that some factor unidentified by the investigator is not responsible both for exposure to the maneuver and good outcomes
- Difficult to achieve blindness to intervention with resulting bias likely (i.e., increased attention to experimental group)
- Difficult to obtain concurrent controls if therapy is in vogue
- Expensive in time, money, and subjects to do well

### Study Design

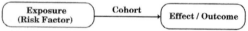

- At least two groups of subjects are studied.
- Entry into these groups is not randomized.
- Both groups of subjects are followed for a period of time to determine the frequency of the outcome in each group.
- The risk of developing the outcome for those exposed and those not exposed will be compared to see if there is a difference.
- To determine whether an association exists between an exposure (risk factor) and a future outcome (health problem).

### Analysis

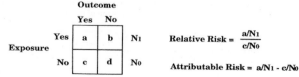

## CASE CONTROL STUDIES

### Advantages

- Useful for health problems that occur infrequently
- Useful for studying health problems with long latent interval
- Less time-consuming and less expensive than cohort studies because of the convenient sampling strategy and relatively short study period

### Disadvantages

- Selection bias—cases and controls are selected from two separate populations
  - Difficult to ensure that they are comparable with respect to extraneous risk factors and other sources of distortion
- Information bias—exposure data is collected from records or by recall after disease occurrence
  - Records may be incomplete and recall of past events is subject to human error and selective recall.
- Inappropriate for determining incidence rates
- Inappropriate for determining the other possible health effects of an exposure

### Study Design

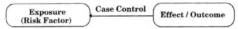

- Two groups of subjects studied: one group that experiences the outcome (cases) and the other that does not (controls).
- Entry into these two groups not influenced by the investigator and therefore cannot be randomized.
- Cases are identified during a given period of time.
- The exposure of the two groups to specific risk factors in the past is investigated.
- The likelihood that the cases were exposed to specific risk factors is then compared to the likelihood that controls were exposed to the same risk factors to see if there is a significant difference.

### Analysis

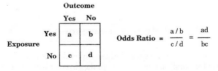

- Proportion that cases and controls represent in the population is unknown.
- Estimate of the relative risk can be obtained by cross-product ratio.
- Odds ratio approximates relative risk if incidence of outcome is <5%.

# EPIDEMIOLOGY

## RANDOMIZED CLINICAL TRIALS

### Advantages

- Controls selection bias effectively
- Balances potential confounding variables
- Allows standardization of eligibility criteria, exposures, and outcome assessments
- Statistically efficient because equal numbers of exposed and unexposed can be studied
- Statistically efficient because statistical power is not lost when confounding is controlled for in the analysis
- Theoretically attractive since many statistical methods are based on random assignment
- Concurrent comparison groups

### Disadvantages

- Design and implementation of an RCT may be complex.
- Extrapolation to the general population may be limited by careful selection criteria employed to conduct RCT.
- Open to ethical challenges: can exposure be ethically withheld from one group.

### Study Design

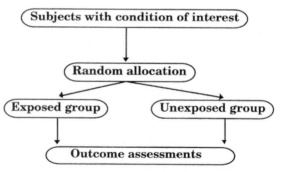

- Two groups of subjects are studied, those exposed to each of two treatments.
- Subjects are randomly assigned to one of the two treatment groups.
- Subjects are analyzed as part of the group to which they were randomized even if they fail to complete therapy (not intuitively obvious).

## Analysis

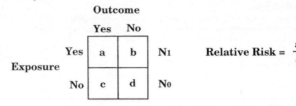

$$\text{Relative Risk} = \frac{a/N_1}{c/N_0}$$

- Essentially same analysis as for cohort study with determination of RR

## STUDY SIZE AND POWER ANALYSIS

### Type I Error (alpha error)

Probability of a study showing a statistically significant difference when no real difference exists (null hypothesis true). A $p$-value of 0.05 indicates a 5% probability of obtaining a difference when there is none.

### Type II Error (beta error)

False-negative result is the probability of failing to show a statistically significant difference when a true difference exists.

### Power

The probability of a study detecting a statistically significant difference when a real difference exists. Complement to Type II error as Power = 1 – beta.

# EPIDEMIOLOGY

## BIAS

### Selection Bias
The persons in one study group are different on some factor other than presence or absence of disease (case control) or exposure (cohort) that was not measured and therefore, cannot be controlled for in the analysis.

### Ascertainment Bias
The information regarding outcome in a cohort study or history of exposure in a case control study has not been obtained in an equal fashion for both subjects and controls.

### Confounding
The two comparison groups differ in some characteristic which is self-associated with both the outcome and exposure being studied but not directly involved in the causal pathway.

### Random Bias
The two comparison groups differ because of chance. Confidence intervals can be computed for the RR estimate thus allowing testing of the null hypothesis.

Special thanks to David Grimes, Ken Schulz, and the Berlex Foundation.

## CESAREAN SECTION

*Preoperative Diagnosis:*
1. 42-week intrauterine pregnancy
2. Failed induction
3. Inability of the fetus to tolerate labor

*Postoperative Diagnosis:* Same

*Procedure:* Primary Low Transverse Cesarean Section via Pfannenstiel

Surgeon:

Assistant:

*Anesthesia:* Epidural

*Complications:* None

*EBL:* 800 cc

*Fluids:* 1500 cc LR

*Urine Output:* 300 cc clear urine at end of the procedure

*Indications:* 20 years old G1P0 at 42 weeks, induced for post-dates, late decels with oxytocin, maximum dilation 2 cm.

*Findings:* Male infant in cephalic presentation. Thick meconium with none below the cords, pediatrics present at delivery, Apgars 6/8, weight 2980 g. Normal uterus, tubes, and ovaries.

*Procedures:* The patient was taken to the operating room where epidural anesthesia was found to be adequate. She was then prepared and draped in the normal sterile fashion in the dorsal supine position with a leftward tilt. A Pfannenstiel skin incision was then made with the scalpel and carried through to the underlying layer of fascia with the bovie. The fascia was incised in the midline and the incision extended laterally with the Mayo scissors. The superior aspect of the fascial incision was then grasped with the Kocher clamps, elevated, and the underlying rectus muscles dissected off bluntly. Attention was then turned to the inferior aspect of this incision which, in a similar fashion, was grasped, tented up with the Kocher clamps, and the rectus muscle dissected off bluntly. The rectus muscles were then separated in the midline, and the peritoneum identified, tented up, and entered sharply with the Metzenbaum scissors. The peritoneal incision was then extended superiorly and inferiorly with good visualization of the bladder. The bladder blade was then inserted and the vesicouterine peritoneum identified, grasped with the pick-ups, and entered sharply with the Metzenbaum scissors. This incision was then extended laterally and the bladder flap created digitally.

The bladder blade was then reinserted and the lower uterine segment incised in a transverse fashion with the scalpel. The uterine incision was then extended laterally with the bandage scissors. The bladder blade was removed and the infant's head delivered atraumatically. The nose and mouth were suctioned with the DeLee suction trap, and the cord clamped and cut. The infant was handed off to the waiting pediatricians. Cord gases were sent.

The placenta was then removed manually; the uterus exteriorized, and cleared of all clots and debris. The uterine incision was repaired with 1-0 chromic in a running, locked fashion. A second layer of the same suture was used to obtain excellent hemostasis. The bladder flap was repaired with 3-0 Vicryl in a running stitch and uterus returned to the abdomen. The gutters were cleared of all clots, and the peritoneum closed with 3-0 Vicryl. The fascia was reapproximated with 0 Vicryl in a running fashion. The skin was closed with staples.

The patient tolerated the procedure well. Sponge, lap, and needle counts were correct times two. Two grams of Cefotetan was given at cord clamp. The patient was taken to the recovery room in stable condition.

# TUBAL LIGATION

*Preoperative Diagnosis:* Multiparity, desires permanent sterilization
*Postoperative Diagnosis:* Same
*Procedure:* Postpartum tubal ligation, Pomeroy method
Surgeon:
Assistant:
*Anesthesia:* Epidural
*Complications:* None
*EBL:* <20 cc
*Fluids:* 500 cc LR

*Indications:* 35 years old G5P4014 s/p NSVD who desires permanent sterilization. Risk/benefits of procedure discussed with patient including risk of failure of 3–5/1000 with increased risk of ectopic gestation if pregnancy occurs.

*Findings:* Normal uterus, tubes, and ovaries

*Procedure:* The patient was taken to the operating room where her epidural was found to be adequate. A small transverse, infraumbilical skin incision was then made with the scalpel. The incision was carried down through the underlying fascia until the peritoneum was identified and entered. The peritoneum was noted to be free of any adhesions and the incision was then extended with the Metzenbaum scissors.

The patient's left fallopian tube was then identified, brought to the incision, and grasped with a Babcock clamp. The tube was then followed out to the fimbria. The Babcock clamp was then used to grasp the tube approximately 4 cm from the cornual region. A 3 cm segment of tube was then ligated with a free tie of plain gut, and excised. Good hemostasis was noted and the tube was returned to the abdomen. The right fallopian tube was then ligated, and a 3 cm segment excised in a similar fashion. Excellent hemostasis was noted, and the tube returned to the abdomen.

The peritoneum and fascia were then closed in a single layer using 3-0 Vicryl. The skin was closed in a subcuticular fashion using 3-0 Vicryl on Keith needle.

The patient tolerated the procedure well. Sponge, lap, and needle counts were correct times two. The patient was taken to the recovery room in stable condition.

*Pathology:* Segments of right and left fallopian tubes.

# OPERATIVE REPORTS

## DILATION & CURETTAGE

*Preoperative Diagnosis:* 8-week intrauterine pregnancy with incomplete abortion

*Postoperative Diagnosis:* Same

*Procedure:* Suction dilation & curettage

*Surgeon:*

*Assistant:*

*Anesthesia:* Paracervical block, IV Fentanyl

*Complications:* None

*EBL:* 50 cc

*Findings:* 8-week–sized anteverted uterus, moderate amounts of products of conception

*Procedure:* The patient was taken to the Special Procedure Room in the Gynecologic Clinic after a deformed gestational sac had been noted on transvaginal ultrasound. A sterile speculum was placed in the patient's vagina and the cervix noted to be 1 cm dilated with products of conception present at the cervical os. The cervix and vagina were then swabbed with Betadine and 2 cc of Xylocaine injected into the anterior lip of the cervix. The single tooth tenaculum was then applied to this location and 5 cc of Xylocaine then injected at 4 o'clock and 7 o'clock to produce a paracervical block.

The uterus was then gently sounded to 9 cm, and an 8 mm suction curette advanced gently to the uterine fundus. The suction device was then activated and the curette rotated to clear the uterus of the products of conception. A sharp curettage was then performed until a gritty texture was noted. The suction curette was then reintroduced to clear the uterus of all remaining products of conception. There was minimal bleeding noted and the tenaculum removed with good hemostasis noted.

The patient tolerated the procedure well. The patient was taken to the recovery area in stable condition.

*Pathology:* Products of conception.

## LAPAROSCOPIC TUBAL LIGATION

*Preoperative Diagnosis:* Multiparity, desires permanent sterilization
*Postoperative Diagnosis:* Multiparity, desires permanent sterilization
*Procedure:* Laparoscopic tubal ligation with Falope rings
*Surgeon:*
*Assistant:*
*Anesthesia:* General endotracheal
*Complications:* None
*EBL:* 25 cc
*Fluids:* 1500 cc LR
*Urine Output:* 100 cc clear urine at end of the procedure

*Findings:* Normal uterus, tubes and ovaries

*Technique:* The patient was taken to the operating room where general anesthesia was obtained without difficulty. The patient was then examined under anesthesia and found to have a small anteverted uterus with normal adnexa. She was then placed in the dorsal lithotomy position and prepared and draped in the sterile fashion. A bivalve speculum was then placed in the patient's vagina and the anterior lip of the cervix grasped with the single toothed tenaculum. A HUMI uterine manipulator was then advanced into the uterus to provide a means to manipulate the uterus. The speculum was removed from the vagina.

Attention was then turned to the patient's abdomen where a 10 mm skin incision was made in the umbilical fold. The veres needle was carefully introduced into the peritoneal cavity at a 45 degree angle while tenting the abdominal wall. Intraperitoneal placement was confirmed by use of a water-filled syringe and drop in intraabdominal pressure with insufflation of $CO_2$ gas. The trocar and sleeve were then advanced without difficulty into the abdomen where intraabdominal placement was confirmed by the laparoscope. Pneumoperitoneum was obtained with 4 liters of $CO_2$ gas and the 10 mm trocar and sleeve were then advanced without difficulty into the abdomen where intraabdominal placement was confirmed by the laparoscope. A second skin incision was made 2 cm above the symphysis pubis in the midline. The second trocar and sleeve were then advanced under direct visualization.

A survey of the patient's pelvis and abdomen revealed entirely normal anatomy. The Falope ring applicator was then advanced through the second trocar sleeve and the patient's left fallopian tube was identified and followed out to the fimbriated end. The ring was applied in the mid-isthmic area with a good knuckle of tube noted and good blanching at the site of application. There was no bleeding in the mesosalpinx. The Falope ring applicator was then reloaded and the patient's right tube manipulated in a similar fashion with easy application of the Falope ring.

The instruments were then removed from the patient's abdomen, and the incision repaired with 3-0 Vicryl. The HUMI was then removed from the vagina with no bleeding noted from the cervix. The patient tolerated the procedure well. Sponge, lap, and needle counts were correct times two. The patient was taken to the recovery room in stable condition.

## TOTAL ABDOMINAL HYSTERECTOMY

*Preoperative Diagnosis:* 1. Hypermenorrhea and Polymenorrhea unresponsive to medical therapy

*Postoperative Diagnosis:* 1. Hypermenorrhea and Polymenorrhea unresponsive to medical therapy

*Procedure:* Total abdominal hysterectomy and bilateral salpingo-oophorectomy

Surgeon:

Assistant:

*Anesthesia:* General endotracheal

*Complications:* None

*EBL:* 150 cc

*Fluids:* 1000 cc LR

*Urine Output:* 200 cc clear urine at end of procedure

*Findings:* EUA: diffusely enlarged uterus. Operative finding: 8 × 7 cm uterus with normal tubes and ovaries bilaterally. On opening the uterus a 2 × 2 cm pedunculated myoma was noted. Frozen section revealed benign tissue. All specimens sent to pathology.

*Procedure:* The risks, benefits, indications, and alternatives of the procedure were reviewed with the patient and informed consent was obtained. The patient was taken to the operating room with IV running and Foley catheter in place.

The patient was placed in the supine position, given general anesthesia, prepared, and draped in the usual sterile fashion. A Pfannenstiel incision was made approximately 2 cm above the symphysis pubis and extended sharply to the rectus fascia. The fascia was then incised bilaterally with the curved Mayo scissors, and the muscles of the anterior abdominal wall were separated in the midline by sharp and blunt dissection.

The peritoneum was grasped between two pick-ups, elevated, and entered sharply with the scalpel. The pelvis was examined with the finding noted above. An O'Connor-O'Sullivan retractor was placed into the incision and the bowel packed away with moist laparotomy sponges. Two Pean clamps were placed on the cornua and used for retraction. The round ligaments on both sides were clamped, transected, and suture ligated with #0 Vicryl. The anterior leaf of the broad ligament was incised along the bladder reflection to the midline from both sides. The bladder was then gently dissected off the lower uterine segment and the cervix with a sponge stick.

# OPERATIVE REPORTS

The infundibulopelvic ligaments on both sides were then doubly clamped, transected, and suture ligated with #0 Vicryl. Hemostasis was visualized. The uterine arteries were skeletonized bilaterally, clamped with Heaney clamps, transected, and suture ligated with #0 Vicryl. Again, hemostasis was assured. The uterosacral ligaments were clamped on both sides, transected, and suture ligated in a similar fashion.

The cervix and uterus were amputated with the cautery. The vaginal cuff angles were closed with figure-of-eight stitches of #0 Vicryl and were transfixed to the ipsilateral cardinal and uterosacral ligaments. The remainder of the vaginal cuff was closed with a series of interrupted #0 Vicryl figure-of-eight sutures. Hemostasis was assured.

The pelvis was irrigated copiously with warmed normal saline. All laparotomy sponges and instruments were removed from the abdomen. The fascia was closed with running #0 Vicryl, and hemostasis was assured. The skin was closed with staples. Sponge, lap, needle, and instrument counts were correct times two. The patient was taken to the PACU, awake and in stable condition.

## VAGINAL HYSTERECTOMY

*Preoperative Diagnosis*: Uterine prolapse
*Postoperative Diagnosis*: Uterine prolapse
*Procedure:* Total vaginal hysterectomy
Surgeon:
Assistant:
*Anesthesia:* General endotracheal
*Complications:* None
*EBL:* 100 cc
*Urine Output*: 200 cc clear urine at end of procedure
*Fluids:* 500 cc LR

*Findings:* EUA: small anteverted uterus with irregular contour. Operative findings: Small 7 × 6 cm irregularly shaped uterus, normal tubes, ovaries not well visualized.

*Procedure:* The risks, benefits, indications, and alternatives of the procedure were reviewed with the patient and informed consent was obtained. The patient was taken to the operating room with IV running and Foley catheter in place. The patient was placed in dorsolithotomy position, prepared, and draped in the usual sterile fashion.

A weighted speculum was placed into the vagina, and the cervix grasped with a toothed tenaculum. The cervix was then injected circumferentially with 1% Xylocaine with 1:200,000 epinephrine. The cervix was then circumferentially incised with the scalpel and the bladder dissected off the pubovesical cervical fascia anteriorly with a sponge stick, and the Metzenbaum scissors. The anterior cul-de-sac was entered sharply. The same procedure was performed posteriorly and the posterior cul-de-sac entered sharply without difficulty.

At this point, a Heaney clamp was placed over the uterosacral ligaments on either side. These were then transected and suture ligated with #0 Vicryl. Hemostasis was assured. The cardinal ligaments were then clamped on both sides, transected and suture ligated in similar fashion.

The uterine arteries and the broad ligament were then serially clamped with Heaney clamps, transected and suture ligated on both sides. Excellent hemostasis was visualized. Both cornua were clamped with Heaney clamps, transected, and the uterus delivered. These pedicles were then suture ligated with excellent hemostasis.

# OPERATIVE REPORTS

The peritoneum was closed with purse-string suture of #0 Vicryl. The vaginal cuff angles were closed with figure-of-eight stitches of #0 Vicryl on both sides and transfixed to the ipsilateral cardinal and uterosacral ligaments. The remainder of the vaginal cuff was closed with figure-of-eight stitches of #0 Vicryl in interrupted fashion.

A Penrose drain was placed into the vaginal cuff between suture ligatures. All instruments were then removed from the vagina, and the patient taken out of dorsolithotomy position and awakened from general anesthesia. The patient was taken to the PACU in stable condition. Sponge, lap, needle, and instrument count was correct times two.

## Numbers

| | | | |
|---|---|---|---|
| one | uno (una) | sixteen | dieciséis |
| two | dos | seventeen | diecisiete |
| three | tres | eighteen | dieciocho |
| four | cuatro | nineteen | diecinueve |
| five | cinco | twenty | veinte |
| six | seis | thirty | trienta |
| seven | siete | forty | cuarenta |
| eight | ocho | fifty | cincuenta |
| nine | nueve | sixty | sesenta |
| ten | diez | seventy | setenta |
| eleven | once | eighty | ochenta |
| twelve | doce | ninety | noventa |
| thirteen | trece | hundred | cien |
| fourteen | catorce | thousand | mil |
| fifteen | quince | | |

## Years

| | |
|---|---|
| 1930 | mil novecientos treinta |
| 1943 | mil novecientos cuarenta y tres |
| 1960 | mil novecientos sesenta |
| 1970 | mil novecientos setenta |
| 1974 | mil novecientos setenta y cuatro |

## Days of the Week

| | |
|---|---|
| Monday | lunes |
| Tuesday | martes |
| Wednesday | miércoles |
| Thursday | jueves |
| Friday | viernes |
| Saturday | sábado |
| Sunday | domingo |

## Times

| | |
|---|---|
| morning | la mañana |
| afternoon | la tarde |
| evening | la tarde |
| night | la noche |
| today | hoy |
| tomorrow | mañana |
| last night | anoche |
| yesterday | ayer |
| day before yesterday | anteayer |

## Months

| | |
|---|---|
| January | enero |
| February | febrero |
| March | marzo |
| April | abril |
| May | mayo |
| June | junio |
| July | julio |
| August | agosto |
| September | septiembre |
| October | octubre |
| November | noviembre |
| December | diciembre |

# SPANISH PRIMER

## Introductions
**Good morning**
Buenos días
**How do you feel?**
Cómo se siente? Cómo esta?
**My name is** _____
Me llamo _____
**Please**
Por favor

## Obstetric and Gynecologic History
**At what age did you begin to menstruate?**
A qué edad empezó su menstruación?

**What was the first day of your last period? (menstruation, period)**
Cuándo fue el primer día de su última regla? (menstruación, período)

**When did you have your last period?**
Cuándo fue su última regla?

**Did you have a normal period?**
Tuvo una regla normal? (Fue esta regla normal?)

**Pregnancy**
Embarazo, encinta, "gorda"

**How many pregnancies have you had?**
Cuántos embarazos ha tenido usted?

**How many children have you had?**
Cuántos niños ha tenido usted?

**Are they all living?**
Estan vivos todos?

**What was the cause of death? At what age?**
Cuál fue la causa de la muerte? A qué edad?

**Have you had any problems with past pregnancies?**
Ha tenido algunos problemas con sus embarazos pasados?

**Bleeding? Hypertension? Toxemia?**
Sangrando (hemorragia)? Alta presión de la sangre? Toxemia?

**Have you had any problems with past deliveries?**
Ha tenido problemas con sus partos pasados?

**What was the duration of your longest (shortest) labor?**
Cuántas horas duró su parto más largo (más corto)?

**What was the date of your last pregnancy?**
Cuál fue la fecha de su último embarazo?

**What was the weight of your largest (smallest) baby at birth?**
Cuánto pesó el bebé más grande (más pequeño) al nacer?

**Were all your pregnancies term?**
Fueron de tiempo (de nueve meses) sus otros niños?

**Were there any problems with the children after birth?**
Después de nacer, tuvo algún o algunos problemas con los niños?

**Have you ever had a miscarriage? Was it the first, second? What date?**
Ha tenido un malparto, aborto? Fue el primero, el segundo? Qué fecha?

**Have you ever had a stillborn?**
Ha tenido un niño que ha nacido muerto?

**Have you ever had a cesarean section? What date?**
Ha tenido usted una operación cesárea? Qué fecha?

## Past Medical and Surgical History

**Have you had any operations? For what? When? In which hospital?**
Ha tenido algunas operaciones? Para qué? Cuándo? En cuál hospital?

**Have you had any major illnesses?**
Ha tenido algunas enfermedades graves?

**Have you had any accidents, fractures?**
Ha tenido algunos accidentes, fracturas?

**Have you ever had a blood transfusion?**
Ha tenido una transfusión (infusión) de sangre?

**Have you been taking any medications?**
Qué medicinas ha estado tomando?

**Are you allergic to medicines or foods?**
Es usted alérgica a medicinas o comidas?

**Do you smoke? How many packs in a day (week)? Cigarettes**
Fuma usted? Cuántos paquetes en un día (una semana)? Cigarillos

# SPANISH PRIMER

## Family History

**Have you or anyone in your family had:**
Usted o alguien en su familia ha tenido:

| | |
|---|---|
| asthma | asma |
| cancer | cáncer |
| convulsions | convulsiones |
| diabetes | diabetes |
| epilepsy | epilepsia |
| gonorrhea | gonorrea |
| syphilis | sífilis |
| hay fever | fiebre del heno |
| heart disease | mala (enfermedad) del corazón |
| hepatitis (liver) | hepatitis (hígado) |
| hypertension | alta presión de la sangre |
| influenza | influenza, gripe |
| jaundice (yellow skin) | ictericia (la piel amarilla) |
| measles | sarampión |
| chickenpox | viruela |
| pneumonia | pulmonía, neumonía |
| rheumatic fever | fiebre reumática |
| scarlet fever | fiebre escarlatina |
| stroke | hemoragia cerebral |
| thyroid | tiroides |
| tuberculosis | tuberculosis |
| tumor | tumor |
| infections of the bladder, kidney | infecciones de la vejiga, de los riñones |
| infections of the chest, lungs | infecciones del pecho o de los pulmones |

## Anatomy

| | | | |
|---|---|---|---|
| head | cabeza | heart | corazón |
| eyes | ojos | **lungs (lung)** | pulmones (pulmón) |
| ears | oídos | **abdomen** | abdomen (vientre) |
| nose | nariz | liver | hígado |
| mouth | boca | intestines | intestinos |
| tongue | lengua | **appendix** | apéndice |
| teeth | dientes | rectum | recto |
| neck | cuello | **bladder** | vejiga |
| arm | brazo | vagina | vagina |
| shoulder | hombro | cervix | cervis |
| hand | la mano | uterus | útero (matriz) |
| fingers | dedos | **fallopian tubes** | las trompas, los tubos |
| axilla | axila | ovaries | ovarios |
| chest | pecho | cyst | quiste |
| breasts | pecho (seno) | | |

## Present Pregnancy

**Why did you come to the hospital (clinic)?**
Porqué ha venido al hospital (a la clínica)?

**Have you been coming to the clinics?**
Ha venido a las clínicas?

**How many times?**
Cuántas veces?

**When was the last time you came to the clinic? What date?**
Cuándo fue la última vez que vinó a la clínica? Qué fecha?

**In what month of your pregnancy did you start prenatal care?**
En qué mes de su embarazo vio al doctor para empezar el cuidado de maternidad?

**Have you had any problems with this pregnancy?**
Ha tenido algunos problemas con este embarazo?

**What is your due date?**
Para cuándo supone será la fecha del nacimiento de su bebé?

**Have you had any bleeding?**
Ha sangrado?

**Have you had any infections? Of what?**
Ha tenido algunas infecciones? De qué?

**Have you had any hypertension?**
Ha tenido alta presión de la sangre?

**Have you had any swelling of the hand, face, legs?**
Se le han hinchado las manos, el rostro (la cara), las piernas?

**How much weight have you gained? How much do you weigh? Your normal weight?**
Cuánto peso ha ganado? Cuánto pesa? Su peso normalmente?

**Have you had spots in front of your eyes?**
Ha tenido manchas enfrente de los ojos?

**Have you had (severe) headaches? How many times in a week?**
Ha tenido dolores (fuertes) de la cabeza? Cuántas veces en una semana?

**Have you had difficulty breathing? Lying down? After working?**
Ha tenido dificultad para respirar? Al acostarse? Después de trabajar?

**Do you tire easily?**
Se cansa facilmente?

# SPANISH PRIMER

**Have you had heart palpitations?**
Ha tenido problemas del corazón?

**Have you had diarrhea? Constipation?**
Ha tenido diarrea? Estreñimiento?

**Have you been vomiting?**
Ha estado vomitando?

**Have you had dysuria?**
Ha tenido dolores al orinar?

## Labor and Delivery

**Are you going to have a baby?**
Va a tener un niño?

**Are you in pain?**
Tiene dolor?

**What time did your pains begin?**
Cuándo empezaron los dolores (las contracciones)?

**What time did they become regular?**
A qué hora fueron (empezaron) regulares (los dolores)?

**How often were they once they became regular?**
Con qué frecuencia cuando empezaron regulares?

**How often are your pains?**
Cada cuándo le dan los dolores?

**How long do they last?**
Cuánto duran?

**Have you had bleeding?**
Ha sangrado?

**Was it pinkish or bright red?**
Fue de color rosado o rojo claro?

**How much? A cupful? A tablespoonful? A teaspoonful?**
Cuánta sangre? Una taza? Una cucharada? Una cucharadita?

**Did your membranes rupture? Has your bag of waters broken?**
Se le revento la bolsa de agua? (Se le) ha roto la bolsa de agua?

**What time did it break?**
A qué hora se le revento?

How much water did you lose? Down the legs?
Cuánta agua perdió? Se le bajó por las piernas?

**Have you felt the baby move today?**
Ha sentido mover el niño?

**Your cervix is not dilated.**
Su cuello no está dilatado.

**Your cervix is dilated to 5 centimeters.**
Su cuello tiene cinco centímetros.

**You are in labor. Your membranes have ruptured.**
Está en trabajo de parto. Sus membranas están rojas.

**The heartrate of the baby is normal.**
El corazón del niño está normal.

**Instructions**
**Take off your clothes.**
Quitese la ropa.

**Take off your panties.**
Quitese su ropa interior.

**I am going to examine you.**
Voy a examinarle.

**Bend your knees.**
Doble las rodillas.

**Open your legs.**
Abra las piernas.

**Put your feet together.**
Junte los pies.

**Relax your body.**
Descanse (relaje) el cuerpo.

**Lie down on your back.**
Acuestese en su espalda. (Acuestese boca arriba.)

**Lie down on your right (left) side.**
Acuestese del lado derecho (izquierdo).

**Move down on the table.**
Bajese.

**607**

# SPANISH PRIMER

**Move.**
Muevase.

**You are going to stay in the hospital.**
Se va a quedar en el hospital.

**You may go home.**
Se puede ir a casa.

**You are in early labor.**
Está en la primera parte del parto.

**Stay at the hospital and walk for two hours.**
Quedese aquí en el hospital y ande por dos horas.

**Don't push.**
No puje.

**Breathe through your mouth.**
Respire por la boca.

**Push with your pains.**
Puje con sus dolores.

**Do you understand?**
Entiende?

**Congratulations. You have a baby boy (girl)!**
Felicitaciones. Es un niño (una niña)!

## STANFORD UNIVERSITY MEDICAL CENTER LABORATORY

### Hematology

| | |
|---|---|
| Hct | 35–47 % |
| Hgb | 11.7–15.7 g/dL |
| Plt | 150–400 K/uL |
| WBC | 4.0–11.0 K/uL |
| Poly | 42.7–73.3 % |
| Bands | 0.0–11.0 % |
| Mono | 2.0–11.0 % |
| Lymph | 12.5–40.0 % |
| Eos | 0.0–7.5 % |
| Baso | 0.0–2.0 % |
| RBC | 3.8–5.2 MIL/uL |
| MCV | 82–98 fl |
| MCH | 27–34 pg |
| MCHC | 32–36 g/dL |
| RDW | 11.5–14.6 % |

### Coagulation

| | |
|---|---|
| PT-seconds | 10.5–13.1 sec |
| PT-INR | 0.89–1.11 INR |
| Coumadin range | |
| Low intensity | 2.0–3.0 INR |
| High intensity | 3.0–5.0 INR |
| APTT | 23–33 sec |
| Thrombin Time | 13–17 sec |
| Fibrinogen | 160–350 mg/dL |
| FSP | 0–10 mcg/mL |
| D-Dimer | 0–200 |

### Drug Levels

| | |
|---|---|
| Carbamazepine | 8–12 mcg/mL |
| Digoxin | 0.5–2.0 mcg/mL |
| Lithium | 0.6–1.2 mEq/L |
| Phenobarb | 10–40 mcg/mL |
| Phenytoin | 10–20 mcg/mL |
| Pro cainamide | 4–8 mcg/mL |
| Quinidine | 2.5–5.0 mcg/mL |
| Theophylline | 5–20 mcg/mL |
| Vancomycin | |
| Peak | 20–30 mcg/mL |
| Trough | 5–10 mcg/mL |
| Gentamicin | |
| Peak | 6–8 ng/mL |
| Trough | <2 ng/mL |

### Chemistry

| | |
|---|---|
| Sodium | 135–148 mEq/L |
| Potassium | 3.5–5.3 mEq/L |
| Chloride | 95–105 mEq/L |
| $CO_2$ | 24–31 mEq/L |
| Anion Gap | 8–16 mEq/L |
| | |
| Osm (serum) | 285–310 mOsm/kg |
| Glucose | 70–110 mg/dL |
| BUN | 5–25 mg/dL |
| Creatinine | 0.5–1.4 mg/dL |
| Calcium | 1.12–1.32 mmol/L |
| Phosphorus | 2.5–4.5 mg/dL |
| Magnesium | 1.5–2.0 mEq/L |
| | |
| Uric Acid | 2.5–7.5 mg/dL |
| Total Protein | 6.3–8.2 g/dL |
| Albumin | 3.9–5.0 g/dL |
| Bilirubin, Total | 0.2–1.3 mg/dL |
| Bilirubin, Direct | 0.0–0.4 mg/dL |
| Alk Phos | 38–126 IU/L |
| AST (SOOT) | 8–39 IU/L |
| ALT (SGPT) | 9–52 IU/L |
| Gamma GT | 8–78 IU/L |
| | |
| Cholesterol | |
| Low Risk | <200 mg/dL |
| Moderate Risk | 200–239mg/dL |
| High Risk | >239 mg/dL |
| Triglyceride | 35–135 mg/dL |
| Amylase | 30–110 IU/L |
| | |
| Ammonia | 9–33 mcmol/L |
| Ferritin | |
| Female 18–50 yrs old | 6–81 ng/mL |
| Female >50 yrs old | 14–186 ng/mL |
| Male | 30–284 ng/mL |
| TIBC | 240–450 % |
| Transferrin | 230–430 mg/dL |
| Haptoglobin | 50–320 mg/dL |

*Source:* Courtesy of H. Sussman, MD, Lab Director, Stanford Health Services

# LABORATORY

## ENDOCRINE LAB VALUES

|  | Conventional Units | Conversion Factor | SI Units |
|---|---|---|---|
| Adrenocorticotropin hormone (ACTH) | | | |
| 6:00 AM | 10–80 pg/mL | 0.2202 | 2.2–17.6 pmol/L |
| 6:00 PM | <50 pg/mL | 0.2202 | <11 pmol/L |
| Androstenedione | 60–300 ng/dL | 0.0349 | 2.1–10.5 nmol/L |
| Cortisol | | | |
| 8:00 AM | 5–25 mcg/dL | 27.9 | 140–700 nmol/L |
| 4:00 PM | 3–12 mcg/dL | 27.9 | 80–330 nmol/L |
| 10:00 PM | <50% of AM value | 27.9 | <50% of AM value |
| Dehydroepiandrosterone sulfate | 80–350 mcg/dL | 0.0027 | 2.2–9.5mcmol/L |
| 11-Deoxycortisol | 0.05–0.25 mcg/dL | 28.86 | 1.5–7.3 nmol/L |
| 11-Deoxycorticosterone | 2–10 ng/dL | 30.3 | 60–300 pmol/L |
| Estradiol | 20–400 pg/mL | 3.67 | 70–1500 pmol/L |
| Estrone | 30–200 pg/mL | 3.7 | 110–740 pmol/L |
| FSH, reproductive years | 5–30 mIU/mL | 1.0 | 5–30 IU/L |
| Glucose, fasting | 70–100 mg/dL | 0.0556 | 4.0–6.0 mmol/L |
| Growth hormone | <10 ng/mL | 1.0 | <10 mcg/L |
| 17-Hydroxyprogesterone | 100–300 ng/dL | 0.03 | 3–9 nmol/L |
| Insulin, fasting | 5–25 mcU/ml | 7.175 | 35–180 pmol/L |
| Insulin-like growth factor-l | 0.3–2.2 U/mL | 1000 | 300–2200 U/L |
| LH, reproductive years | 5–20 mIU/mL | 1.0 | 5–20 IU/L |
| Progesterone | | | |
| Follicular phase | <3 ng/mL | 3.18 | <9.5 nmol/L |
| Secretory phase | 5–30 ng/mL | 3.18 | 16–95 nmol/L |
| Prolactin | 1–20 ng/mL | 44.4 | 44.4–888 pmol/L |
| Testosterone, total | 20–80 ng/dL | 0.0347 | 0.7–2.8 nmol/L |
| Testosterone, free | 100–200 pg/dL | 0.0347 | 35–700 pmol/L |
| Thyroid stimulating hormone (TSH) | 0.35–6.7 mcU/mL | 1.0 | 3.5–6.7 mU/L |
| Thyroxine, free T4 | 0.8–2.3 ng/dL | 1.29 | 10–30 nmol/L |
| Triiodothyronine, T3, total | 80–220 ng/dL | 0.0154 | 1.2–3.4 nmol/L |
| Triiodothyronine, T3, free | 0.13–0.55 ng/dL | 15.4 | 2.0–8.5 pmol/L |
| Triiodothyronine, reverse | 8–35 ng/dL | 15.4 | 120–540 pmol/L |

*Source: Speroff L, Glass RH, Kase NG. Clinical Assays. In: Clinical Gynecologic Endocrinology and Infertility. 5th ed. Baltimore: Williams & Wilkins, 1994. Reproduced with the permission of the publisher.*

# REFERENCES

**Alberman E.** The epidemiology of repeated abortion. In Beard RW, Sharp F. *Early Pregnancy Loss: Mechanisms and Treatment.* New York: Springer-Verlag, 1988:9.

**Amar AP, Couldwell WT,** et al. Predictive value of serum prolactin levels measured immediately after transsphenoidal surgery. *J Neurosurg.* 2002;97(2):307.

**Ayvaliotis B, Bronson R,** et al. Conception rates in couples where autoimmunity to sperm is detected. *Fertil Steril.* 1985;43(5):739.

**Baillargeon JP, Jakubowicz DJ,** et al. Effects of metformin and rosiglitazone, alone and in combination, in nonobese women with polycystic ovary syndrome and normal indices of insulin sensitivity. *Fertil Steril.* 2004;82(4):893.

**Bajekal N, Li TC.** Fibroids, infertility and pregnancy wastage. *Hum Reprod Update.* 2000;6(6):614.

**Bates G.W, Jr., Hill JA.** Autoimmune ovarian failure. *Infertil Reprod Med Clinics NA.* 2002;13(1):65.

**Blake D, Proctor M,** et al. Cleavage stage versus blastocyst stage embryo transfer in assisted conception. *The Cochrane Database of Systematic Reviews.* Issue 2, 2002.

**Breitkopf DM, Frederickson RA,** et al. Detection of benign endometrial masses by endometrial stripe measurement in premenopausal women. *Obstet Gynecol.* 2004;104(1):120.

**Brenner B, Sarig G,** et al. Thrombophilic polymorphisms are common in women with fetal loss without apparent cause. *Thromb Haemost.* 1999;82(1):6.

**Burrow GN, Wortzman G,** et al. Microadenomas of the pituitary and abnormal sellar tomograms in an unselected autopsy series. *N Engl J Med.* 1981;304(3):156.

**Buttram VC, Jr.** Mullerian anomalies and their management. *Fertil Steril.* 1983;40(2):159.

**Canonico M.** Hormone therapy and venous thromboembolism among postmenopausal women: impact of the route of estrogen administration and progestogens: the ESTHER study. *Circulation.* 2007;115(7):840-845.

**Carr B, Breslau N,** et al. Oral contraceptive pill, GnRH agonists, or use in combination for treatment of hirsutism. *J Clin Endocrinol Metab.* 1995;80(4):1169.

**Catarci T, Fiacco F,** et al. Empty sella and headache. *Headache.* 1994;34(10):583.

**Cermik D, Arici A, Taylor HS.** Coordinated regulation of HOX gene expression in myometrium and uterine leiomyoma. *Fertil Steril.* 2002;78(5):979-984.

**Christiansen OB, Pedersen B,** et al. A randomized, double-blind, placebo-controlled trial of intravenous immunoglobulin in the prevention of recurrent miscarriage: evidence for a therapeutic effect in women with secondary recurrent miscarriage. *Hum Reprod.* 2002;17(3):809.

# REFERENCES

Ciccarelli E, Camanni F. Diagnosis and drug therapy of prolactinoma. *Drugs*. 1996;51(6):954.

Ciotta L, Cianci A, et al. Clinical and endocrine effects of finasteride, a 5 α-reductase inhibitor, in women with idiopathic hirsutism. *Fertil Steril*. 1995;64(2):299.

Clarke GN, Elliott PJ, et al. Detection of sperm antibodies in semen using the immunobead test: a survey of 813 consecutive patients. *Am J Reprod Immunol Microbiol*. 1985;7(3):118.

Col NF, Pauker SG. The discrepancy between observational studies and randomized trials of menopausal hormone therapy: did expectations shape experience? *Ann Intern Med*. 2003;139(11):923.

Colao A, Di Sarno A, et al. Withdrawal of long-term cabergoline therapy for tumoral and nontumoral hyperprolactinemia. *N Engl J Med*. 2003;349(21):2023.

Colao A, Di Somma C, et al. Prolactinomas in adolescents: persistent bone loss after 2 years of prolactin normalization. *Clin Endocrinol (Oxf)*. 2000;52(3):319.

Copperman AB, Wells V, Luna M, et al. Presence of hydrosalpinx correlated to endometrial inflammatory response in vivo. *Fertil Steril*. 2006;86(4):972-976.

Dabirashrafi H, Bahadori M, et al. Septate uterus: new idea on the histologic features of the septum in this abnormal uterus. *Am J Obstet Gynecol*. 1995;172(1 Pt 1):105.

Daniely M, Aviram-Goldring A, et al. Detection of chromosomal aberration in fetuses arising from recurrent spontaneous abortion by comparative genomic hybridization. *Hum Reprod*. 1998;13(4):805.

Davis OK, Berkeley AS, et al. The incidence of luteal phase defect in normal, fertile women, determined by serial endometrial biopsies. *Fertil Steril*. 1989;51(4):582.

Dewan S, Puscheck EE, Coulam CB, et al. Y-chromosome microdeletions and recurrent pregnancy loss. *Fertil Steril*. 2006;85:441-445.

di Nisio M, Peters L, Middeldorp S. Anticoagulants for the treatment of recurrent pregnancy loss in women without antiphospholipid syndrome. *Cochrane Review*. 2005;(2):CD004734.

Djahanbakhch O, McNeily AS, et al. Changes in plasma levels of prolactin, in relation to those of FSH, oestradiol, androstenedione and progesterone around the preovulatory surge of LH in women. *Clin Endocrinol (Oxf)*. 1984;20:463.

Dorn C, Mouillet JF, et al. Insulin enhances the transcription of luteinizing hormone-beta gene. *Am J Obstet Gynecol*. 2004;191(1):132.

Dunaif A. Insulin resistance and the polycystic ovary syndrome: mechanism and implications for pathogenesis. *Endocr Rev*. 1997;18(6):774.

**Dunaif A, Segal KR, Futterweit W, et al.** Profound peripheral insulin resistance, independent of obesity, in polycystic ovary syndrome. *Diabetes.* 1989;38:1165-1174.

**Dunaif A, Segal KR, Shelley DR, et al.** Evidence for distinctive and intrinsic defects in insulin action in polycystic ovary syndrome. *Diabetes.* 1992;41:1257-1266.

**Dunaif A, Zia J, et al.** Excessive insulin receptor serine phosphorylation in cultured fibroblasts and in skeletal muscle. A potential mechanism for insulin resistance in the polycystic ovary syndrome. *J Clin Invest.* 1995;96(2):801.

**Eagleson CA, Gingrich MB, et al.** Polycystic ovarian syndrome: evidence that flutamide restores sensitivity of the gonadotropin-releasing hormone pulse generator to inhibition by estradiol and progesterone. *J Clin Endocrinol Metab.* 2000; 85(11):4047.

**Edmonds DK, Lindsay KS, et al.** Early embryonic mortality in women. *Fertil Steril.* 1982;38(4):447.

**Eisenhardt S, Schwarzmann N, Henschel V, et al.** Early effects of metformin in women with polycystic ovary syndrome: a prospective randomized, double-blind, placebo-controlled trial. *J Clin Endocrinol Metab.* 2006;91(3):946-952.

**Elias KA, Weiner RI.** Direct arterial vascularization of estrogen-induced prolactin-secreting anterior pituitary tumors. *Proc Natl Acad Sci U S A.* 1984;81(14): 4549.

**Espeland MA, Rapp SR, et al.** Conjugated equine estrogens and global cognitive function in postmenopausal women: Women's Health Initiative Memory Study. *JAMA.* 2004;291(24):2959.

**Farquhar CM, Lethaby A, et al.** An evaluation of risk factors for endometrial hyperplasia in premenopausal women with abnormal menstrual bleeding. *Am J Obstet Gynecol.* 1999;181(3):525.

**Fassnacht M, Schlenz N, et al.** Beyond adrenal and ovarian androgen generation: increased peripheral 5 alpha-reductase activity in women with polycystic ovary syndrome. *J Clin Endocrinol Metab.* 2003;88(6):2760.

**Ferriman D, Gallway JD.** Clinical assessment of body hair growth in women. *J Clin Endocrinol Metab.* 1961;21:1440.

**Foka ZJ, Lambropoulos AF, et al.** Factor V Leiden and prothrombin G20210A mutations, but not methylenetetrahydrofolate reductase C677T, are associated with recurrent miscarriages. *Hum Reprod.* 2000;15(2):458.

**Foulk RA, Martin MC, et al.** Hyperreactio luteinalis differentiated from severe ovarian hyperstimulation syndrome in a spontaneously conceived pregnancy. *Am J Obstet Gynecol.* 1997;176(6):1300; discussion, 1302.

**Freedman RR, Roehrs TA.** Lack of sleep disturbance from menopausal hot flashes. *Fertil Steril.* 2004;82(1):138.

# REFERENCES

Fritz B, Hallermann C, et al. Cytogenetic analyses of culture failures by comparative genomic hybridisation (CGH)-Re-evaluation of chromosome aberration rates in early spontaneous abortions. *Eur J Hum Genet.* 2001;9(7):539.

Fruzzetti F, Bersi C, et al. Treatment of hirsutism: comparisons between different antiandrogens with central and peripheral effects. *Fertil Steril.* 1999;71:445.

Fujimoto VY, Clifton DK, et al. Variability of serum prolactin and progesterone levels in normal women: the relevance of single hormone measurements in the clinical setting. *Obstet Gynecol.* 1990;76(1):71.

Gilbert C, Valois M, Koren G. Pregnancy outcome after first-trimester exposure to metformin: a meta-analysis. *Fertil Steril.* 2006;86:658-663.

Gillam MP. *Endo Reviews.* 2005;27(5):485-534.

Girardi G, Redecha P, Salmon JE. Heparin prevents antiphospholipid antibody-induced fetal loss by inhibiting complement activation. *Nature Medicine.* 2004; 10:1222-1226.

Glueck CJ, Wang P, et al. Pregnancy outcomes among women with polycystic ovary syndrome treated with metformin. *Hum Reprod.* 2002;17(11):2858.

Gnoth C, Godehardt E, Frank-Herrmann P, et al. Definition and prevalence of subfertility and infertility. *Hum Reprod.* 2005;20(5): 1144-1147.

Gnoth C, Godehardt D, et al. Time to pregnancy: results of the German prospective study and impact on the management of infertility. *Hum Reprod.* 2003;18(9): 1959.

Goodarzi MO, Shah NA, Antoine HJ, et al. Variants in the 5alpha-reductase type 1 and type 2 genes are associated with polycystic ovary syndrome and the severity of hirsutism in affected women. *J Clin Endocrinol Metab.* 2006;91: 4085-4091.

Guzick DS, Overstreet JW, et al. Sperm morphology, motility, and concentration in fertile and infertile men. *N Engl J Med.* 2001;345(19):1388.

Hansen LM, Batzer FR, et al. Evaluating ovarian reserve: follicle stimulating hormone and oestradiol variability during cycle days 2–5. *Hum Reprod.* 1996;11 (3):486.

Hansen M. Assisted reproductive technologies and the risk of birth defects—a systematic review. *Hum Reprod.* 2005;20(2):328.

Harborne LR, Sattar N, Norman JE, Fleming R. Metformin and weight loss in obese women with polycystic ovary syndrome: comparison of doses. *J Clin Endocrinol Metab.* 2005;90:4593-4598.

Hassold TJ. A cytogenetic study of repeated spontaneous abortions. *Am J Hum Genet.* 1980;32(5):723.

Haynes PJ, Hodgson H, et al. Measurement of menstrual blood loss in patients complaining of menorrhagia. *Br J Obstet Gynaecol.* 1977;84(10):763.

Heard MJ, Pierce A, et al. Pregnancies following use of metformin for ovulation induction in patients with polycystic ovary syndrome. *Fertil Steril.* 2002;77(4):669.

Heck KE, Schoendorf KC, et al. Delayed childbearing by education level in the United States, 1969–1994. *Matern Child Health J.* 1997;1(2):81.

Hellmuth E, Damm P, et al. Oral hypoglycaemic agents in 118 diabetic pregnancies. *Diabet Med.* 2000;17(7):507.

Herman-Giddens ME, Slora EJ, et al. Secondary sexual characteristics and menses in young girls seen in office practice: a study from the Pediatric Research in Office Settings network. *Pediatrics.* 1997;99(4):505.

Hobbs L, Ort R, et al. Synopsis of laser assisted hair removal systems. *Skin Therapy Lett.* 2000;5(3):1.

Hofle G, Gasser R, Mohsenipour I, Finkenstedt G. Surgery combined with dopamine agonists versus dopamine agonists alone in long-term treatment of macroprolactinoma: a retrospective study. *Exp Clin Endocrinol Diabetes.* 1998.

Isik AZ, Gulekli B, et al. Endocrinological and clinical analysis of hyperprolactinemic patients with and without ultrasonically diagnosed polycystic ovarian changes. *Gynecol Obstet Invest.* 1997;43(3):183.

Jaffe R, Jauniaux E, et al. Maternal circulation in the first-trimester human placenta—myth or reality? *Am J Obstet Gynecol.* 1997;176(3):695.

Jain T, Soules MR, Collins JA. Comparison of basal follicle-stimulating hormone versus the clomiphene citrate challenge test for ovarian reserve screening. *Fertil Steril.* 2004;82:180-185.

Jakimiuk AJ, Weitsman SR, et al. Luteinizing hormone receptor, steroidogenesis acute regulatory protein, and steroidogenic enzyme messenger ribonucleic acids are overexpressed in thecal and granulosa cells from polycystic ovaries. *J Clin Endocrinol Metab.* 2001;86(3):1318.

Jakubowicz DJ, Iuorno MJ, et al. Effects of metformin on early pregnancy loss in the polycystic ovary syndrome. *J Clin Endocrinol Metab.* 2002;87(2):524.

Jasonni VM, Raffelli R, et al. Vaginal bromocriptine in hyperprolactinemic patients and puerperal women. *Acta Obstet Gynecol Scand.* 1991;70(6):493.

Jeng GT, Scott JR, et al. A comparison of meta-analytic results using literature vs individual patient data. Paternal cell immunization for recurrent miscarriage. *JAMA.* 1995;274(10):830.

Jivraj S, Rai R, Underwood J, Regan L. Genetic thrombophilic mutations among couples with recurrent miscarriage. *Hum Reprod.* 2006;21(5):1161-1165.

Johnson NP, Mak W, et al. Laparoscopic salpingectomy for women with hydrosalpinges enhances the success of IVF: a Cochrane review. *Hum Reprod.* 2002;17(3):543.

# REFERENCES

**Kamel HS, Darwish AM, et al.** Comparison of transvaginal ultrasonography and vaginal sonohysterography in the detection of endometrial polyps. *Acta Obstet Gynecol Scand*. 2000;79(1):60.

**Kaplowitz PB, Oberfield SE.** Reexamination of the age limit for defining when puberty is precocious in girls in the United States: implications for evaluation and treatment. Drug and Therapeutics and Executive Committees of the Lawson Wilkins Pediatric Endocrine Society. *Pediatrics*. 1999;104(4 Pt 1):936.

**Kaufman RH, Adam E, et al.** Continued follow-up of pregnancy outcomes in diethylstilbestrol-exposed offspring. *Obstet Gynecol*. 2000;96(4):483.

**Khorram O, Helliwell JP, Katz S, Bonpane CM, Jaramillo L.** Two weeks of metformin improves clomiphene citrate-induced ovulation and metabolic profiles in women with polycystic ovary syndrome. *Fertil Steril*. 2006;85:1448-1451.

**Kleinhaus K, Perrin M, Friedlander Y, et al.** Paternal age and spontaneous abortion. *Obstet Gynecol*. 2006;108:369-377.

**Kodama H, Fukuda J, et al.** Characteristics of blood hemostatic markers in a patient with ovarian hyperstimulation syndrome who actually developed thromboembolism. *Fertil Steril*. 1995;64:1207.

**Kouides PA, Phatak PD, et al.** Gynaecological and obstetrical morbidity in women with type I von Willebrand disease: results of a patient survey. *Haemophilia*. 2000;6(6):643.

**Kovalevsky G, Gracia CR, Berlin JA, et al.** Evaluation of the association between hereditary thrombophilias and recurrent pregnancy loss: a meta-analysis. *Arch Intern Med*. 2004;164(5):558-563.

**Kriplani A, Agarwal N.** Effects of metformin on clinical and biochemical parameters in polycystic ovary syndrome. *J Reprod Med*. 2004;49(5):361.

**Kruger TF, Coetzee K.** The role of sperm morphology in assisted reproduction. *Hum Reprod Update*. 1999;5(2):172.

**Kundsin RB, Driscoll SG, et al.** Ureaplasma urealyticum incriminated in perinatal morbidity and mortality. *Science*. 1981;213(4506):474.

**Lanigan SW.** Incidence of side effects after laser hair removal. *J Am Acad Dermatol*. 2003;49(5):882.

**Legro RS, Barnhart HX, Schlaff WD, et al.** Clomiphene, metformin, or both for infertility in the polycystic ovary syndrome. *New Engl J Med*. 2007;356(6):551-566.

**Levi AJ, Raynault MF, et al.** Reproductive outcome in patients with diminished ovarian reserve. *Fertil Steril*. 2001;76(4):666.

**Lipscomb GH, Bran D, et al.** Analysis of three hundred fifteen ectopic pregnancies treated with single-dose methotrexate. *Am J Obstet Gynecol*. 1998;178:1354.

**Lipscomb GH, Givens VA, et al.** Previous ectopic pregnancy as a predictor of failure of systemic methotrexate therapy. *Fertil Steril*. 2004;81(5):1221.

Lipscomb GH, McCord ML, et al. Predictors of success of methotrexate treatment in women with tubal ectopic pregnancies. *N Engl J Med.* 1999;341:1974.

Lipscomb GH, Stovall TG, et al. Nonsurgical treatment of ectopic pregnancy. *N Engl J Med.* 2000;343(18):1325.

Lo JC, Schwitzgebel VM, et al. Normal female infants born of mothers with classic congenital adrenal hyperplasia due to 21-hydroxylase deficiency. *J Clin Endocrinol Metab.* 1999;84(3):930-936.

Lobo R, Shoupe D, et al. The effects of two doses of spironolactone on serum androgens and anagen hair in hirsute women. *Fertil Steril.* 1985;43(2):200.

Looker AC, Orwoll ES, et al. Prevalence of low femoral bone density in older U.S. adults from NHANES III. *J Bone Miner Res.* 1997;12(11):1761.

Lord JM, Flight IH, et al. Insulin-sensitising drugs (metformin, troglitazone, rosiglitazone, pioglitazone, D-chiro-inositol) for polycystic ovary syndrome. *Cochrane Database Syst Rev.* 2003;(3):CD003053.

Lucidi RS, Pierce JD, Kavoussi SK, et al. Prior fertility in the male partner does not predict a normal semen analysis. *Fertil Steril.* 2005;84(3):793-794.

Mahabeer S, Naidoo C, et al. Metabolic profiles and lipoprotein lipid concentrations in non-obese patients with polycystic ovarian disease. *Horm Metab Res.* 1990;22(10):537.

Makris M. Hyperhomocysteinemia and thrombosis. *Clin Lab Haematol.* 2000;22(3):133.

Many A, Elad R, et al. Third-trimester unexplained intrauterine fetal death is associated with inherited thrombophilia. *Obstet Gynecol.* 2002;99(5 Pt 1):684.

Markee JE. Menstruation in intraocular endometrial transplants in the rhesus monkey. *Contrib Embryol.* 1940;177:221.

Marshall WA, Tanner JM. Variations in pattern of pubertal changes in girls. *Arch Dis Child.* 1969;44(235):291.

Martinelli I, Mannucci PM, et al. Different risks of thrombosis in four coagulation defects associated with inherited thrombophilia: a study of 150 families. *Blood.* 1998;92(7):2353.

McDonough PG. Puberty. In *Precis, Reproductive Endocrinology: an Update in Obstetrics and Gynecology.* Washington, DC: American College of Obstetricians and Gynecologists, 1998:32.

Naftolin F, Taylor HS, et al. The Women's Health Initiative could not have detected cardioprotective effects of starting hormone therapy during the menopausal transition. *Fertil Steril.* 2004;81(6):1498.

Navot D, Scott RT, Droesch K, et al. The window of embryo transfer and the efficiency of human conception in vitro. *Fertil Steril.* 1991;55:114-118.

Nestler JE. Metformin and the polycystic ovary syndrome. *J Clin Endocrinol Metab.* 2001;86(3):1430.

# REFERENCES

Nestler JE, Powers LP, et al. A direct effect of hyperinsulinemia on serum sex hormone-binding globulin levels in obese women with the polycystic ovary syndrome. *J Clin Endocrinol Metab.* 1991;72(1):83.

New MI. Extensive clinical experience: nonclassical 21-hydroxylase deficiency. *J Clin Endocrinol Metab.* 2006;91(11):4205-4214.

Ng EH, Chan CC, Tang OS, et al. Comparison of endometrial and subendometrial blood flows among patients with and without hydrosalpinx shown on scanning during in vitro fertilization treatment. *Fertil Steril.* 2006;85:333-338.

Ober C, Karrison T, et al. Mononuclear-cell immunisation in prevention of recurrent miscarriages: a randomised trial. *Lancet.* 1999;354(9176):365.

Ogasawara M, Aoki K, et al. Embryonic karyotype of abortuses in relation to the number of previous miscarriages. *Fertil Steril.* 2000;73(2):300.

Orio F, Jr., Palomba S, et al. The cardiovascular risk of young women with polycystic ovary syndrome: an observational, analytical, prospective case-control study. *J Clin Endocrinol Metab.* 2004;89(8):3696.

Pagotto U, Marsicano G, et al. Normal human pituitary gland and pituitary adenomas express cannabinoid receptor type 1 and synthesize endogenous cannabinoids: first evidence for a direct role of cannabinoids on hormone modulation at the human pituitary level. *J Clin Endocrinol Metab.* 2001;86 (6): 2687.

Papanikolaou EG, Tournaye H, et al. *Early Pregnancy Outcome Is Impaired in Early Ovarian Hyperstimulation Syndrome (OHSS) Comparing to Late OHSS.* St. Louis: American Society for Reproductive Immunology, 2004.

Patton PE, Burry KA, Thurmond A, et al. Intrauterine insemination outperforms intracervical insemination in a randomized, controlled study with frozen, donor semen. *Fertil Steril.* 1992;57(3):559-594.

Pearlstone AC, Fournet N, et al. Ovulation induction in women age 40 and older: the importance of basal follicle-stimulating hormone level and chronological age. *Fertil Steril.* 1992;58(4):674.

Pellestor F, Andreo B, et al. Maternal aging and chromosomal abnormalities: new data drawn from in vitro unfertilized human oocytes. *Hum Genet.* 2003;112(2): 195.

Pierpoint T, McKeigue PM, et al. Mortality of women with polycystic ovary syndrome at long-term follow-up. *J Clin Epidemiol.* 1998;51(7):581.

Polson DW, Adams J, et al. Polycystic ovaries—a common finding in normal women. *Lancet.* 1988;1(8590):870.

Poppe K, Glinoer D, et al. Assisted reproduction and thyroid autoimmunity: an unfortunate combination? *J Clin Endocrinol Metab.* 2003;88(9):4149.

Preston FE, Rosendaal FR, et al. Increased fetal loss in women with heritable thrombophilia. *Lancet.* 1996;348(9032):913.

Price TM, Allen S, et al. Lack of effect of topical finasteride suggests an endocrine role for dihydrotestosterone. *Fertil Steril.* 2000;74(2):414.

# REFERENCES

Proctor JA, Haney AF . Recurrent first trimester pregnancy loss is associated with uterine septum but not with bicornuate uterus. *Fertil Steril.* 2003;80(5): 1212.

Ray NF, Chan JK, et al. Medical expenditures for the treatment of osteoporotic fractures in the United States in 1995: report from the National Osteoporosis Foundation. *J Bone Miner Res.* 1997;12(1):24.

Rey E, Kahn SR, et al. Thrombophilic disorders and fetal loss: a meta-analysis. *Lancet.* 2003;361(9361):901-908.

Ridker PM, Miletich JP, et al. Factor V Leiden mutation as a risk factor for recurrent pregnancy loss. *Ann Intern Med.* 1998;128(12 Pt 1):1000.

Rivera JL, Lal S, et al. Effect of acute and chronic neuroleptic therapy on serum prolactin levels in men and women of different age groups. *Clin Endocrinol (Oxf).* 1976;5(3):273.

Robertson L, Wu O, Langhorne P, et al. Thrombophilia in pregnancy: a systematic review. *Br J Haematol.* 2006;132(2):171-196.

Roque H, Paidas MJ, Funai EF, et al. Maternal thrombophilias are not associated with early pregnancy loss. *Thromb Haemost.* 2004;91(2):290-295.

Rubinek T, Hadani M, et al. Prolactin (PRL)-releasing peptide stimulates PRL secretion from human fetal pituitary cultures and growth hormone release from cultured pituitary adenomas. *J Clin Endocrinol Metab.* 2001;86(6):2826.

Salat-Baroux J. [Recurrent spontaneous abortions]. *Reprod Nutr Dev.* 1988;28 (6B):1555.

Sam S, Legro RS, Essah PA, et al. Evidence for metabolic and reproductive phenotypes in mothers of women with polycystic ovary syndrome. *Proc Natl Acad Sci U S A.* 2006;103(18):7030-7035.

Sanson BJ, Friederich PW, et al. The risk of abortion and stillbirth in antithrombin, protein C-, and protein S-deficient women. *Thromb Haemost.* 1996;75(3):387.

Sargent IL, Wilkins T, et al. Maternal immune responses to the fetus in early pregnancy and recurrent miscarriage. *Lancet.* 1988;2(8620):1099.

Schlechte J, Dolan K, et al. The natural history of untreated hyperprolactinemia: a prospective analysis. *J Clin Endocrinol Metab.* 1989;68(2):412.

Scott RT, Opsahl MS, et al. Life table analysis of pregnancy rates in a general infertility population relative to ovarian reserve and patient age. *Hum Reprod.* 1995;10(7):1706.

Seki K, Kato K, et al. Parallelism in the luteinizing hormone responses to opioid and dopamine antagonists in hyperprolactinemic women with pituitary microadenoma. *J Clin Endocrinol Metab.* 1986;63(5):1225.

Sharara FI, Scott RT, Jr., et al. The detection of diminished ovarian reserve in infertile women. *Am J Obstet Gynecol.* 1998;179(3 Pt 1):804.

Shumaker SA, Legault C, et al. Conjugated equine estrogens and incidence of probable dementia and mild cognitive impairment in postmenopausal women: Women's Health Initiative Memory Study. *JAMA.* 2004;291(24):2947.

# REFERENCES

Slayden SM, Azziz R. The role of androgen excess in acne. In Azziz R, Nestler JE, Dewailly D. *Androgen Excess Disorders in Women.* Philadelphia: Lippincott–Raven Publishers: 131, 1997.

Sluijmer AV, Lappohn RE. Clinical history and outcome of 59 patients with idiopathic hyperprolactinemia. *Fertil Steril.* 1992;58(1):72.

Speiser PW, White PC. Congenital adrenal hyperplasia. *N Engl J Med.* 2003; 349(8):776.

Stein ZA. A woman's age: childbearing and child rearing. *Am J Epidemiol.* 1985;121 (3):327.

Steiner AZ, Chang L, et al. 3alpha-hydroxysteroid dehydrogenase type III deficiency: a novel cause of hirsutism (O-307). *J Soc Gynecol Invest.* 2004;11 (2S):307.

Strandell A, Lindhard A, Eckerlund I. Cost-effectiveness analysis of salpingectomy prior to IVF, based on a randomized controlled trial. *Hum Reprod.* 2005; 20(12):3281-3292.

Strandell A, Lindhard A. Why does hydrosalpinx reduce fertility? The importance of hydrosalpinx fluid. *Hum Reprod.* 2002;17(5):1141.

Strandell A, Lindhard A, Waldenstrom U, Thorburn J. Hydrosalpinx and IVF outcome: cumulative results after salpingectomy in a randomized controlled trial. *Hum Reprod.* 2001a;16(11):2403.

Strandell A, Lindhard A, Waldenstrom U, Thorburn J. Prophylactic salpingectomy does not impair the ovarian response in IVF treatment. *Hum Reprod.* 2001b;16(6):1135.

Sun L, Peng Y, Sharrow AC, et al. FSH directly regulates bone mass. *Cell.* 2006;125:247-260.

Tartagni M, Schonauer MM, et al. Intermittent low-dose finasteride is as effective as daily administration for the treatment of hirsute women. *Fertil Steril.* 2004;82(3):752.

Thatcher SS, Jackson EM. Pregnancy outcome in infertile patients with polycystic ovary syndrome who were treated with metformin. *Fertil Steril.* 2006;85:1007-1009.

Toner JP. Age = egg quality, FSH level = egg quantity. *Fertil Steril.* 2003;79(3):491.

Trio D, Strobelt N, et al. Prognostic factors for successful expectant management of ectopic pregnancy. *Fertil Steril.* 1995;63:469.

van Montfrans JM, Dorland M, et al. Increased concentrations of follicle-stimulating hormone in mothers of children with Down's syndrome. *Lancet.* 1999; 353(9167):1853.

Velazquez E, Acosta A, et al. Menstrual cyclicity after metformin therapy in polycystic ovary syndrome. *Obstet Gynecol.* 1997;90:392.

# REFERENCES

Verhelst J, Abs R, et al. Cabergoline in the treatment of hyperprolactinemia: a study in 455 patients. *J Clin Endocrinol Metab.* 1999;84(7):2518.

Waggoner W, Boots LR, et al. Total testosterone and DHEAS levels as predictors of androgen-secreting neoplasms: a population study. *Gynecol Endocrinol.* 1999;13(6):394.

Walker-Bone K, Dennison E, et al. Epidemiology of osteoporosis. *Rheum Dis Clin North Am.* 2001;27(1):1.

Wang X, Chen C, et al. Conception, early pregnancy loss, and time to clinical pregnancy: a population-based prospective study. *Fertil Steril.* 2003;79(3):577.

Warburton D. De novo balanced chromosome rearrangements and extra marker chromosomes identified at prenatal diagnosis: clinical significance and distribution of breakpoints. *Am J Hum Genet.* 1991;49(5):995.

Warburton D, Fraser FC. Spontaneous abortion risks in man: data from reproductive histories collected in a medical genetics unit. *Am J Hum Genet.* 1964;16:1.

Wild S, Pierpoint T, et al. Cardiovascular disease in women with polycystic ovary syndrome at long-term follow-up: a retrospective cohort study. *Clin Endocrinol (Oxf).* 2000;52(5):595.

Wong IL, Morris RS, et al. A prospective randomized trial comparing finasteride to spironolactone in the treatment of hirsute women. *J Clin Endocrinol Metab.* 1995;80(1):233.

World Health Organization. *WHO Laboratory Manual for the Examination of Human Semen and Semen-Cervical Mucus Interaction.* New York: Cambridge University Press, 1999.

Yates J, Barrett-Connor E, et al. Rapid loss of hip fracture protection after estrogen cessation: evidence from the National Osteoporosis Risk Assessment. *Obstet Gynecol.* 2004;103(3):440.

Young RL, Goldzieher JW, et al. The endocrine effects of spironolactone used as an antiandrogen. *Fertil Steril.* 1987;48(2):223.

Yucelten D, Erenus M, et al. Recurrence rate of hirsutism after 3 different antiandrogen therapies. *J Am Acad Dermatol.* 1999;41(1):64.

# SUBJECT INDEX

# SUBJECT INDEX

# SUBJECT INDEX

## SUBJECT INDEX

# SUBJECT INDEX

# SUBJECT INDEX

# SUBJECT INDEX

# SUBJECT INDEX

# SUBJECT INDEX

# SUBJECT INDEX

**649**

# SUBJECT INDEX

# SUBJECT INDEX

# DRUG INDEX

# DRUG INDEX

Corticosteroid(s)
    for acute severe asthma
            exacerbation, 105
    FHR effects of, 89
Cortisone, 410
Coumarin derivatives, as teratogen,
    211
COX-2 inhibitors, in low back pain
        management, 36
Cromolyn, for asthma, 104
Cromolyn cream, for vulvodynia,
    298
Cryselle, 233, 244
Cyclessa, 235
Cyclooxygenase inhibitors, for preterm
        labor, Cochrane reviews
        of, 150
Cyclophosphamide, 405
Cyproterone acetate
    in PCOS management, 501
    pharmacologic profiles of, 231

## D

Danazol, for mastalgia, 436
Daunorubicin, for chemotherapy
        extravasation injury,
        407
Delavirdine, 232
Demulen, 234
Doxorubicin, 404
Depo-Provera, 239
Depo-subQ Provera, 239
DES. *See* Diethylstilbestrol (DES)
Desogen, 233
Desogestrel
    in combination estrogen-progestin
        oral contraceptives, 228
    pharmacologic profiles of, 231
Dexamethasone, 410
    for preterm labor, 147

Dicloxacillin, for mastitis, 306
Dicyclomine, for urinary incontinence,
    291
Didanosine, in prevention of mother-
        to-child transmission of
        HIV, 325
Dienestrol, 474
Dienogest, pharmacologic profiles of,
    231
Diethylstilbestrol (DES)
    exposure to, infertility due to, 550
    as teratogen, 212
Diflunisal, for postoperative pain, 289
Digoxin, for maternal valvular heart
        disease, 111
Dihydroergotamine mesylate, for
        migraines, 32
Diltiazem, for hypertension, 126
Dimethisterone, in combination
        estrogen-progestin oral
        contraceptives, 228
Dinoprostone, attributes of, 52–53
Diphenhydramine, for nausea and
        vomiting in pregnancy,
        47
Diuretic(s)
    botanical interactions with, 43
    effects on lower urinary tract
        function, 293
    in hypertension management, 23–24
    for maternal valvular heart disease,
        110
    thiazide, for hypertension, 126
DNA intercalators, for
        chemotherapy
        extravasation injury, 407
Docetaxel, 404
Dopamine agonists, for
        hyperprolactinemia, 518
Doxepin, for migraines, 33

# DRUG INDEX

# DRUG INDEX

# DRUG INDEX

# DRUG INDEX

# DRUG INDEX

**NOTES**

**NOTES**

# NOTES